Delivery
Systems for
Peptide Drugs

NATO ASI Series

Advanced Science Institutes Series

A series presenting the results of activities sponsored by the NATO Science Committee, which aims at the dissemination of advanced scientific and technological knowledge, with a view to strengthening links between scientific communities.

The series is published by an international board of publishers in conjunction with the NATO Scientific Affairs Division

A	**Life Sciences**	Plenum Publishing Corporation
B	**Physics**	New York and London
C	**Mathematical and Physical Sciences**	D. Reidel Publishing Company Dordrecht, Boston, and Lancaster
D	**Behavioral and Social Sciences**	Martinus Nijhoff Publishers
E	**Engineering and Materials Sciences**	The Hague, Boston, Dordrecht, and Lancaster
F	**Computer and Systems Sciences**	Springer-Verlag
G	**Ecological Sciences**	Berlin, Heidelberg, New York, London,
H	**Cell Biology**	Paris, and Tokyo

Recent Volumes in this Series

Volume 119—Auditory Frequency Selectivity
edited by Brian C. J. Moore and Roy D. Patterson

Volume 120—New Experimental Modalities in the Control of Neoplasia
edited by Prakash Chandra

Volume 121—Cyst Nematodes
edited by F. Lamberti and C. E. Taylor

Volume 122—Methods for the Mycological Examination of Food
edited by A. D. King, Jr., J. I. Pitt, L. R. Beuchat,
and Janet E. L. Corry

Volume 123—The Molecular Basis of B-Cell Differentiation and Function
edited by M. Ferrarini and B. Pernis

Volume 124—Radiation Carcinogenesis and DNA Alterations
edited by F. J. Burns, A. C. Upton, and G. Silini

Volume 125—Delivery Systems for Peptide Drugs
edited by S. S. Davis, Lisbeth Illum, and E. Tomlinson

Volume 126—Crystallography in Molecular Biology
edited by Dino Moras, Jan Drenth, Bror Strandberg,
Dietrich Suck, and Keith Wilson

Series A: Life Sciences

Delivery Systems for Peptide Drugs

Edited by

S. S. Davis

University of Nottingham
Nottingham, England

Lisbeth Illum

The Royal Danish School of Pharmacy
Copenhagen, Denmark

and

E. Tomlinson

Ciba-Geigy Pharmaceuticals
Horsham, England

Plenum Press
New York and London
Published in cooperation with NATO Scientific Affairs Division

Proceedings of a NATO Advanced Research Workshop on
Advanced Drug Delivery Systems for Peptides and Proteins,
held May 28–June 1, 1986,
in Copenhagen, Denmark

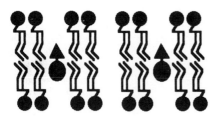

ISBN 0-306-42496-7

Recent years have seen enormous advances in the field of protein and peptide engineering and a greater understanding in the way in which biological response modifiers function in the body. It is now possible through the use of recombinant DNA techniques, or by solid phase protein synthesis, to produce significant quantities of a wide variety of regulatory agents that are therapeutically applicable. The list of these response modifiers expands almost daily to include interferons, macrophage activation factors, neuropeptides and agents that may have potential in cardiovascular disease, inflammation, contraception etc. Prospects to use some of these materials in medicine have reached the stage where products have either been approved by regulatory authorities or are the subject of applications as investigatory drugs or as new therapeutic agents. In some uses the pertinent agent will be administered on an acute basis in the form of a simple injection, as, for example, the use of a tissue plasminogen activator for the treatment of coronary infarct. In other cases regulatory proteins and peptides are indicated for chronic therapy and here they will need to be administered by an appropriate delivery system. Unfortunately, the research on delivery systems for peptides and proteins has not kept pace with the rapid progress in biotechnology and, consequently, there are presently few systems that are entirely appropriate for the administration of macromolecular drugs according to complex dosage regimens, (eg intermittent and pulsed therapy). Furthermore essential pharmacokinetic and pharmacodynamic data may be missing. For example, questions like where and how does the peptide function?, how much is needed and how often should it be dosed? Thus, so far, the construction of delivery systems for peptides and proteins has been largely based upon conjecture rather than sound rationale.

In order to correct this inbalance, groups or individuals, charged with the role of developing delivery systems for peptides and proteins have become established within biotechnology companies and large pharmaceutical organisations. Pharmaceutical researchers in academia are also turning their attention to this complex problem. With this background in mind we considered that a useful role would be served by bringing together the leaders in the field in a workshop where advanced delivery systems for peptides and proteins could be discussed. A three-day meeting (Advanced Science Workshop), sponsored by the NATO Science Foundation and various pharmaceutical and biotechnology companies, was held in Copenhagen during May 28-June 1 1986 and this book comprises the various contributions presented.

The book considers first the overall pharmaceutical considerations for the rational design of delivery systems for peptides and proteins, to include relevant aspects of the production of peptides and proteins by biotechnology, pharmacokinetic analysis and strategies for chemical modification. The major routes of access into the body are examined in turn, and include parenteral, oral, rectal, nasal, buccal and transdermal. In each case attention is given to relevant physiology and the critical role of biological barriers to drug uptake to include membranes and enzymes. Attention is focused on the role of absorption enhancers for the oral and nasal routes. A number of important and representative regulatory peptides are then selected for more detailed examination as case histories. These include calcitonin, insulin, enkephalins, somatostatin, TPA, macrophage activation factors etc.

The penultimate Chapter reviews the regulatory implications relevant to the delivery of peptides and proteins and the requirements that might be demanded by regulatory authorities.

The participants at the meeting were allocated to small syndicate groups, and each syndicate was given two topics to discuss and report upon at the conclusion of the workshop. The deliberations of the syndicate sessions have been summarised in the final Chapter of the book.

We wish to express our appreciation to the NATO Science Foundation for financial support of the workshop as part of the Double Jump Programme and to the various pharmaceutical and biotechnology companies who also provided assistance.

September 1986

S.S. Davis
Lisbeth Illum
E. Tomlinson

SPONSORSHIP

Apotekernes Laboratories, Oslo (N)
Bayer AG, Leverkusen (D)
Beecham Pharmaceuticals, Brentford (GB)
Biogen S.A., Geneva (CH)
Boehringer Ingelheim GmbH (D)
Bristol-Myers, New York (USA)
California Biotechnology Inc., Mountain View (USA)
Carlbiotech, Copenhagen (DK)
Ciba-Geigy, Horsham (GB)
Cilag AG, Schaffhausen (CH)
Ferring AB, Malmø (S)
FMC Corporation, Philadelphia (USA)
Glaxo Group Research, Ware (GB)
Hoechst Ltd., Milton, Keynes (GB)
Hoffmann-La-Roche, Basle (CH)
Hässle AB, Göteborg (S)
ICI Plc., Pharmaceuticals Division, Macclesfield (GB)
Johnson & Johnson, New Brunswick (USA)
KabiVitrum, Stockholm (S)
Lilly Research Laboratories, Indianapolis (USA)
Merck, Sharp & Dohme, Hoddesdon (GB)
Merrell Dow Research Institute, Egham (GB)
Nordisk Insulin, Gentofte (DK)
Norwich Eaton Pharmaceuticals Inc., New York (USA)
Novo Industry, Bagsværd (DK)
Nycomed, Oslo (N)
Organon International BV, BH Oss (NL)
Ortho Pharmaceutical Corporation (USA)
PA Technology, Royston (GB)
Penwalt Corporation Pennsylvania (USA)
Pfizer Central Research, Sandwich (GB)
Pharmacia, Uppsala, (S)
Reckitt and Coleman, Hull (GB)
Rorer Group Inc.,Tuckahoe, NY (USA)
Rousell Uclas, (F)
Sandoz AG, Basle (CH)
R.P. Scherer Corporation, Troy (USA)
Schering Corporation, Kenilworth (USA)
Searle Research & Development, Skokie (USA)
Smith Kline & French Laboratories, Philadelphia (USA)
Sterling Winthrop, London (GB)
Syntex Research, Palo Alto (USA)
TAP Pharmaceuticals, North Chicago (USA)
Travenol Laboratories Inc., Morton Grove (USA)
Upjohn Co. Kalamazoo (USA)
Warner-Lambert, Ann Arbor (USA)
Wellcome Research Laboratories, Beckenham (GB)

CONTENTS

ADVANCED DELIVERY SYSTEMS FOR PEPTIDES AND PROTEINS - PHARMACEUTICAL

CONSIDERATIONS

S. S. Davis

Department of Pharmacy
University of Nottingham
University Park
Nottingham NG7 2RD, UK

Presently, a wide variety of routes of administration and delivery systems exists for drug substances, but by far the most popular approach is oral delivery where the drug is intended to be absorbed from the gastrointestinal tract. Injectable systems (that include implants), suppositories and transdermal devices, have a more limited place in current therapy. Some of these administration systems can be employed directly for the delivery of peptides and proteins, however, others cannot be used in their present form and will require extensive modification. In particular, the delivery of peptides and proteins via the gastrointestinal tract will be especially difficult because of the inherent instability of such materials and the poor permeability of the intestinal mucosa to high molecular weight substances. Indeed it can be claimed that the process of evolution, over many thousands of years, has resulted in the gastrointestinal tract being impermeable to large molecular weight molecules in the adult mammal and that serious immunological consequences could arise if such materials happened to be taken up intact. This point will be discussed further below. In future the less well known routes of administration, namely nasal, vaginal and buccal, could play a more important role in the delivery of peptides and proteins because of their superior permeability characteristics or the fact that the dosage form can be retained at the site of administration for a prolonged period of time to maximise absorption.

Those reading popular fiction may have been led to believe that the problem in delivering peptides had already been solved. To quote from Arthur Hailey's book entitled 'Strong Medicine' (Hailey, 1984) one learns that

"The way in which the drug would be ingested .... was important. We've researched this exhaustively and recommend delivery by nasal spray. This is the modern coming system .... Peptide 7 will be in an inert saline solution mixed with a detergent (that) assures the best absorption rate .... The best non-toxic (detergent) creating no irritation of nasal membranes had been found".

If only it was so easy! While it is true that certain peptides are well taken up via the nasal route (Su, 1986), totally innocuous absorption enhancers have yet to be discovered and the implications of long term therapy on possible damage to the mucosa need to be resolved.

1

A universal delivery system for peptides and proteins is neither possible nor perhaps desirable, largely because the types of materials being considered for therapeutic application comprise a diverse range of biological response modifiers (Table 1). They have different physical and chemical characteristics (molecular size, stability, conformation etc) as well as different sites and modes of action within the body. For example a delivery system for tumour necrosis factor or an interleukin by necessity, will be rather different from that for insulin or calcitonin. Furthermore, unlike conventional low molecular weight drugs, biological response modifiers are often involved in complex processes where a whole group of regulatory materials can be involved. The "classical" situation of a single pharmacodynamic agent acting independently on one particular receptor type may not necessarily pertain. For example, it is known that materials such as interferon can act to prime or "up-regulate" the action of another material (Aggarwal et al, 1985). Similarly, the action of one agent may lead to a whole process of actions, often in the form of a cascade process. Consequently the resultant biological response may be determined by an alteration in a delicate balance between a number of inter-related regulatory materials. Clearly, in the development of any potential therapeutic agent and its delivery system it will be essential that such aspects of molecular and biochemical pharmacology are elucidated. The complexity of the properties and actions of regulatory peptides and proteins will mean that the successful development of pharmaceutically elegant delivery systems for peptides and proteins will be a multidisciplinary venture, to include input from disciplines such as biochemistry (the action of enzymes), physiology (membrane permeability), immunology (immunogenicity), physical chemistry (molecular characteristics; solubility, stability).

The main emphasis of the present contribution will be to consider the possibilities and problems for peptide and protein delivery and the different options available for rational drug delivery systems. By necessity comment will also be made on the pharmacokinetics of peptide systems, their assay and preformulation studies and the possibilities of immunogenic reactions.

Kinetic profiles

In many cases the simplest form of a delivery system for peptides and proteins will be the hypodermic syringe containing the drug in a buffered aqueous solution. The appropriate dose of agent is then injected intravenously or subcutaneously according to the desired time pattern. This mode of administration, although ideal from the standpoint of clinical pharmacology, is obviously limited in its widespread applicability to the patient population at large. Even for a simple system (and especially for complex systems providing sustained therapy), essential information is necessary. This includes the dose, dose frequency and the site of action of the drug. Generally speaking, natural peptides and proteins acting as agonists are short-lived in their action and are rapidly metabolised. Furthermore, the body provides these agents as pulses rather than continuously to a particular receptor site (Knobil, 1980; Urquhart et al, 1984). From the outset, the ability to mimic such a pattern of delivery using a novel delivery system will present substantial challenges to the pharmaceutical scientist. Moreover, it is often found that the desired pharmacokinetic profile for a regulatory material in man has yet to be determined since animal models, although useful, may not be entirely suitable. An obvious starting point is studies with infusion pump systems in animal models and more recently the implantable osmotic pump (Alzet) has been employed to provide a response without the necessity of tethering the animal (Obie et al, 1979; Knobil, 1980; Lynch et al, 1980; Ewing et al, 1983). This

Table 1. Selected polypeptides and proteins (and analogues) with potential for therapeutic use

PEPTIDE	AA	ORAL*	NASAL*	BRAIN
Adrenocorticotrophic hormone (ACTH)	39	X	X	X
Atrial natriuretic factor				
Calcitonin	32	X	X	
Cholecystekinin (CCK)	33			X
Colony stimulating factor				
DDAVP	9	X		X
Delta sleep inducing peptide				X
β Endorphin	31			X
Enkephalin	5		X	X
Fibroblast growth factor				
Glucagon	29		X	
Growth hormone				
Growth hormone releasing factor	40-44			
Insulin	51	X	X	
Inhibin				
Interferon			X	
Interleukin 2				
Leuprolide		X	X	
Leutinising hormone releasing hormone (LHRH)	10		X	X
Lipmodulin				
Melanocyte inhibiting factor I	3	X		X
Melanocyte stimulating hormone			14	
Muramyl dipeptide	2	X		X
Migration inhibiting factor				

(continued)

Table 1 (continued)

PEPTIDE	AA	ORAL*	NASAL*	BRAIN
Oxytocin		9		X
Parathyroid hormone				
Relaxin				
Somatostatin	14	X		X
Superoxide dismustase			X	
Thyrotropic releasing hormone	3	X	X	X
Tissue plasminogen activator				
Tumour necrosis factor				
Vasopressin		9		X

* Activity following oral or nasal administration of peptide or analogue (Samanen, 1985; Lee, 1986; Su, 1986).

Table 2. Analytical methods for peptides. Studies carried out on a peptide (Somatostatin-14) prior to use in man (after Wunsch, 1983 and Wada, 1983)

A. Chromatographic methods

1. Amino acid analysis of acid and enzymatic hydrolysates

2. Gas chromatographic analysis of derivitised acid hydrolysate for postsynthetic chiral analysis

3. TLC on normal and high performance plates in different solvent systems

4. HPLC using different reversed phase supports and eluant systems

5. Electrophoresis on supports or free flow systems to characterise homogeneity

6. Micropreparative gel filtration to detect polymeric species

B.   Spectroscopic Methods

    1.   UV measurements

    2.   NMR (^{1}H and ^{13}C) to detect possible synthetic side products or residual protecting groups

    3.   IR to detect possible contamination by column material from repeated chromatographic steps

    4.   MS (chemical ionisation, field desorption and fast-atom bombardment) to characterise enzymatic fragments or entire molecule for sequence

    5.   Fluorescence methods to detect contaminants from solvents, resins etc

C.   Enzymatic Methods

    1.   Amino-peptidase-M digest

    2.   Trypsin digest followed by chromatographic separation

    3.   Dipeptidyl-peptidase digest followed by chromatographic separation

D.   Biological Methods

    1.   In vitro assay

    2.   In vivo assay

    3.   Toxicological evaluation

E.   Immunological Methods

    1.   Cross-reactivities with various antisera

F.   Other methods

    1.   Circular dichroism to study conformation changes

    2.   Light scattering to follow aggregation

device, originally developed to provide a zero order input of drug, can also be used to provide the necessary driving force for pulsed delivery (Ewing et al, 1983). This is achieved by attaching the pump to a reservoir where boluses of the agent are separated by placebo. For example, thin plastic tubing filled with alternate doses of drug dissolved in water and separated by vegetable or mineral oil has been employed for the delivery of melatonin.

The pulsed delivery of peptides and proteins may well be the desired mode of delivery for therapeutic effect rather than the more conventional steady state levels that have been popular with conventional drug molecules. In many cases the continuous administration of a regulatory material can result in the phenomenon of tolerance or "down-regulation" (Catt et al, 1979; Obie et al, 1979; Koch and Lutz-Bucher, 1985). That is, the continual presence of the agent at a receptor site can lead to a reduction of activity. Here again osmotic pumps have been a useful aid. Continuous infusion and resultant steady state levels of an agent, while not necessarily desirable for agonist action, may be entirely appropriate for antagonist action.

In therapy a pulsed delivery pattern could be achieved by a programmed series of injections and possibly by nasal administration. Programmable, transportable pump systems, although bulky and inconvenient to use, have been developed and are used in clinical practice. For example, a device developed in Sweden (the Ferring product Zyklomat) has been used to deliver LHRH in order to induce ovulation. The pump contains a 10 day supply and is active every 90th minute for one minute duration delivering on each occasion 50 ug of drug. More complex patterns of delivery on a daily, weekly or even monthly basis are presently beyond the capabilities of conventional pharmaceutical dosage forms.

Preformulation studies

An essential part in the development of a delivery system for a peptide and protein, as for any other drug molecule, will be extensive preformulation studies to establish the physicochemical characteristics of the agent and possible limitations in terms of stability etc. Methods for examining the physicochemical properties of peptides are given in Table 2. High molecular weight proteins and peptides present some unique difficulties because of their molecular properties. For example, a peptide or protein may demonstrate aggregation and changes in conformation (unfolding and denaturation) (Dodson et al, 1983; Toniolo et al, 1986). Flexibility within a molecule can have a direct bearing upon biological response and such flexibility can arise in amino acid side chains, within certain parts of the molecule itself or in separate domains that are separated by more rigid covalent bonds (Glover et al, 1983). Immunoglobulin G is a good example of a molecule that has two flexible domains that are believed to be important in antigen binding. Such subtle changes may not only lead to a loss of biological activity (Goldenberg et al, 1983) but could also lead to immunogenic reactions. Self-association can involve intermolecular H-bonds and hydrophobic interactions and will lead to a decrease in the solubility of the peptide. The degree of aggregation will be controlled by the mean chain length, the solvent and the concentration of the peptide. Other external factors such as pH, metal ions, ionic strength, temperature and agitation have been implicated. It can be minimised by incorporation of residues promoting folding (Toniolo et al, 1986).

Insulin is a good example of a molecule where extensive studies have been undertaken to ascertain its properties in solution, the phenomenon of aggregation, polymerisation of the molecule (gelling in solution) and how this can be controlled by pharmaceutical means through the addition of stabilising agents, eg nonionic surfactants (Dodson et al, 1983). The sites in the molecule responsible for aggregation have also been determined.

Peptide molecules can also change their structure and aggregation behaviour depending upon the environment in which they are placed. For example gramicidin A can undergo different conformational arrangements, depending on whether it is for example within a phospholipid bilayer (helical dimer structure) or a nonpolar solvent (double helix structure) (Wallace, 1983). Small changes in peptide sequences in a molecule can alter dramatically the physicochemical properties of such a species. These modifications can occur through instability or can be induced deliberately into a peptide molecule to improve its characteristics both for delivery and biological response (Samanen, 1985).

Proteins and peptides may cause special difficulties in their handling characteristics; particularly adsorption onto surfaces to include glass and plastic. Such adsorptive behaviour can lead to a significant loss in the amount of material available for delivery. Interestingly these properties can be exploited and the adsorption of peptides to microporous polyethylene has been used as a way of developing a controlled release system for the delivery of Vasopressin. The adsorbed material provides a reservoir effect and consequently pseudo zero order kinetics for the drug material (Kruisbrink and Boer, 1984).

Conventional preformulation studies such as those on stability-pH profile, solubility-pH profiles etc need to be supplemented with investigations involving the action of enzymes (proteases and peptidases) (Wunsch, 1983; Tobey et al, 1985). Peptides and proteins are particularly susceptible to hydrolysis of amide bonds (catalysed by peptidases) and oxidation of disulphide bonds (Carone et al, 1982). There are various ways in which the molecular structure might be altered to provide enhanced stability (Wunsch, 1983; Samanen, 1985). Table 3 (after Samanen, 1985) lists a variety of possible options. Proteins modified by the covalent attachment of carbohydrate and polyoxyethylene derivatives also possess enhanced stability characteristics and a higher resistance to proteolysis (Abuchowski and Davis, 1981).

Table 3. Modification to peptide backbone to reduce peptide degradation

- olefin substitution

- carbonyl reduction

- D-amino acid substitution

- N α-methyl substitution

- C α-methyl substitution

- C α C'-methylene insertion

- dehydro amino acid substitution

- retro-inverso modification

- N-terminal to C-terminal cyclisation

- thiomethylene modification

Design of delivery systems

As mentioned above, the appropriate delivery system for a particular peptide or protein will depend upon the nature of the agent being delivered, the clinical application and the site of drug action. The two main areas for concern are the entry of the drug into the body and passage across critical organ barriers (Samanen, 1983). Obvious advantages would accrue if it was possible to deliver peptides efficiently via the oral route. However, as will be discussed further, this is probably impossible in many cases. Early investigations are essential to establish whether a given material has any significant uptake from the proposed absorption site, whether this can be modified by the use of absorption enhancers or enzyme inhibitors or by the addition of a non-pharmacologically active enzyme substrate. Similar studies should determine metabolic fate, in particular whether the material is transported across cells or is degraded within the lysosomal compartment of the cell. The immunological consequences of delivery also need to be established. For instance, the molecule may be taken up into the systemic circulation or reach tissue sites in suitably high concentrations, but may lead not only to a biological response but also to an immunogenic reaction. In such situations it may be necessary to modify the molecule in order to mask immunogenic groups or to attach the molecule to a so-called tolerogen, such as polyethylene glycol, dextran, albumin etc (Abuchowski et al, 1977; Abuchowski and Davis, 1981; Lissi et al, 1982; Wileman et al, 1986). In addition, this strategy can lead to an increased stability both in vitro and in vivo; the latter demonstrated by an increase in the circulation time of the molecule following IV injection.

Routes of administration

Other chapters in this book consider in detail the possibilities of administering peptides and proteins via a variety of routes to include the nose, gastrointestinal tract, parenteral formulations and even the skin. Consequently this contribution will consider the more general aspects that pertain to peptide and protein delivery. At the outset, the simplicity of the intravenous, subcutaneous and intramuscular routes of administration should not be overlooked for the apparent greater convenience, but far greater complexity of implants, nasal delivery systems etc especially when some form of pulsed therapy is required. Insulin represents a molecule that has been studied extensively over many years, yet is still delivered via injection. Here is an example of a regulatory agent that is required at a basal level and then pulsed in relation to food intake. Presently investigators are exploring the use of various pumps, sensors and feedback devices (Albin et al, 1985; Jeong et al, 1985), but it is interesting to note that the Novo company in Denmark have developed an elegant device that simplifies subcutaneous administration of pulses of insulin. The so-called Novopen has been well received by diabetics in that it provides an unobtrusive way of delivering a programmed quantity of insulin on demand without the complexity of filling syringes and associated paraphenalia.

Parenteral administration of peptides and proteins

Those wishing to avoid serial injections on a daily, weekly or even monthly basis have been attracted by the concept of polymer implants for peptide delivery. While this approach is attractive in principle, it is limited by the number of available materials that are presently acceptable for such a purpose (Brown et al, 1983; Sidman et al, 1983; Siegel and Langer, 1984). Pulsed systems based upon magnetic inclusions have been described (Langer et al, 1980; Siegel and Langer, 1984).

Simple implants can be based upon waxes and fats and of the synthetic polymers, polylactides and polyglycolides represent some of the few materials that are recognised by regulatory authorities as being acceptable in terms of biocompatibility, biodegradation and tissue response (Langer et al, 1985). Commercial peptide delivery systems have now been developed based upon monolithic implants, microcapsules and microsphere systems are presently under active evaluation (Williams et al, 1984; Schally and Reading, 1985; Visscher et al, 1985). With microsphere systems it is not always possible to provide a well defined or controlled release pattern and indeed drug release can be rapid for a period subsequent to administration with a second burst after the microspheres have undergone substantial biodegradation. Notwithstanding this less than optimal pattern of delivery the microsphere can still represent a beneficial means of delivery for a drug with a wide therapeutic index.

Liposomes and microsphere systems administered into the vascular and lymphatic systems could be an important means of delivering peptides (Fukunga et al, 1984) particularly for activation of macrophages in the treatment of cancer or for the delivery of colony stimulating factors. Here special regard has to be given to the fate of the administered material. It is well known that intravenously administered colloids are removed rapidly and effectively by the cells of the reticuloendothelial system (mononuclear phagocyte systems). The Kupffer cells in the liver and circulating blood monocytes are especially effective in this regard. Both types of cells can be activated by a number of different agents in order to kill tumour cells. This process of activation has the advantage that there is no need for specificity and has shown to work both in vitro and in vivo. It could be useful in combination therapy, especially for low tumour burdens and the treatment of metastases. The problem in delivery is presently one of activating the appropriate macrophage population (Juliano and Posnansky, 1984). In the case of interleukin 2 treatment in cancer chemotherapy the blood monocytes are activated ex vivo and then returned to the patient (Rosenberg et al, 1985). Clearly, it would be an advantage if this could be achieved by targeting the delivery system to the appropriate macrophage following a simple intravenous injection. Preliminary studies conducted by Poste and others (Poste, 1985) have shown that this effect can be achieved to a limited extent using liposomes with appropriate surface characteristics that are taken up preferentially into lung tissue. Here the liposomes were thought to be ingested by monocytes that could leave the circulation to become alveolar macrophages. This approach should be helpful for the treatment of tumours within the lung and recent in vivo data are encouraging (Saiki et al, 1985).

The non-specific targeting of colloidal carriers to the Kupffer cells of the liver presents a major obstacle to the use of colloidal particles in therapy (Poste, 1985). However, recently work conducted by our own group has shown that it is possible to prevent the uptake of colloidal carriers in the liver by the use of appropriate surface coatings (Illum and Davis, 1983). Block copolymers, based upon polyoxyethylene and polyoxypropylene can be used either to divert colloidal particles away from the liver to the bone marrow to keep administered colloidal particles almost totally within the vascular compartment (Illum et al, 1986). In the latter case the particles could be given an appropriate attached label (homing device) that would allow them to be recognised and taken up by circulating monocytes. In this way it should be possible to deliver macrophage activating factors and colony stimulating factor in a more rational manner.

Blood-brain barrier

A number of regulatory peptides have a central effect (Samanen, 1985) (Table 1). However, the short half life and hydrophilicity of such compounds means that brain concentrations greater than a few percent are difficult, if not impossible, to achieve. Claims that liposome formulations are beneficial in delivering higher concentrations across the blood-brain barrier have been published (Postmes et al, 1980; Yagi et al, 1982). One recent contribution has the distinction of reporting the uptake of intact liposomes in the brain following rectal administration! (Gabev et al, 1985). The delivery of small lipophilic molecules to the brain would seem to be problem enough (Juliano and Posnansky, 1984). Current opinion could indicate that liposomes are not taken up intact from the gastrointestinal tract. Instability within the vascular compartment together with capture by the reticuloendothelial system constitute other barriers (Davis and Illum, 1986).

Gastrointestinal tract

Certain peptide and protein materials will be used in severe clinical conditions such as cancer or for the treatment of acute cardiac infarction etc where convenience of delivery is of secondary importance. However, if peptides are to compete with the conventional orally administered drug molecules used in therapy for hypertension, depression, rheumatoid arthritis, methods will need to be found whereby macromolecules can be taken up from the gastrointestinal tract in a reliable manner to provide sufficient concentration within the blood or at the site of action (Michaels, 1985). Without doubt this is an important but difficult objective. By design the gastrointestinal tract is very efficient at preventing the uptake of intact polypeptides and proteins. Thus biological response modifiers delivered by the oral route are usually unstable to the acid of the stomach and are degraded by various digestive enzymes present in the lumen or brush border. Furthermore, active molecules have characteristics that do not normally lend themselves to good transport across biological membranes. They are large in size and tend to be polar in nature and the poor permeability of the gastrointestinal mucosa is not unexpected. Rarely do peptides and proteins have structures that would be recognised by some natural active transport processes and even if materials are taken up into cells intact there is the very likely possibility that the macromolecule will undergo storage or metabolism within the cell without being transferred to the systemic circulation (Gabev and Foster, 1983; Lecce, 1984). If the molecule can get this far intact it may well be metabolised by the liver (first pass effect) or be excreted into the bile (Renston et al, 1980). Experiments with in situ gut loops (rat) can be used to assess the magnitude of some of these factors.

Notwithstanding major difficulties, the advantages in being able to deliver a peptide or protein via the gastrointestinal tract will encourage many to explore this route for possible avenues. Some indicators for future exploitation include the fact that dietary dipeptides and tripeptides can be absorbed by active transport processes and that these processes are involved with a number of drug substances (eg the amino cephalosporins etc). Limited quantities of peptides (less than 1%) have been shown to be taken up from the gastrointestinal tract in animal models and in man (Table 1) and that the use of so-called absorption enhancers can increase this uptake (Yoshikawa et al, 1985; Takada, 1985; Miyake et al, 1985). In some situations rectal administration can be a better alternative because of the lack of dilution effects, low levels of peptidases and the ability to hold the agent close to the absorptive surface for long periods of time. The last factor is important, if advantage is to be taken of an absorption enhancer. Other pointers to possible routes for exploitation include the interesting behaviour of the M-cells located in the Peyers Patches within the small intestine and the fact that materials such as botulism toxin with a molecular weight of nearly 1 million can be taken up apparently intact (via the lymphatic system?) (O'Hagan et al, 1986). The involvement of Intrinsic Factor in the absorption of vitamin B12 represents another interesting area for potential exploitation (Sennett et al, 1981; Steinman et al, 1983). The good bioavailability of orally administered cyclosporin A, a cyclic polypeptide consisting of 11 amino-acids, is also worthy of note.

Recently we have reviewed the literature on the absorption of peptides and proteins from the gastrointestinal tract to include a detailed consideration of colloidal carriers (O'Hagan et al, 1986). We have examined the absorption processes from the standpoints of drug delivery and the delivery of oral allergens and antigens to the gut associated lymphoid tissue (oral immunisation). For the latter case the M-cells appear to have a critical role. Macromolecules are taken up selectively by those cells from the gastrointestinal lumen and are presented to the underlying lymphoid tissues. Interestingly, from the standpoint of transcellular trafficking the M-cells seem to be largely devoid of lysosomes and therefore the molecules are transported intact (Owen et al, 1982). Successful immunisation via the oral route clearly raises the question of possible presensitisation and immunogenic response to the chronic administration of regulatory peptides and proteins via the oral route. On the one hand it would be an advantage to identify the antigenic peptide sequences (Sela, 1983) and to understand the importance of conformation and configuration so that the effect could be enhanced by modifications to the molecule or by attachment to a macromolecular carrier or to the surface of a colloidal particle. On the other hand it will be necessary to mask immunogenic determinants (Artursson et al, 1986).

Modification to gastrointestinal transit could hold some advantages. Normally the transit of dosage forms through the small intestine and past the most likely sites for protein and peptide absorption is quite rapid (Davis et al, 1986a). Methods for the retention of a dosage form in the stomach, or reduction of transit rate in the intestine are presently being explored for conventional controlled release dosage forms. Successful developments could find application to suitable candidate peptides and proteins.

Future approaches to drug delivery via the gastro-intestinal tract can perhaps be best categorised into two different types; the mechanistic, those that will rely upon a far better understanding of cell biology and intracellular processing; and the pragmatic, those that will rely upon an empirical approach using absorption enhancers, enzyme inhibitors etc, and even liposomes (Beahon and Woodley, 1984; Woodley, 1986), to modify membrane permeability and peptide stability without necessarily understanding the processes involved. Each of these approaches will be considered here briefly with examples.

Transcytosis mechanisms

Macromolecules can be taken up into and across cells by different processes (Juliano and Posnansky, 1984). The phenomenon of pinocytosis allows macromolecules to be taken up into cells but normally the macromolecule will find its way into an endocytic vesicle and then following fusion of this vesicle with the lysosome the macromolecule will be degraded or stored. As a consequence the major part of material taken up into the cell does not find its way across into underlying tissues and thence to the blood circulation. For example, studies on the uptake of horseradish peroxidase have shown that about 97% of the material taken up from the gastrointestinal lumen travels via the lysosomal pathway and is therefore metabolised (Heyman et al, 1982). Lysosomal metabolism can be inhibited by drugs such as monesin. It is interesting to note that certain viruses and micro-organisms gain entry into cells by riding the endocytic pathway but are not degraded within the lysosomal compartment. Some micro-organisms and parasites actually live within the lysosomal compartment while others can find their way into the cytoplasm through processes that may involve changes in lysosomal pH or the presence of certain groups and structures on membrane surfaces (Armstrong and Herd, 1971; Rikihisa et al, 1978). It would be most interesting if mechanisms could be found whereby peptides and proteins (or their conjugates with carrier molecules or even colloidal carriers) could exploit these processes.

Materials can also be taken across cells through receptor mediated processes in mechanisms known collectively as transcytosis (Juliano and Posnanski, 1984; Mostov and Simister, 1985). For the horseradish peroxidase example given above about 3% of the dose is believed to find its way across the cell by the transcytosis mechanism. Other complex materials are transported intact across cells and are not degraded by the lysosomes. Immunoglobulin G is a well known example. Low density lipoprotein also has two methods of uptake, one involving coated pits on the surface of cells and the transfer of LDL to the lysosome and a secondary process of transcytosis that allows the delivery of LDL (and the cholesterol contained therein) to underlying tissues (Juliano and Posnansky, 1984).

In polarised cell types such as the intestinal epithelium (and hepatocytes), endocytic vacuoles move continuously from the apical (or sinusoidal) to basolateral surface delivery solutes (Steinman et al, 1983; Kondor-Koch, 1985). In spite of such transcellular movement two chemically distinct membrane domains are maintained. The pathways followed by an endocytic vacuole can vary depending upon the cell type and applied stimulus or tracer. Endocytosed contents can be delivered to the lysosome or across cells (or even to the Golgi apparatus). Such observations suggest that transcytosis, endocytosis and the transport of membrane proteins to the correct cell surface are interconnected pathways in a network of membrane traffic. To follow the correct route the protein must contain signal sequences that are recognised at the various stages (intersections) (Gilmore et al, 1982). A key question is what region of the protein contains such information? since this could provide a means of controlling the fate and disposition of suitably designed regulatory peptide analogues intended for therapeutic effect (De Roberts, 1983; Evans et al, 1986; Holland and Drickamer, 1986).

Absorption enhancers

The approach of using absorption enhancers to enhance the uptake of peptides and proteins in the gastrointestinal tract, albeit empirical, could lead to early successful clinical applications. The major problems remaining to be resolved are the long term chronic effects of such materials on the integrity of the membrane being modified and the consequences of poor selectivity permitting the uptake of immunogenic materials (Yoshikawa et al, 1985; Morimoto et al, 1985; Muranishi, 1985).

Many studies have been conducted on the use of absorption enhancers for improving the rectal and intestinal delivery of a variety of molecules to include various high molecular weight materials such as peptides and proteins. Generally speaking, use of salicylates and bile salts can enhance the uptake of peptides and proteins from the tract (Fergundes-Neto et al, 1981) although the increase expressed in terms of the percent of dose absorbed is still quite small. An interesting range of absorption enhancers has been examined in rats by Japanese workers for the peptide eel calcitonin (Miyake et al, 1985) (Table 4). The bioavailability data shows the dramatic effects that can be achieved with absorption enhancers that are believed to modify the properties (fluidity?) of membranes and are not surface active in nature. Interestingly, the reported effects for eel calcitonin show a considerable discrimination between the various absorption enhancers, whereas a simpler cephalosporin molecule (cefoxamine) indicates that the absorption enhancers have similar abilities in changing the characteristics of the rectal mucosa.

Table 4. Rectal absorption of eel calcitonin in rats. The effect of adjuvants (dose 800 u/kg)

(Miyake et al, 1985)

Adjuvant	$\dfrac{AUC(Ad)}{AUC(cont)}$[1]	
Sodium alginate (1%)	3.2	
Diethyleneoxymethylene malonate (0.17M)	186	(11.5)[2]
Phenylalanine enamine of ethylacetoacetate	214	(10.7)
Sodium salicylate (0.6M)	25	(10.6)

[1] Area under plasma curve 0-2 h for adjuvant (Ad) and no adjuvant (cont)

[2] Relative data for absorption (%) of cefmatazole

We have conducted one of the few reported studies on absorption enhancers in human volunteers, using the model material cefoxitin (Davis et al, 1985). By employing a mixture of sodium salicylate and a nonionic surfactant (Brij 37) we increased the bioavailability from about 5% to nearly 30% in a non-optimised suppository formulation. Considerable intra- and inter-subject variation was demonstrated but it is interesting to note that it was possible to achieve a similar blood level-time profile via rectal administration to that normally achieved by intramuscular injection. The volunteers did not report any adverse reactions or side effects to the suppositories in terms of irritation but the long term acceptability of such absorption enhancers for chronic administration have yet to be evaluated. Questions on the mechanism of action of such absorption enhancers and whether it could be possible to open up the mucosa to allow absorption of undesirable materials have yet to be answered in detail. The same considerations would apply to the use of absorption enhancers for improving the nasal delivery of drugs.

Lymphatic delivery

The role of the lymphatic system in the uptake of high molecular weight materials (to include peptides and proteins) may have been underestimated (Muranishi, 1985). Normally, with low molecular weight drug, the majority of the administered dose is taken up via the portal circulation and lymphatic delivery is considered to be of little consequence except for highly lipid soluble materials that are transported in association with the fat digestion pathway. However, certain large molecular weight toxins such a botulism toxin have been found in significant levels in lymph. In a series of experiments Katayama and Fujita (1972) have examined the intestinal absorption of three enzymatic proteins. The absorption of each molecule was low (0.05 to 2.06% of total dose) but the role of the lymphatic vessels varied considerably. One protein, a coenzyme, was largely (80%) recovered in the lymph. The authors concluded that absorption into the lymph was dependent on the physico-chemical properties of the macromolecules. In more recent studies in Japan by Muranishi and others (Yoshikawa et al, 1983, 1984) have indicated that the lymphatic delivery and total bioavailability of drugs can be enhanced by their attachment to high molecular weight dextran carriers. Exploitation of the lymphatic pathway could be especially important for peptides and proteins, since the molecules will find their way into the circulation without passing through the liver, thereby avoiding first pass metabolism and excretion into the bile. On the other hand the well-known involvement of the lymphatic system in the immune response could militate against successful applications unless the administered molecule was rendered non-immunogenic by suitable modification or derivatisation.

Nasal delivery

As is mentioned in the introduction, the nasal route of administration has been heralded as being the most likely means for the successful delivery of peptides (and proteins) in the near future. This would certainly seem to be the case, notwithstanding the problems of delivery to a nose with a pathological condition (eg rhinitis etc) (Su, 1986). A variety of drugs of peptide origin have been shown to be well absorbed from the nasal mucosa with bioavailabilities (compared to IV or subcutaneous administration) approaching 100%. Poorly bioavailable materials can be enhanced by the addition of absorption enhancers. Bile salts and their derivatives and non-ionic surfactants have been popular in this respect (Gordon et al, 1985; Salzman et al, 1985). The choice of animal model in studies on the nasal administration of peptides and proteins may be important. Data obtained in rats, dogs and even sheep may not necessarily be relevant to the situation in man.

One thing clear is that the nasal mucosa has very different absorption characteristics to the gastrointestinal tract and polar molecules of quite high molecular weight can be taken up to significant extents. We have recently conducted studies investigating the relationship between molecular weight and molecules administered to the rat and their absorption from the nasal mucosa into the systemic circulation (Fisher et al, 1986) (Figure 1).

In nasal delivery, mucociliary clearance could be an important factor. Advantages may be gained in keeping the dosage form in contact with the absorptive surface for extended periods of time and reports have described the use of gels (Nagai, 1985) as well as microsphere systems for this purpose (Davis et al, 1986). As with the gastrointestinal tract, the optimal concomitant delivery of efficient and innocuous absorption enhancers could be a means of providing effective delivery of peptides and proteins in clinical practice.

CONCLUSIONS

The successful delivery of regulatory peptides and proteins presents an enormous challenge to the pharmaceutical scientist. The treatment and prevention of diseases with the new molecules available through biotechnology await the development of new delivery systems. Before this can happen a thorough understanding of temporal, biophysical, biochemical, immunological and physiological determinants will be required.

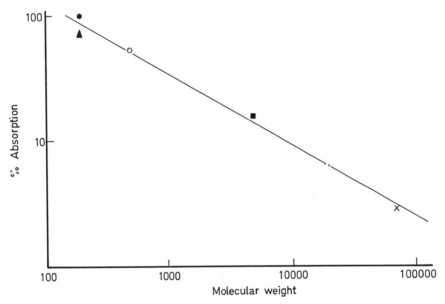

Fig. 1.   The effect of molecular weight on nasal absorption (from Fisher et al, 1986)

REFERENCES

Abuchowski, A. and Davis, F.F., 1981, Soluble polymer-enzyme adducts, in: "Enzymes as Drugs", J.S. Holcenberg and J. Roberts, eds., Wiley, New York, p367.

Abuchowski, A., Van Es, T., Palczuk, N.C. and Davis, F.F., 1977, Alteration of immunological properties of bovine serum albumin by covalent attachment of polyethylene glycol, J. Biol. Chem., 252: 3578.

Aggarwal, B.B., Eessalu, T.E. and Hass, P.E., 1985, Characterisation of receptors for human tumour necrosis factor and their regulation by γ-interferon, Nature, 318: 665.

Albin, G., Horbett, T.A. and Ratner, B.D., 1985, Glucose sensitive membranes for controlled delivery of insulin: insulin transport studies, J. Control. Rel. 2: 153.

Armstrong, J.A. and Herd, P.D., 1971, Response of cultured macrophages to myobacterium tuberculosis with observations on the fusion of lysosomes with phagosomes, J. Expl. Med. 134: 713.

Artursson, P., Mårtensson, I.C. and Sjöholm, I., 1986, Biodegradable microspheres. IV. Some immunological properties of polyacyl starch microparticles, J. Pharm. Sci. in press.

Beahon, S.J. and Woodley, J.F., 1984, The uptake of macromolecules by adult rat intestinal columnar epithelium and Peyer's patch tissue in vitro, Biochem. Soc. Trans., 1088.

Brown, L.R., Wei, C.L. and Langer, R., 1983, In vivo and in vitro release of macromolecules from polymeric drug delivery systems, J. Pharm. Sci., 72: 1181.

Carone, F.A., Peterson, D.R. and Flouret, G., 1982, Renal tubular processing of small peptide hormones, J. Lab. Clin. Med., 100: 1.

Catt, K.J., Harwood, J.P., Aguilera, G. and M.L. Dufau, 1979, Hormonal regulation of peptide receptors and target cell responses, Nature 280: 109.

Davis, S.S., Burnham, W.R., Wilson, P. and O'Brien, J., 1985, The use of adjuvants to enhance the rectal absorption of cefoxitin in human volunteers, Antimicrob. Agents Chemother., 28: 211.

Davis, S.S., Fara, J. and Hardy, J.G., 1986a, The intestinal transit of pharmaceutical dosage forms, Gut, in press.

Davis, S.S. and Illum, L., 1986, Colloidal delivery systems: opportunities and challenges, in: "Site Specific Delivery", E. Tomlinson and S.S. Davis, eds., Wiley, London, in press.

De Robertis, E.M., 1983, Nucleocytoplasmic segregation of proteins and RNAs, Cell, 32: 1021.

Dodson, E.J., Dodson, G.G., Hubbard, R.E. and Reynolds, C.D., 1983, Insulin's structural behaviour and its relation to activity, Biopolymers, 22: 281.

Evans, E.A., Gilmore, R. and Blobel, G., 1986, Purification of microsomal signal peptidase as a complex, Proc. Natl. Acad. Sci. USA, 83: 581.

Ewing, L.L., Wing, T.Y., Cochran, R.C., Kromann, N. and Zirkin, B.R., 1983, Effect of luteinizing hormone on Leydig cell structure for testosterone secretion, Endocrinology, 112: 1763.

Fagundes-Neto, U., Teichberg, S., Bayne, M.A., Morton, B. and Lifshitz, F., 1981, Bile salt-enhanced rat jejunal absorption of a macromolecular tracer, Lab. Invest., 44: 18.

Fisher, A.N., Brown, K., Davis, S.S., Parr, G.D. and Smith, D.A., 1986, The effect of molecular size on the nasal absorption of water soluble compounds by the albino rat, In preparation.

Fukunga, M., Miller, M.M., Hostetler, K.Y. and Deftos, L.J., 1985, Liposome entrapment enhances the hypercalcaemic action of parenterally administered calcitonin, Endocrinol., 115: 757.

Gabel, C.A. and Foster, S.A., 1986, Lysosomal enzyme trafficking in mannose 6-phosphate receptor-positive mouse L-cells: demonstration of a steady state accumulation of phosphorylated acid hydrolases, J. Cell Biol., 102: 943.

Gabev, E.E., Suilenov, D.K., Poljakakova-Krusteva, O.T. and Vassilev, I., 1985, Brain, liver and spleen detection of liposomes after rectal administration, J. Microencaps., 2: 85.

Gilmore, R., Blobel, G. and Walter, P., 1982, Protein translocation across the endoplasmic reticulum. Detection in the microsomal membrane of a receptor in the signal recognition particle, J. Cell Biol., 95: 463.

Glover, I., Haneef, I., Pitts, J., Wood, S., Moss, D., Tickle, I. and Blundell, T., 1983, Conformational flexibility in a small globular hormone: X-ray analysis of avian pancreatic polypeptide at 0.98 A resolution, Biopolymers, 22: 293.

Goldenberg, D.P., Smith, D.H. and King, J., 1983, Genetic and biochemical analysis of in vivo protein folding and subunit assembly, Biopolymers, 22: 125.

Gordon, G.S., Moses, A.C., Silver, R.D., Flier, J.S. and Carey, M.C., 1985, Nasal absorption of insulin: enhancement by hydrophobic bile salts, Proc. Natl. Acad. Sci. USA, 82: 7419.

Hailey, A., 1984, "Strong Medicine", Michael Joseph Ltd, London.

Heyman, M., Ducroc, R., Desjeux, J.F. and Morgat, J.L., 1982, Horseradish peroxidase transport across adult rabbit jejunum in vitro, Am. J. Physiol., 242: G558.

Holland, E.C. and Drickamer, K., 1985, Signal recognition particle mediates the insertion of a transmembrane protein which has a cytoplasmic NH_2 terminus, J. Biol. Chem., 261: 1286.

Illum, L. and Davis, S.S., 1984, The organ uptake of intravenously administered colloidal particles can be altered using a non-ionic surfactant (Poloxamer 338), FEBS Letters, 167: 79.

Illum, L., Davis, S.S., Muller, R.H., Mak, E. and West, P., 1986, The organ distribution and circulation time of intravenously injected carriers sterically stabilised with a block copolymer, To be submitted to Science.

Jeong, S.Y., Kim, S.W., Holmberg, D.L. and McRea, J.C., 1985, Self-regulating insulin delivery systems, J. Controll. Rel., 2: 143.

Katayama, K. and Fujita, T., 1972, Studies on biotransformation of elastase. II. Intestinal absorption of ^{131}I-labelled elastase in vivo, Biochim. Biophys. Acta, 288: 181.

Knobil, E., 1980, The neuroendocrine control of the menstrual cycle, Recent Prog. Hormone Res., 36: 53.

Koch, B. and Lutz-Bucher, B., 1985, Specific receptors for vasopressin in the pituitary gland: evidence for down-regulation and desensitisation to adrenocorticotropin-releasing factors, Endocrinology, 116: 671.

Kondor-Koch, C., Bravo, R., Fuller, S.D., Cutler, D. and Garoff, H., 1985, Exocytic pathways exist to both the apical and the basolateral cell surface of the polarized epithelial cell MDCK, Cell, 43: 297.

Kruisbrink, J. and Boer, G.J., 1984, Controlled long-term release of small peptide hormones using a new microporous polypropylene polymer. Its application for vasopressin in the Brattleboro rat and potential perinatal use, J. Pharm. Sci., 73: 17.

Langer, R., Lund, D., Leong, K. and Folkman, J., 1985, Controlled release of macromolecules: biological studies, J. Controll. Rel., 2: 331.

Langer, R., Rhine, W., Hsleh, D.S.T. and Folkman, J., 1980, Control of release kinetics of macromolecules from polymers, J. Membr. Sci., 7: 333.

Lecce, J.G., 1984, Absorption of macromolecules by mammalian epithelium, in: "Intestinal Toxicology", C.M. Schiller, ed., Raven Press, New York.

Lisi, P.J., Van Es, T., Abuchowski, A., Palczuk, N.C. and Davis, F.F., 1982, Enzyme therapy. I. Polyethylene glycol: -glucuronidase conjugates as potential therapeutic agents in acid mucopolysaccharidosis, J. Appl. Biochem., 4: 19-33.

Lynch, H.J., Rivest, R.W. and Wurtman, R.J., 1980, Artificial induction of melatonin rhythms by programmed microinfusions, Neuroendocrinol., 31: 106.

Michaels, A.S., 1985, Controlled release: challenges and opportunities for the next decade, J. Controll. Rel., 2: 405.

Miyake, M., Nishihata, T., Nagano, A., Kyobashi, Y. and Kamada, A., 1985, Rectal absorption of [Asu^{1,7}]-eel calcitonin in rats, Chem. Pharm. Bull., 33: 740.

Morimoto, K., Akatsuchi, H., Morisaka, K., Kamada, A., 1985, Effect of non-ionic surfactants in a polyacrylic acid gel base on the rectal absorption of [Asu^{1,7}]-eel calcitonin in rats, J. Pharm. Pharmacol., 37: 759.

Mostov, K.E. and Simister, N.E., 1985, Transcytosis, Cell, 43: 389.

Muranishi, S., 1985, Modification of intestinal absorption of drugs by lipoidal adjuvants, Pharmaceutical Research, 108.

Nagai, T., 1985, Adhesive topical drug delivery system, J. Controll. Rel., 2: 121.

Obie, J.F. and Cooper, C.W., 1979, Loss of calcemic effects of calcitonin and parathyroid hormone infused continuously into rats using the Alzet osmotic mini-pump, J. Pharm. Expl. Ther., 209: 422.

O'Hagan, D.T., Palin, K.J. and Davis, S.S., 1986, Intestinal absorption of proteins and macromolecules and the immunological response, CRC Critical Reviews in Therapeutic Drug Carrier Systems in press.

Owen, R.L., Pierce, N.F., Apple, R.T. and Cray, W.D., 1982, Phagocytosis and transport by M-cells of intact vibrio-cholerae into rabbit Peyer's patch follicles, J. Cell Biol., 95: 446A.

Posnansky, M.J. and Juliano, R.L., 1984, Biological approaches to the controlled delivery of drugs: a critical review, Pharmacol. Rev., 36: 277.

Poste, G., 1985, Drug targeting in cancer chemotherapy, in: Receptor Mediated Targeting of Drugs", G. Gregoriadis, G. Poste, J. Senior and A. Trouet, eds., Plenum Press, New York, p427.

Postmes, Th.J., Hukkelhoven, M., van den Bogaard, A.E.J.M., Holders, S.G. and Coegracht, J., 1980, Passage through blood-brain barrier of thyrotopin releasing hormone encapsulated in liposome, J. Pharm. Pharmac., 32: 722.

Renston, R.H., Maloney, D.G., Jones, A.L., Hradek, G.T., Wong, K.Y. and Goldfine, I.D., 1980, Bile secretory apparatus: evidence for a vesicular transport mechanism for proteins in the rat, using horseradish peroxidase and [^{125}I] insulin, Gastroenterol., 78: 1373.

Rikihisa, Y. and Mizuna, D., 1978, Different arrangements on phagolysosomal membranes which depend upon the particles phagocytised. Observations on the markers of the two sides of the plasma membranes, Expl. Cell Res., 111: 437.

Rosenberg, S.A., Lotze, M.T., Muul, L.M., Leitman, S., Chang, A.E., Ettinghausen, S.E., Matory, Y.L., Skibber, J.M., Shiloni, E., Vetto, J.T., Seipp, C.A., Simpson, C. and Reichert, C.M., 1985, Observations on the systemic administration of autologous lymphokine-activated killer cells and recombinant interleukin-2 to patients with metastatic cancer, New Engl. J. Med., 313: 1485.

Rowland, R.N. and Woodley, J.F., 1981, Uptake of free and liposome-entrapped horseradish peroxidase by rat intestinal sacs in vitro, FEBS Letters, 123: 41.

Saiki, I., Sone, S., Fogler, W.E., Kleinerman, E.S., Lopez-Berestein, G. and Fidler, I.J., 1985, Synergism between human recombinant gamma interferon and muramyl dipeptide encapsulated in liposomes for activation of antitumor properties in human blood monocytes, Cancer Research, 45: 6188.

Salzman, R., Manson, J.E., Griffing, G.T., Kimmerle, R., Ruderman, N., McCall, A., Stoltz, E.I., Mullin, C., Small, D., Armstrong, J. and Melby, J.C., 1985, Intranasal aerosolized insulin. Mixed meal studies and long-term use in Type I diabetes, New Engl. J. Med., 1078.

Samanen, J.M., 1985, Polypeptides as Drugs, in: "Polymeric Materials in Medication", C.G. Gebelein and C.E. Carraher, eds., Plenum Press, New York, p227.

Schally, A.V. and Redding, T.W., 1985, Combination of long-acting microcapsules of the D-tryptophan-6 analog of luteinizing hormone-releasing hormone with chemotherapy: investigation in the rat prostate cancer model, Proc. Natl. Acad. Sci. USA, 82: 2498.

Schlessinger, J., 1983, Lateral and rotational diffusion of EGF-receptor complex: relationship to receptor-mediated endocytosis, Biopolymers, 22: 347.

Sela, M., 1983, From synthetic antigens to synthetic vaccines, Biopolymers, 22: 415-424.

Sennett, C. and Rosenberg, L.E., 1981, Transmembrane transport of cobalamin in prokaryotic and eukaryotic cells, Ann. Rev. Biochem., 50: 1053.

Siegel, R.A. and Langer, R., 1984, Controlled release of polypeptides and other macromolecules, Pharmaceutical Research, 2.

Sidman, K.R., Steber, W.D., Schwope, A.D. and Schnaper, G.R., 1983, Controlled release of macromolecules and pharmaceuticals from synthetic polypeptides based on glutamic acid, Biopolymers, 22: 547.

Steinman, R.M., Mellman, I.S., Muller, W.A. and Cohn, Z.A., 1983, Endocytosis and the recycling of plasma membrane, J. Cell Biol., 96: 1.

Su, K.S.E., 1986, Intranasal delivery of peptides and proteins, Pharm. Int., 7: 8.

Takada, K., Shibata, N., Yoshimura, H., Masuda, Y., Yoshikawa, H., Muranishi, S. and Oka, T., 1985, Promotion of the selective lymphatic delivery of cyclosporin A by lipid-surfactant mixed micelles, J. Pharmacobio-Dyn., 8: 320.

Tobey, N., Heizer, W., Yeh, R., Huang, T-I. and Hoffner, C., 1985, Human intestinal brush border peptidases, Gastroenterol., 88: 913.

Toniolo, C., Bonora, G.M., Stavropoulos, G., Cordopatis, P. and Theodoropoulos, D., 1986, Self-association and solubility of peptides: solvent-titration study of N-protected C-terminal sequences of substance P, Biopolymers, 25: 281.

Urquhart, J., Fara, J.W. and Willis, K.L., 1984, Rate-controlled delivery systems in drug and hormone research, Ann. Rev. Pharmacol. Toxicol., 24: 199.

Visscher, G.E., Robison, R.L., Maudling, H.V., Fong, J.W., Pearson, J.E. and Argentieri, G.J., 1985, Biodegradation of and tissue reaction to 50:50 poly(DL-lactide-coglycolide) microcapsules, Biomed. Materials Res., 19: 349.

Wada, A., Saito, Y. and Ohogushi, M., 1983, Multiphasic conformation transition of globular proteins under denaturating perturbation, Biopolymers, 22: 93.

Wallace, B.A., 1983, Gramicidin A adopts distinctly different conformations in membranes and in organic solvents, Biopolymers, 22: 397.

Wileman, T.E., Foster, R.L. and Elliott, P.N.C., 1986, Soluble asparaginase-dextran conjugates show increased circulatory persistance and lowered antigen reactivity, J. Pharm. Pharmacol., 38: 264.

Williams, G., Kerle, D., Griffin, S., Dunlop, H. and Bloom, S.R., 1984, Biodegradable polymer luteinising hormone releasing hormone analogue for prostatic cancer: use of a new peptide delivery system, Brit. Med. J., 289: 1580.

Woodley, J.F., 1986, Liposomes for oral administration of drugs, CRC Critical Reviews in Therapeutic Drug Carrier Systems, 2: 1.

Wunsch, E., 1983, Peptide factors as pharmaceuticals: criteria for applications, Biopolymers, 22: 493.

Yagi, K., Naoi, M., Sakai, H., Abe, H., Konishi, H. and Arichi, S., 1982, Incorporation of enzyme into the brain by means of liposomes of novel composition, J. Appl. Biochem., 4: 121.

Yoshikawa, H., Sezaki, H. and Muranishi, S., 1983, Mechanism for selective transfer of bleomycin into lymphatics by a bifunctional delivery system via the lumen of the large intestine, Int. J. Pharmac., 13: 321.

Yoshikawa, H., Takada, K. and Muranishi, S., 1984, Molecular weight dependence of permselectivity to rat small intestinal blood-lymph barrier for exogenous macromolecules absorbed from the lumen, J. Pharm. Dyn., 7: 1.

Yoshikawa, H., Takada, K., Satoh, Y., Naruse, N. and Muranishi, S., 1985, Potentiation of enteral absorption of human interferon alpha and selective transfer into lymphatics in rats, Pharm. Res., 249.

BIOTECHNOLOGY AND PROTEIN PRODUCTION

Spencer Emtage

Molecular Biology Division
Celltech Limited, 250 Bath Road
Slough SL1 4DY, Berks, England

INTRODUCTION

A recent review of the Biotechnology Industry listed 48 small companies (Genentech being the largest of these) and 9 Pharmaceutical majors in this field. The areas being investigated ranged from Immune Modifiers and anti-Cancer agents through Blood Proteins and Hormones to Vaccines and Anti-infectives. Indeed, a number of these products, namely human insulin, human growth hormone and interferon alpha are now being marketed while others such as tissue plasminogen activator and hepatitis B vaccine are in advanced trials.

In all cases so far the products on the market are sold as injectables. Insulin and growth hormone are replacement products and so this method of administration is not questioned at present. Interferon is being used to treat hairy-cell leukaemia and again an injection is acceptable. Indeed injections will probably be acceptable in most situations where life is threatened; a good example of this is the use of tissue plasminogen activator on patients with coronary thrombosis. But what of products that are not aimed at life threatening diseases or situations, those that may reduce pain in arthritis sufferers or reduce the incidence of fractures associated with osteoporosis. What will patient compliance be if these have to be injected frequently? Is there any alternative to injections?

The answer to the last question is yes. There are two main strategies that are being pursued. The first is to develop novel systems to deliver these new protein and peptide drugs. This concept is not really new. What is new is the type of molecule under consideration. In general these are molecules with relatively high molecular weights and probably low stability. The problem is how to get them absorbed efficiently and this is really the subject of this meeting. The second strategy is more radical and long term. Here the proteins and peptides are seen as a means to an end rather than an end in themselves. It is accepted that delivery of large proteins is difficult and that a solution may not be found. Instead the proteins and their effects are analysed in detail in the belief that an understanding of protein-protein interactions will allow the rational design of small chemical molecules that will mimic those actions of the particular protein and be orally active.

Which of these approaches is better cannot be stated at present. What is clear however is that for either to even begin, a source of protein or peptide is needed and this is where Biotechnology comes in. The Biotechnologist now has available to him a choice of systems for producing proteins. These have evolved over the last four or five years as knowledge has accumulated and some of the problems become clearer. The remainder of this paper will review these systems and discuss some of the problems and their implications. References to original papers have not been included in this discussion. If required they can be found in reviews by Harris (1983), Harris and Emtage (1986), Carter et al (1986) and Bebbington and Hentschel (1986).

THE SYSTEMS

Gene expression means taking the genetic information stored in DNA and decoding it so that a protein molecule is produced. This is done by transcribing the DNA into RNA and translating the RNA into protein. Three types of cell are currently used for protein production by expression of foreign genes. These are Escherichia coli, the yeast Saccharomyces cerevisiae and various mammalian cells. Although the general requirements for gene expression do not vary greatly among these cells, the specific mechanisms of transcription and translation are quite different. Thus there are specific transcriptional and translational barriers between the three types of cells mentioned above. The important conclusion from this is that to optimally express, for example, a gene from a human cell in E.coli, one must mimic and/or exploit the features of E.coli genes that result in high levels of both transcription and translation. Usually this is done by creating for the foreign gene a molecular biological environment as similar as possible to that of the genes from the host cell itself. From this comes the concept of an 'expression cassette' for the different cell types into which different genes may be placed. It is comprised of three main features, a region of DNA capable of binding RNA polymerases and initiating transcription (the promoter), the gene itself and a region downstream of the gene that is involved either in transcription termination (for E.coli and yeast) or mRNA maturation and polyadenylation (mammalian cells)

It is beyond the scope of this paper to describe the details of either prokaryotic and eukaryotic promoters or transcription termination. Suffice it to say that many systems are now available and that moving from E.coli through yeast to the higher eukaryotic cells results in increased complexity and choice of system. In E.coli the situation is quite simple; promoters are well characterised and function effectively in most E.coli strains. In yeast, strain differences start to become important. For example the α-factor promoter functions in $\underline{\alpha}$ cells but not in $\underline{a}$ cells or a/α cells. In animal cells the situation is even more complex and the final choice of cell type and expression cassette will depend on whether one is trying to establish permanent cell lines, whether the DNA should be maintained episomally or integrated into the chromosome, whether a suspension cell is favoured over an anchorage dependent one and whether the protein will be correctly modified by one particular cell.

ESCHERICHIA COLI

There are two general strategies for obtaining expression of the foreign genes in E.coli. Either the protein is produced as a fusion by cloning the foreign gene downstream of and in frame with a bacterial coding sequence or as a 'native' protein by direct expression of the gene.

Fusion Proteins

Why should one wish to express a eukaryotic gene as part of a fusion protein? There is one very good reason for doing this. Our experience is that small peptides are turned over very rapidly by E. coli proteolytic enzymes, making it very difficult to accumulate large quantities of these molecules. If however they are produced, as part of a fusion protein, by fusing the gene in the correct translational reading frame to an E. coli gene that is known to be efficiently expressed, then they are stabilised. Of course, since it is the peptide that is required rather than the fusion protein itself, a strategy must exist for cleaving the fusion to liberate the peptide.

The somatostatin experiment was the first report of the designed expression of a small eukaryotic gene in E. coli as part of a fusion protein. It is still a good paradigm of this type of experiment as it also demonstrates the use of chemically synthesised oligonucleotides in gene assembly as well as the subsequent cleavage of the β-galactosidase- somatostatin fusion by cyanogen bromide to form the native hormone.

With this success, very similar strategies were followed for the production of the A and B chains of insulin, for the neuropeptide β-endorphin and others. The main differences were in methods used to liberate the peptides from the fusions and these reflected the amino acid compositions of the peptides themselves. For example, those peptides lacking methionine can be synthesised as β-gal-met-peptide and cleaved chemically with cyanogen bromide while those lacking arginine or lysine can be produced as β-gal-lys (or arg)-peptide and cleaved with trypsin. Other proteases that may be used are clostripain, which cleaves preferentially after arginine and S. aureus V8 protease which cleaves after glutamic acid residues. The rather limited number of proteases and the requirements for the absence of certain amino acids from the peptide of interest has stimulated a search for cleavage strategies that are more generally applicable. Two of these have recently been reported based on the enzymes enterokinase and Factor Xa (Table 1).

Table 1 Strategies for Cleaving Fusion Proteins

Enzyme or Chemical	Specificity
Cyanogen bromide	-met↓
Acid	-asp↓pro-
Trypsin	-lys↓; -arg↓
V8 protease	-glu↓
Clostripain	-arg↓
Enterokinase	-(asp)$_4$-lys↓
Factor Xa	-ile-glu-gly-arg↓
Collagenase	-pro-x↓gly-pro-y↓

Direct Expression of Eukaryotic Genes

As already mentioned, the requirements for efficient gene transcription in E. coli are now well understood and, in general, achieving efficient production of mRNA from heterologous genes is not usually a major hurdle. Ho·ever the determinants of the translation initiation process have not been completely elucidated and it is these, especially the ribosome binding site, to which careful attention must be given.

The ribosome binding site (RBS) is defined as the region of the mRNA protected by the ribosome from nucleolytic digestion. The RBS has only two semi-conserved sequences, as initiator AUG and the Shine Dalgarno (SD) sequence. The SD sequence consists of a 3-9 nucleotide long, purine-rich sequence which is complementary to the 3' end of 16 S ribosomal RNA. There is genetic and biochemical evidence that this SD sequence plays a role in the selection of sites for translational initiation by 30 S ribosomal subunits. The SD sequence is found between 6 and 11 nucleotides upstream of the AUG initiation codon in most E. coli mRNAs.

The efficiency of initiation seems to be controlled in at least three ways: the extent of complementarity between the SD sequence and 16 S RNA, the distance between the SD sequence and AUG, and the structural environment of the SD sequence and AUG. Experimental evidence for the first two of these is now overwhelming. Evidence for the third is however only circumstantial as the existance of predicted secondary structures has never been proven.

Protein Products

A major advantage of E. coli as an expression host is that gene expression in the cytoplasm can accumulate to levels of up to 20% of total cell protein. A major disadvantage of E. coli as an expression host is that it is now clear that the majority of eukaryotic proteins synthesised in this organism are insoluble and hence inactive. Some of these insoluble products form dense aggregates, called inclusion bodies, which can be easily seen in the phase-contrast light microscope. Under the electron microscope they are seen as amorphous aggregates not enclosed by or in contact with membranes.

The means by which inclusions form is poorly understood. In part, it may be due to the presence of abnormally high concentrations of a single protein in the cell. Thus, normal E. coli proteins like β-galactosidase will accumulate in insoluble form when synthesised at high levels. This cannot be the whole story however, since many eukaryotic proteins are insoluble even when expressed at low levels. The main reason for the insolubility probably relates to the nature of the eukaryotic proteins themselves and the environment of the cell in which they are being produced.

Many of the eukaryotic proteins that are found to be insoluble in the E. coli cytoplasm, are normally secreted after synthesis and have structures that include specific disulphide bridges which form between cysteine residues during the process of secretion. The cytoplasm of E. coli however is very reducing and thus unsuitable for disulphide formation. In keeping with this, few if any E. coli cytoplasmic proteins have disulphide bonds and, for one of the secreted E. coli proteins (β-lactamase) that does have a disulphide bond, there is clear evidence that its intracellular precursor does not have this linkage.   Its formation is concomitant with processing and secretion into the periplasmic space.

With this in mind it is very likely that, when large eykaryotic proteins are synthesised in E. coli, the disulphide bridges are not formed.   The result of this may be an incorrectly folded polypeptide that precipitates from solution and aggregates as a result of hydrophobic, ionic or covalent interactions between the protein molecules.   Then, on exposure to air during cell lysis the formation of both inter- and intra-molecular disulphide bridges may take place.

A consequence of the insolubility is that after cell lysis the protein sediments with cell debris on centrifugation.   On the positive side this offers a partial purification which can be made even better with certain washing procedures.   A negative aspect is that this fraction is also rich in lipopoly-saccharide.   Purification however is not the major difficulty;   that is the process of going from insoluble aggregation to soluble, active protein.   In most cases this is a multistep process, the precise details of which will differ from protein to protein.   The first task is to denature the proteins completely using agents such as 8M Urea, 6M guanidine-HCl, high pH or organic solvents all of which will disrupt hydrogen bonds and ionic or hydrophobic interactions and leave the polypeptide completely unfolded.   In this state the proteins may be purified further by, for example, gel filtration in the presence of guanidine-HCl or ion exchange chromatography in the presence of 8M urea.

Renaturation may also be accomplished in a variety of ways. The denaturant may be dialysed away or diluted out;   it may be done in a stepwise fashion where guanidine HCl is exchanged for urea which in turn is dialysed away.   The message is that there is no one method that is suitable for all proteins and that many combinations and permutations may have to be tried before a suitable one is found. Even then, careful testing will be needed to verify that all molecules are correctly folded and that no conformational variants are present.   Indeed, for very large, complex proteins such as tPA it may prove impossible to achieve acceptable yields of biologically active protein.

So far, attention has been given only to insoluble proteins. There are a number of proteins that are produced in a soluble, active form in E. coli.   It must be stated however that whether all or only a proportion of these proteins are soluble is not clear from the data given.   Examples of these include human and bovine interferon alpha, human lymphotoxin and human tumour necrosis factor.   In the soluble form these proteins can be purified by conventional methods.

A final question concerns the nature of the N-terminus of the molecule.   For example, when human growth hormone is synthesised in E. coli, the primary protein product contains an N-terminal formyl methionine residue.   The formyl group is removed by the endogenous formylase but the methionine group remains.   With bovine growth hormone the situation is different in that more than 93% of the molecules had the methionine removed.   The reason for this variation probably lies in the specificity of the methionyl aminopeptidase, the enzyme responsible for cleavage of the N-terminal methionine.   This shows a preference for alanine, threonine or glycine in juxtaposition to the methionine.   In bovine growth hormone the second residue is alanine while in human growth hormone the second residue is phenylalanine.   The presence of an N-terminal methionine on many

eukaryotic proteins produced in E. coli is a potential problem as it
may be immunogenic or cause other side effects when administered to
humans.

Final Considerations

Although E. coli has been widely used to date, it is clear that
it is not universally suited as a host organism for producing proteins
or peptides for pharmaceutical use. Host/vector systems are well
developed and many groups now have considerable experience of working
at medium to large scale. The real problems and difficulties arise
with downstream processing - cell harvesting and breakage, isolation
of inclusion bodies, denaturation/ renaturation and purification.
Many of the renaturation protocols involve large dilution steps and
therefore involve very big volumes. The combination of these
procedures leads to a very complicated and expensive process and
produces products which, as already stated may contain a methionine at
the N-terminus, may be contaminated with endotoxins and may contain
conformational isomers.

Some of these problems may be overcome in the future with the
development of easily scaled up reactivation protocols.
Alternatively, some of the interesting work in progress at present on
secretion of proteins into the periplasm or even into he medium may
lead to processes that are simpler and, at the same time, produce
properly folded proteins with correct amino termini. If these
advances are made then it seems likely that E.coli will remain an
important host for expressing many recombinant proteins. The major
exceptions will probably be proteins that need specific
post-translational modifications, such as glycosylation, before use.
A summary of these factors is given in Table 2.

Table 2   E.coli as a Host Organism

Advantages	Problems at Present	Future
1. Genetics and molecular biology are well researched. 2. Good host/vector systems are available 3. It is capable of rapid growth in cheap defined medium.	1. It is at potential source of endotoxins 2. Proteins are insoluble leading to tedious and difficult processes. 3. Some intracellular proteins contain an N-terminal methionine. 4. Proteins are not glycosylated. 5. Proteins are not usually secreted.	1. Easily scaled up reactivation processes may be developed. 2. Secretion into the periplasm may lead to a simpler process as well as correctly folded protein with an authentic N-terminus. 3. The potential for continuous processes.

SACCHAROMYCES CEREVISIAE

The first attempt to express a foreign gene in yeast was with a genomic clone of the rabbit β-globin gene using a vector based on the yeast 2-micron plasmid. It was found that the mammalian promoter was not used normally and that the introns in the mRNA transcript were not excised. Further experiments have confirmed that yeast is unable to splice the mRNA transcripts of higher eukaryotes and as a result, in the more recent experiments either cDNA's or synthetic genes have been used to provide coding information. These genes are "sandwiched" between promoters and terminators of yeast genes that are normally expressed at high levels.

A considerable number of genes have now been expressed in yeast so that the protein accumulates intracellularly. It is a general observation however that the heterologous genes are expressed much less efficiently than the yeast gene from which the expression signals were derived. For example, interferon alpha is synthesised from the PGK promoter on a 2-micron based plasmid as 1-3% of total cell protein. If the PGK gene is expressed instead, then PGK is present at over 50% of total cell protein. Clearly much work is still required to define the factors that limit accumulation of foreign proteins and so maximise the potential of yeast as a host system. In spite of these difficulties, at least one potential product from yeast, a vaccine to hepatitis B virus has already entered clinical trials.

As well as intracellular expression, a number of laboratories are investigating the use of yeast to secrete proteins and peptides into the medium and really, this may ultimately be the best use for the organism. On the scientific side, an attraction of secretion is that the mechanism has been well studied and is known to be similar to that of higher eukaryotes, that is, there is also the potential for protein glycosylation. Thus, proteins destined for secretion pass into the lumen of the endoplasmic reticulum where signal sequences are removed and core glycosylation takes place. From there they pass to Golgi-like vesicles where further glycosylation takes place. After secretion into the periplasm, the proteins are then transported via secretory granules to the plasma membrane. Whether this ability to glycosylate is really a blessing or will turn out to be a burden is not yet clear since there is a very significant difference between the carbohydrate moieties found on yeast and mammalian proteins.

On the practical side, the attraction of secretion is that downstream processing and purification should be simplified since yeast cells naturally secrete very few proteins into the medium. A number of higher eukaryotic proteins have now been secreted from yeast using their natural signal sequences. Examples are interferons alpha and gamma and mouse and wheat α-amylases. The evidence available is indicative of processing of signal sequences but, except for interferon alpha where 64% of the secreted molecules were correctly processed, the accuracy is unknown.

Some success has also been achieved using endogenous yeast signal sequences such as those from the acid phosphatase and invertase genes. However, perhaps the most interesting signal to be used for secretion of both peptides and proteins is the leader region of the precursor of the yeast mating pheromone alpha factor.

α-Factor is synthesised from a 165 amino acid precursor that consists of a signal sequence, a "pro" sequence with three glycosylation sites and four repeats of the 13 amino acid α-factor peptide. The repeats are separated by the dipeptide, lysine-arginine, followed by two or three dipeptides which consist of either glutamic acid-alanine or aspartic acid-alanine. Mature α-factor is excised from the precursor by cleavage after the lysine-arginine by a trypsin-like enzyme, followed by removal of the N-terminal dipeptides with dipeptidyl aminopeptidase and removal of the C-terminal basic residues by carboxypeptidase B.

A number of foreign genes have been placed after the sequences coding either for the first lysine-arginine or for the first glutamic acid-alanine dipeptide repeat. For example, when the sequence for human epidermal growth factor (EGF) was inserted in these positions nearly all of the EGF peptide synthesised was secreted. Furthermore, this secreted EGF was biologically active, although sequence analysis showed that authentic EGF was only produced when the coding sequence was adjacent to the lysine-arginine residues. Very similar results were obtained when a gene for interferon alpha was used in place of EGF.

Not all peptides and proteins examined using the α-factor system are correctly processed however and, in addition, internal cleavages at lysine residues have also been observed. Presumably the conformation of different proteins may affect the susceptibility of the cleavage sites. Clearly the α-factor system has great potential for the future.

As with E.coli, there are still questions to be asked for yeast. Will it be possible to design linkages with the pre-pro α-factor sequence so that the correct cleavage patterns for proteins and peptides are always seen? How well will larger proteins be secreted using this system? Will the different glycosylation patterns referred to above present an immunological problem for recombinant proteins derived from yeast and used as therapeutic agents? A summary of the advantages, present and potential future situation for the organism is given in Table 3

Table 3   Yeast as a Host Organism

Advantage	Problems at Present	Future
1.Genetics, molecular biology and physiology well researched. 2.It is non-pathogenic and acceptable to food industry. 3.There is extensive fermentation experience. 4.The mechanism of secretion is well researched. 5.Some heterologous proteins accumulate intracellularly in a soluble form.	1. Expression levels are generally low. 2. Glycosylation not the same as in higher eukaryotes. 3. Not all secreted peptides are processed properly. 4. Large proteins are poorly secreted. 5. Commercial processes for expression are still to be fully established.	1. Factors affecting expression will be better understood. 2. Expression levels can be regulated. 3. Processing mechanisms better understood. 4. Supersecreting mutants will be available. 5. Production systems for low cost proteins.

MAMMALIAN CELLS

Academic work aimed at understanding the mechanism of gene transcription and expression in many mammalian systems was advancing rapidly at the time that the insolubility of many eukaryotic proteins in E.coli was becoming apparent. These problems have since led to many of the specialist biotechnology companies putting a special emphasis on eukaryotic cells for protein production. Two systems have emerged from this work as good candidates for use in industrial processes.

The first of these is based on gene amplification after the DNA is integrated into the chromosome. The phenomenon of gene amplification arose from the observation that if cultured cells were grown in the presence of increasing concentrations of certain drugs, then variant clones could be isolated with higher resistance to the drug than the wild type cells. In most cases the increased resistance was due to the overproduction of an essential enzyme whose activity was inhibited by the drug. Further investigation confirmed that overproduction was due to an increase in the copy number of the gene coding for the enzyme.

From this it was speculated that it might be possible to overproduce a non-selectable protein if its gene was introduced into the cell with another gene that was capable of being amplified. This speculation has proved to be correct and the use of co-amplification is now well established. The best characterised of these systems uses the Chinese hamster ovary (CHO) cell as recipient and the gene for the enzyme dihydrofolate reductase (DHFR) for selection and amplification. The strategy favoured by most groups is to transfect the CHO cells with DNA that contains the DHFR gene linked to the gene for expression. At the laboratory and development levels this approach has been very successful and cell lines producing considerable quantities (up to 50pg per cell per day) of tPA, Hepatitis β surface antigen and interferon beta have been reported,

In the second system that is quite widely used, the newly introduced DNA is maintained episomally in the cell rather than integrated into the chromosome. This is achieved by constructing vectors that contain an origin of replication as an intergral part. Many of these origins of replication are obtained from the DNA of animal viruses such as the monkey virus SV40 and bovine papillomavirus (BPV). An advantage of these systems is that since these viruses are present in multiple copies in each cell, then vectors based on them should provide an easy means of achieving increased gene copy number. Of the two viruses mentioned above, BPV is the most useful in producing stable cell lines and vectors containing either the whole virus genome or subgenomic fragments have been produced for introduction into recipient cells such as the mouse fibroblast line C127. Together with a strong promoter-enhancer combination, this system has proved very effective for the production of some proteins, for example human growth hormone.

Whether these cell lines will be stable to prolonged culture in the absence of selection is not clear as stability may depend on the protein being produced. If stability does prove to be a problem it may eventually be necessary to develop ways of controlling gene expression.

As well as removing the insolubility problems often encountered with E.coli, the mammalian cell systems offer other very significant advantages. The protein is secreted into the medium, from where it can be recovered with relative ease, and will have a correct amino terminus. However, most importantly perhaps there is the probability of having correct post-translational modifications, such as glycosylation, carried out. For some other modifications, such as gamma- carboxylation of proteins like the blood-clotting Factor IX, it may be necessary to use selected cell lines known to produce the carboxylase enzyme.

Table 4 Mammalian Cells as Hosts

Advantages	Problems at Present
1. Produces the natural protein.	1. Relatively high cost to grow cells.
2. Product is secreted into the medium.	2. Molecule biology still being worked out.
3. Serum-free media available for some cells.	3. Long term stability of some cell lines not clear
4. High yields achieved for products.	4.Some concern by regulatory authorities about, for example, viruses.
5. Correct post-translational modifications carried out.	

In spite of producing authentic proteins, mammalian cell systems also have difficulties associated with them and they may not be the panacea that they appear to be. Stability of cell lines has already been mentioned. Another concern is the presence of viruses or DNA in the final product. This concern will presumably grow if human cells are used instead of animal cells. A list of advantages and some of the difficulties with animal cells is given in Table 4.

CONCLUSIONS

A multiplicity of systems are now available for producing human proteins that have therapeutic potential. At present not all of these systems produce authentic proteins and this, coupled with other properties that may be introduced by the difficult downstream processing required in some cases, may give rise to products with undesirable characteristics, some of which may cause immunogenic reactions (Table 5). However, such is the pace of this technology that no sooner has a problem arisen than a potential solution has been found. For example, the insolubility of proteins encountered in E.coli may be overcome by using either E.coli or yeast vectors designed for secretion and the lack of protein glycosylation by using mammalian cells.

In the future, each system may have its own niche. E.coli and yeast for proteins that do not need post-translational modifications, especially if secretion is possible. These systems will come into their own when large quantities of product are required. Yeast at present also looks especially attractive for peptide production while the animal cell systems (and maybe human cells at some stage) will be needed for the more complex proteins that require glycosylation or other modifications either for activity or to overcome immunogenic reactions.

Table 5 Factors that could contribute to
immunogenicity of recombinant DNA
derived proteins

1.   Denatured protein or conformations isomers

2.   Aggregates

3.   Presence of an N-terminal methionine

4.   Incorrect glycosylation or lack of glycosylation

5.   Amino acid substitutions or deletions

REFERENCES

Bebbington, C., and Hentschel, C.C., 1986, The expression of recombinant
    DNA products in mammalian cells, Trends in Biotechnology, 3:314
Carter, B.L.A., Doel, S., Goodey, A., Piggott, J., and Watson, M.E.W.,
    1986, Secretion of mammalian polypeptides from yeast, Microbio-
    logical Sciences, 3:23.
Harris, T.J.R., 1983, Expression of eykaryotic genes in E.coli, in:
    Genetic Engineering, vol 4, R. Williamson, ed., Academic Press,
    London
Harris, T.J.R., and Emtage, J.S., 1986, Expression of heterologous genes
    in E.coli, Microbiological Sciences, 3:28

PEPTIDE ANALYSIS: CRITICAL TECHNOLOGY FOR EVALUATING DELIVERY APPROACHES

Larry A. Sternson and Thomas R. Malefyt

Smith Kline & French Laboratories
709 Swedeland Road
Swedeland, PA   19479

Peptides and proteins are emerging as an increasingly important chemical class of drugs as they become more readily available through improvements in recombinant DNA technology and approaches to their chemical synthesis.

Their development and production as drugs present daunting scientific challenges. The rigor of the analytical methods that are adopted to characterize and evaluate this group of substances will not only help define our understanding of their chemical and biological properties, but will likely impact on their regulatory approval and the success and safety of the resulting products.

In a recent review (de Vlaminck, 1984), it was suggested that the level of analysis necessary to support regulatory filing of recombinant DNA products should include: in-process monitoring of the DNA sequence of the micro-organism producing the protein; HPLC tryptic mapping of in-process materials and final products; sensitive techniques to evaluate purity; and biological properties evaluated through clinical trials. The vagueness and simplicity of this list reflects the current uncertainty within the Industry regarding the subtleties and complexities involved in developing peptide/protein drug substances into safe and efficacious products. Indeed, it appears that regulatory approval of Protropin (human growth hormone) was based on analytical methods that gave relatively little information on absolute identity and purity of the drug substance. Other than routine tests for color, appearance, pH, sterility, pyrogenicity and general safety, the only tests performed for batch release were determination of protein concentrations (using Lowry's method), identity confirmed by silver stained SDS PAG electrophoretograms, amino acid analysis and HPLC of the tryptic digest, and therapeutic potency evaluated in terms of relative rates of growth of treated and untreated hypophysectomized rats. Similar approaches to analysis were found in the NDA approval for human insulin - Humanlin. The need for analytical methodology that can provide more information regarding drug identity and purity is clear.

Several properties of peptides and proteins present particular challenges to their analysis. The biological potency characteristic of these molecules requires methods that are exquisitely sensitive. Additionally, the striking similarity in structure between analyte, degradates, impurities and matrix components places tremendous demands for selectivity on analytical methodology. Such methods must also consider the relationship between the purity and activity of the analyte. Whereas for small molecules, physical chemical identity and purity assessment is sufficient to guarantee therapeutic potency; peptides and proteins, due to their complexity, also require an independent evaluation of activity. Purity must reflect not only chemical composition, but also chirality, conformation and physical states of aggregation of the analyte. Consideration must be given to the fact that, in some cases, loss of purity measured in terms of these criteria may not impact on biological activity, while in other cases, deficiencies in the scope of available analytical methodology cause impurities that do influence biological activity not to be recognized.

Peptides and proteins may exist in several active forms (i.e., they exhibit microheterogeneity). Portions of the backbone termini may be lost through proteolytic degradation, without compromising drug potency. For example, variants ("clipped products") of tissue plasminogen activator (in which the N-terminus is serine [1]) have been reported where the N-terminus amino acid is glycine [-3] (Wallen et al., 1983), valine [4] (Jornvall et al., 1983) or a more dramatic loss of about 3000 daltons (Ranby et al., 1982), which represents the loss of about 27 amino acids from the N-terminus. All of these species have apparently identical thrombolytic activity. Similarly, the extent and nature of post-translational modifications (e.g., glycosylation) may vary over a range among the naturally occurring active molecules without affecting activity. It is likely that peptide and protein samples will contain a number of active compositions and forms that will have to be individually understood before a precise assessment of drug purity can be made.

The activity of larger polypeptides (>10,000 daltons) usually resides in their tertiary and quaternary structure and thus, depends on maintaining certain conformation(s). This fragile property may be the only feature that distinguishes an active from an inactive material. Thus, it is important to recognize factors that can alter conformation and have analytical methods at hand to sense such subtle changes in form.

Analytical methods for the determination of peptides and proteins can be divided into four types: bioassays, immunoassays, enzyme assays and physical/chemical assays. The distinction is somewhat artificial, since many methods are hybrids of two or more of these categories. However, within a category, the methods share common properties making these divisions useful for discussion.

Bioassay

Historically, most proteinaceous materials are evaluated by bioassay. The inactivation of such molecules is frequently chemically invisible and samples appear by all chemical/instrumental methods to be completely homogenous. Thus, activity measured in terms of biological response divided by total protein concentration (i.e., specific activity) has proven to be a useful measure of purity.

Most bioassays are difficult to use in an analytically rigorous program of drug substance evaluation. They are generally highly variable, very time consuming, economically unsound and not suitable for automation. They are, therefore, impractical for formulation optimization tasks in which a variety of excipients and experimental conditions must be evaluated. Assay reproducibility is generally on the order of ± 20-50% due to variabilities in the assay system itself, as well as uncertainties as to the role of "impurities" or degradates in modulating the biological endpoint. The high degree of variability inherent in bioassays makes assignment of shelf life based on such methodology difficult and often results in a severe under-estimation of drug stability. Furthermore, multiple replication of assays, and the use of extensive standards, blanks and controls is essential if data are to be interpreted with reasonable statistical confidence. With the advent of recombinant technology and improvements in peptide synthesis, however, more stringent criteria for acceptance, approaching the criteria for "small" molecules, is anticipated. Thus, more convenient, economically sound analytical approaches are needed to supplement bioassays, although bioassays are essential for validating the relevance of (bio)chemically-based assays which will be discussed in the remainder of this chapter. In fact, correlations between assays based on chemical and biological endpoints will likely be required to define "protein concentration" in terms of drug purity, stability and pharmacokinetics. The confidence gained by such correlations is illustrated in the evaluation of the bioavailability of the vasopressin antagonist, SK&F 101926, when administered intranasally (Liversidge et al., 1986). Bioavailability determined independently by HPLC analysis (of drug concentration in plasma) and in terms of increased urine output and urine osmolality both approximated 20% (at doses of 100 ug/kg) in the dog.

Immunoassays

The specific and tight association of antibody with drug substance antigens can be exploited to determine very low concentrations of peptide/protein drugs in a variety of complex matrices. Such methods are routinely used to monitor the drug in the host cell medium and its fate in metabolism studies. But because an antibody recognizes a relatively small portion of a macromolecular antigen, these assays may be neither purity nor activity indicating. Although this limitation does not affect their usefulness in the above mentioned applications, immunoassays may be of little value in establishing drug substance and product release criteria unless (a) antibodies can be made to recognize conformationally dependent epitopes that correlate with drug potency, (b) panels of antibodies are employed to recognize the entire structure of the drug substance (in assessment of purity) or (c) immunoassays are combined with other analytical techniques that provide added assurance of specificity (e.g., SDS PAGE or HPLC).

The specificity of immunoassays is determined by the cross-reactivity of the antibody used in the analysis, i.e., its binding constant for analyte relative to its association constant toward other species present in the sample. Sensitivity is also dependent on antigen (analyte)-antibody binding constant as well as on the instrumental sensitivity of the selected "reporter" group. Three types of reporter groups are commonly used: radioisotopic labels, fluorescent moieties and enzyme conjugates.

Two basic strategies have been adopted in the design of immunoassays: competitive and direct. Competitive immunoassays allow a small amount of labeled antigen (otherwise identical to the analyte) to equilibrate with the antibody and the analyte. The greater the concentration of analyte in the sample, the less the amount of labeled antigen that will be bound to antibody. Experimentally determining the ratio of free to bound forms of the labeled analyte compared to a standard curve will allow the determination of analyte concentration. It is implicitly assumed that the incorporation of the reporter group into the antigen does not alter its binding affinity for the antibody. When radioisotopes are used, this is a more valid assumption than when enzyme or fluorescent reporter groups are used. In instances where reporter groups influence binding characteristics to antibody, analytical confidence and sensitivity will be compromised. All of these methods described so far require physical separation of free and bound forms of analyte. The most common approaches to achieve such separation include adsorption of the free fraction to dextran-coated charcoal or precipitation of the bound fraction using solvent, salt, immunochemical (second antibody), or Protein A from S. aureus (Ying, 1981). Thus, while more convenient than bioassays, such heterogenous immunoassays require significant manual manipulations and the use of fresh standard curves for each analytical run due to irreproducibility of reagents, conditions and quality of separation.

A number of homogenous competitive immunoassays have been developed to enhance the convenience and marketability of immunoassays. The need to separate the free and bound forms of the labeled antigen is eliminated by exploiting a change induced in the label on binding. Such assays employ fluorescent, spin label or enzyme reporter groups.

Fluorescence polarization immunoassays, for example, are based on the differential rates of fluorescence depolarization for small (i.e., free molecule) and large (i.e., associated molecular complex) species and allow the ratio of the free and bound labeled antigens to be determined without a separation step (Blecka, 1983; Jolley, 1981a; Jolley et al., 1981b). This approach does not appear applicable to macromolecular analytes, however, whose depolarization rates in free solution are not significantly different from their rates of depolarization in the bound form.

Avoidance of a separation step can also be achieved with enzyme reporter groups, since enzyme activity may be inhibited by steric restrictions imposed by association with an antibody (Conander, 1967). Rubenstein et al. (1969) described a method for determination of morphine, based on this concept in which morphine conjugated with lysozyme was used as the labeled probe, i.e., lysozyme activity was related to morphine levels.

All of the immunochemical approaches discussed to this point are based on competitive association of labeled and non-labeled antigen for antibody binding sites. More recently, direct immunoassays, also referred to as immunoradiometric procedures, have been developed which are not based on a competitive binding principle and require that the antibody be labeled with a high specific activity reporter group. The ELISA (enzyme linked immunoabsorbent assays) is the most notable example of such procedures (Engvall and Perlman, 1971). Direct analysis is achieved by allowing analyte to first associate with a stationary support phase and then adding a labeled antibody that associates with complementary antigen. Excess antibody is washed away before the measurement (i.e., enzyme activity in the case of ELISA) is completed. A comparison of radioimmunoassay vs. immunoradiometric assay has been made for human growth hormone and a common specific antibody to the antigen (Wilson et al., 1981). The immunoradiometric assay showed a 13 fold increase in sensitivity and a 6 fold increase in assay range over the RIA procedure.

Although variations on the concept of immunoassays have increased their reliability and convenience, specificity limitations remain inherent obstacles to their general acceptance. Their value, however, is greatly enhanced by using them in conjunction with separation techniques such as electrophoresis or HPLC. Furthermore, the development of monoclonal antibodies now offers the opportunity for obtaining antibodies which adhere to the same rigorous standards of purity and homogeneity that have been established for more traditional analytical reagents. Such species, potentially specific for a single epitope, offer a level of discrimination that allow detection of conformational changes in an antigen (although the antibody is still responsive to only a portion of the antigen [Bachi et al., 1985; Yewdell et al., 1983]).

The production of monoclonal antibodies (Kohler and Milstein, 1975) will play a very important role in the development of protein and peptide drugs (Staehelin et al, 1981; Schwarz et al, 1985). Their specificity for particular antigens makes them ideal affinity column ligands in the purification of crude protein preparations (Secher and Burke, 1980) and in the development of immunoassays with directed specificity. It is possible to generate and select monoclonal antibodies with a sufficiently high degree of selectivity that they can discriminate between the desired protein form and species differing by point mutation or single residue alteration or conformation. Stability-indicating assays can be developed from the monoclonal antibodies specific to difference in conformation or residues critical to bioactivity. If the altered protein is known to form under conditions encountered in storage or formulation, this immunoassay can be used to monitor the extent of activity loss. A panel of these monoclonal antibodies could be prepared against other known inactive species. When used in concert, these antibodies would give a multidimensional characterization of the state of specific protein regions impacting on bioactivity. Strategies have been developed for the production and selection of such monoclonal antibodies (Schonherr and Houwink, 1984).

The active sites of many proteins frequently are present in regions of the molecule where the polypeptide chain has folded back onto itself, and the residues that participate in the active site are located between 3-dimensionally juxtaposed portions of the protein backbone. Monoclonal antibodies directed against the active site can be identified by their ability to block normal protein function and may be selected based on their ability to recognize a conformationally dependent epitope and thus may be activity-indicating (Ivanyi, 1982).

Enzyme Assays

Drug molecules that are enzymes or that inhibit or stimulate enzyme activity may be quantitated by methodology based on kinetic measurement of enzyme activity. When suitable substrates are provided and the catalytic component(s) added under controlled conditions, the rate of formation of product (or cofactor loss) can be related to drug concentration through a standard curve. For the relatively few drug substances that are enzymes or that can influence enzyme activity, there are distinct advantages to this type of analysis. The biochemical action of catalytic molecules or molecules specifically inhibiting or accelerating catalysis is likely to relate to their in vivo activity giving enzymatic assays good correlation to therapeutic potency. Enzyme assays are generally suitable for automation, are of inherently high specificity and can be made very sensitive. The generation of many product molecules per molecule of enzyme amplifies the analytical signal and may provide the basis for achieving very low detection limits. This amplification concept has been further extended by the introduction of "enzyme cycling" assays for a number of biochemicals (Lowry and Passonneau, 1972). Such procedures have claimed amplification factors of 400,000,000 and the ability to measure 10^{-18} moles of certain cellular metabolites. The possibility of creating specific and sensitive geometrically-amplified enzyme cycles has been proposed, but has not been fully developed

(Sternson and Malefyt, 1985a, 1985). Since the bioactivity of many drugs amenable to enzyme analysis are related to their catalytic properties or their effect on enzyme kinetics, assays based on enzyme activity often offer close correlation to therapeutic potency.

The most serious concern regarding enzyme assays lies with the possible influence of co-analytes in the sample on enzyme activity and viability. Even slight modulations in enzyme kinetics produced by impurities, degradates or matrix components could result in large analytical inaccuracies. This again introduces elements of uncertainties in analysis based on enzyme activity.

A number of proteinaceous drugs are proteases or effect proteases and have been analyzed by observing the rate of degradation of synthetic substrates specifically designed based on the amino sequence at the protease cleavage sites and which produce a chromophoric or fluorophoric product on hydrolysis (Kiss et al., 1985; Svendsen et al., 1983; Tang et al., 1984; Fareed et al., 1983; Messmore et al., 1981; Ohno et al., 1981; Witt et al., 1981a,1981b). Among these are plasma proteases responsible for hemostasis which normally exist in their zymogenic form and can be activated to promote thrombolysis or fibrinolysis. Enzyme assays exploiting this property have been developed for drugs such as strepto-kinase, urokinase and tissue plasminogen activator (tPA). The chromgenic substrate D-val-L-leu-L-lys-p- nitroanilide (S-2251) has been used in a coupled assay to measure the concentration of plasminogen activators. For every mole of plasminogen activator present in the sample, many molecules of plasmin are formed; and for every mole of plasmin formed, many molecules of chromophoric p-nitroaniline are subsequently produced. The method provides high sensitivity by geometric amplification of the mass of analyte that is ultimately monitored spectrophotometrically (as p-nitroaniline).

Plasminogen   activator protease ⟶ Plasmin

S-2251   plasmin ⟶ p-nitroaniline

Physical/Chemical Assays

Conventional drugs have traditionally been analyzed by physical/ chemical methods. The size and complexity of peptides and proteins has severely limited the application of such techniques to macromolecular species. However, with the commercialization of such materials as drugs, the need to extend classical methodology to peptides and proteins is recognized. Such methods are now employed to determine (a) total protein concentration, (b) separation and visualization of different molecular species, (c) amino acid composition, (d) absolute and confirmation of anticipated amino acid sequence and (e) conformational analysis (of polypeptides and proteins).

Determination of total protein concentration is essential as a specification of drug substance and product as well as for establishing mass balance in a sample that is to be further analyzed to determine component composition. If the aromatic residue content of the peptide is sufficiently high, the method of choice is direct absorbance measurement. The molar absorptivity is calculated by dividing the observed absorbance at 280 nanometers by the protein concentration determined by amino acid analysis or, more reliably, micro Kjeldahl nitrogen analysis of a pure sample of known molecular composition. When the concentration is too low to be measured directly or interfering substances may be present, any of several colorimetric (Lowry et al., 1951; Bradford, 1976; Smith et al., 1985) or HPLC methods may be used. However, it should be recognized that even these methods are subject to interference. Both the Lowry and Bradford methods give erroneous readings in the presence of surfactants (Peterson, 1979) and the bicinchoninic acid method is sensitive to any species that can reduce Cu^{+2} to Cu^+.

Amino acid composition analysis is also an essential regulatory component of peptide/protein characterization for identity and purity. Because there may be several forms of a protein with equal activity (microheterogeneity), deviations observed from theoretical composition may, therefore, not be a meaningful indicator of product purity. Variations of 10% are typically observed even for pure protein samples.

Further characterization of peptides/proteins includes determination of primary amino acid sequence. Traditionally, this involves sequential degradation from the N-terminus of the polypeptides. Derivatization with phenylisothiocyanate (or other reagent) followed by acid treatment liberates the (N-1) polypeptide and a thiohydantoin derivative characteristic of the amino acid from which it is derived (Edman, 1950; Zimmerman et al., 1977). This procedure can be repeated to determine each N-terminal residue in succession. Small losses of polypeptide on each turn of the cycle limit the number of residues that can be analyzed to about 30. Methods using carboxypeptidase Y have been developed for C-terminal analysis, but are limited to 5 or 6 residues.

Although useful for single component analysis, conventional amino acid analysis cannot be readily used to evaluate mixtures of peptides or their post-translational adducts. Fast atom bombardment mass spectrometry (FAB-MS [Barbet et al., 1981]) of tryptic digests of peptides or proteins has, however, proven highly useful in peptide mapping. FAB mass spectra of trypsin-generated peptide fragments and FAB-MS of the Edman degradates of these fragments can be compared to a library of anticipated fragments to make unambiguous assignments of the observed peaks to portions of the anticipated sequence. Other enzymes and reagents that allow predictable and reproducible fragmentation (with specificities different than trypsin) can be used to generate fragments that will overlap the tryptic fragments and extend the portion mapped. Peptide fragments containing residues that were post-translationally modified will appear to be missing in the FAB-MS analysis, because the anticipated mass of the backbone peptide will not be observed. The absence of such peaks is only an indication of post-translational modification. Verification can be gained following further treatment of the tryptic digest (Carr and Roberts, 1986). For example, a sample containing a putative glycopeptide can be treated with peptide:N-glycosidase F to cleave asparagine linked glycosyl adducts across the linking amide bond. This cleavage gives an aspartic acid in place of the original asparagine and results in the appearance of a spectral signal at one mass unit greater than the anticipated fragment ($-CONH_2 < -COOH$). This is conclusive proof of asparagine linked glycosylation occurring within the peptide. New peaks in the spectra can provide additional information regarding the composition of the original carbohydrate adduct.

Peptide analysis is generally complicated by the complex matrix in which the analyte resides and the presence of impurities or degradates which closely resemble the analyte of interest. In many instances, it is not only the drug that must be monitored but also degradates or "metabolites". For such applications, the availability of separation techniques capable of resolving proteinaceous components within mixtures is necessary.

Electrophoretic methods have been widely used for protein and peptide separations (Reghetti and Drysdale, 1975; Gordon, 1975; Allen and Maurer,

1974; Arbuthnot and Beeley, 1975). The most common of these techniques separates a reduced and sodium dodecyl sulfate (SDS)-solubilized sample on a SDS polyacrylamide gel (PAG). Silver staining of SDS-PAGE gels is the currently accepted method of protein sample purity determination. Separation is based on molecular size. High resolution separations can be achieved using gradient or isoelectric focusing techniques. The major limitations of electrophoretic methods include their unsuitability for automation, limited resolving capabilities, limited sensitivity and difficulties in quantitating components (generally attempted by densitometric measurements of stained gels). Western blotting of polyacrylamide gels followed by detection of specific protein bands using antibodies and protein A-enzyme conjugates or ^{125}I protein A will allow visualization of sub-microgram quantities. Resolution capability has been significantly improved using an adaptation of conventional electrophoresis - capillary zone electrophoresis. By carrying out separations in very narrow tubes at high field strengths, chromatographic efficiency approaching that seen with modern HPLC is realized (Lukacs and Jorgenson, 1981; Jorgenson, 1983). However, this technique is not at a stage of development where it can be broadly applied, nor does it at present provide opportunity for sensitive detection of eluting components.

Chromatographic strategies have also been applied to peptide/protein analysis, including the use of size exclusion, adsorption, ion exchange and partition approaches (see Hearn et al., 1983a for review). Newer, controlled porosity mechanically-resilient supports and improved chemically-bonded microparticulate silicas (using various elution modes) now allow high resolution separation of proteins to be achieved. Reversed phase and hydrophobic interaction partition chromatography have been of particular value, where elution of analytes is achieved from an aqueous eluent modulated in strength by varying pH, organic modifier (type and concentration) or electrolyte composition (salt type, ionic strength, use of ion pairing agents).

Detection of peptides/proteins in chromatographic eluents has been achieved spectrophotometrically, refractometrically or fluorometrically. Such approaches are limited to quantitation of species present in relatively high concentration. Chemical derivatization approaches have been used to enhance detectability with limited success. These approaches have primarily focused on conversion of peptides to fluorescent (Schlabach and Wehr, 1983) products (although dinitrophenyl derivatives have been prepared for spectrophotometric monitoring [Sanger, 1975]). Derivatization with fluorescamine or o-phthalaldehyde (OPA) (the latter reacting only with free lysine residues) either pre- or post-column produces fluorophores that can be detected at pg/ml levels with conventional detector technology at even lower levels with laser-based detectors. Recently, Sternson and co-workers (1985b,c) described several analogs of OPA, that produce more stable products (than those produced with OPA) and react with a broader spectrum of peptides (i.e., not only at lys residues).

The first of these analogs, o-acetylbenzaldehyde, 1b, (Sternson, et al., 1985c) confers a >100% improvement in the stability of the resulting isoindole derivative, 2b (in comparison with 2a) without altering the reactivity profile of the reagent or the fluorescent intensity of the product. Blocking the 1-position of the isoindole with a methyl group reduces the proclivity for auto-oxidation (which is initiated by hydrogen abstraction in the OPA analog) to a series of carbonyl-containing non-fluorescent products (Stobaugh, et al., 1984).

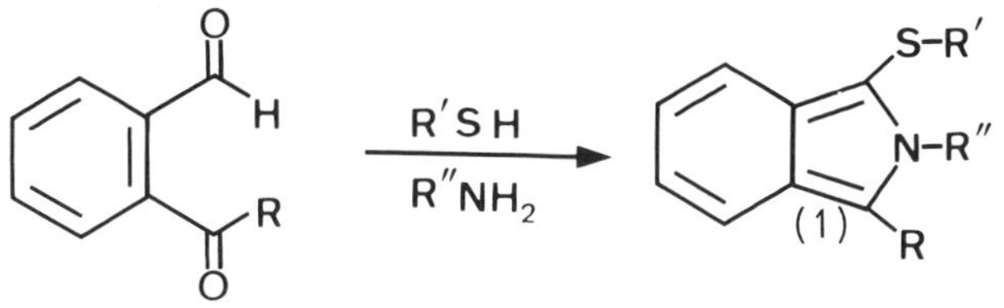

1a   R=H (OPA)
1b   R=CH$_3$

2

More recently, further improvements in OPA-like fluorogenic reagents have been achieved with the synthesis of a naphthalene analog of OPA, 3, (Sternson, et al., 1985b,c).

Unlike 1, 3 does not form measurable products following reaction with amine in the presence of thiol. However, if cyanide is substituted for the thiol, a benzisoindole, 4, is formed which provides a vast improvement in stability ($t_{1/2}$, ~ 24 h) over its OPA analogs (1a and 1b do not form stable isoindoles in the presence of cyanide; the thiol-containing adducts have $t_{1/2}$ < 1 h). The increase in planar surface area and extended conjugation (over that found in 2 and related isoindoles) characteristic of 4 and the increase in quantum yield from 0.11 (in 2) to 0.70 (as observed in 4) provide the basis for the significant improvement in sensitivity which is attained with the reagent.

Furthermore, unlike OPA and its mononuclear analogs, 3 also reacts with non-lys-containing peptides (to date, reactivity has been demonstrated with peptides of ≤ 8 amino acid residues) to produce products with fluorescent intensity approaching that of its component amino acids (Sternson, et al., 1985b,c). This represents a significant broadening of the spectrum of reactivity over that offerred by 1a and 1b, which fail to produce fluorescent products with the α-amine of an α-amino acid that has been esterified or in which the carboxylate has been converted to a carboxamide (as is the case with peptides). Although reagents such as 3 offer significant improvements in capabilities to detect peptides, further advances in derivatization technology are needed to provide the selectivity and sensitivity that will be required to evaluate peptide drugs. Means of extending this sensitivity-enhancing technology to larger peptides and proteins is also necessary.

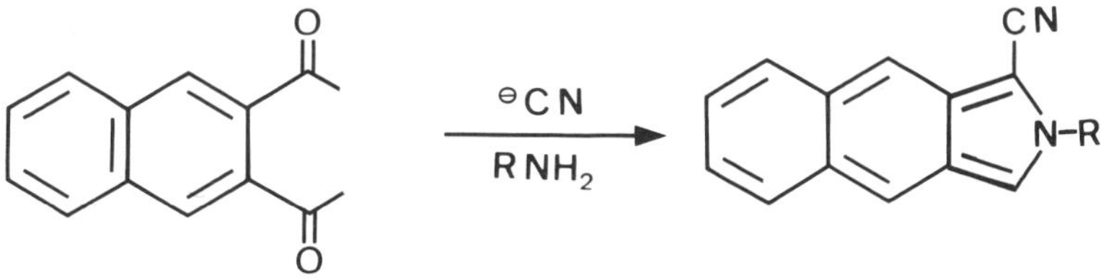

3   4

Conclusion

The need for reliable, selective and highly sensitive analytical methodology that is applicable to peptides and proteins is clear. Methodology suitable for various facets of development of proteinaceous drugs is complicated by analyte size and complexity and the yet to be resolved definition of purity as related to biological activity. These complexities will likely require that future analytical strategies include components of each of the types of methods described in this article as well as others not enumerated. Furthermore, batteries of analytical tests will likely be required to assess all the aspects pertinent to the description of identity and purity of such drugs and their degradates in a variety of matrices (e.g., fermentation broths, formulations, biological fluids, etc.).

References

Allen, R.C. and Maurer, H.R., 1974, "Electrophoresis and Isoelectric Focusing in Polyacrylamide Gel", Walter deGruyter, New York.

Arbuthnot, J.P. and Beeley, J.A., 1975, "Isoelectric Focusing, Butterworths, London.

Bachi, T., Gernard, W. and Yewdell, J.W., 1985, Monoclonal Antibodies Detect Different Forms of Influenza Virus Hemagglutinin During Viral Penetration and Biosynthesis, J.Virol., 55:307-313.

Barber, M., Bordoli, R.S., Garner, G.V., Gordon, D.B., Sedgwick, R.D., Tetler, L.W. and Tyler, A.N., 1981, Fast-Atom-Bombardment Mass Spectra of Enkephalins, Biochem.J., 197:401.

Blecka, L.J., 1983, Fluorescence Polarization Immunoassay: A Review of Methodology and Applications, Amer.Assoc.Clin.Chem., March 1.

Bradford, M., 1976, A Rapid and Sensitive Method for the Quantitation of Microgram Quantities of Protein Utilizing the Principle of Protein Dye Binding, Anal.Biochem., 72:248.

Carr, S.A. and Roberts, G.D., 1986, Carbohydrate Mapping by Mass Spectrometry. A Novel Method for Identifying Attachment sites in Asn-linked Sugars in Glycoproteins, manuscript in preparation.

Cinander, B., 1967, Antibodies to Biologically Active Molecules, in: "Proceedings of the Second Meeting of the Foundation of European Biochemical Societies, Vienna, Pergamon Press, Oxford.

deVlaminck, W., 1984, FDA's Role in Approval and Regulation of Recombinant DNA Drugs, in: "Recombinant DNA Products: Insulin, Interferon and Growth Hormone", A.P. Bollen, ed., CRC Press Inc., Boca Raton.

Edman, P., 1950, Method for Determination of the Amino Acid Sequence in Peptides, Acta.Chem.Scand., 4:283.

Engvall, E. and Perlman, P., 1971, Enzyme Linked Immunosorbant Assay (ELISA) Quantitative Assay of Immunoglobulin G, Immunochem., 8:871.

Fareed, J., Walenga, H.L., Messmore, E.W. and Bermes, E.W., 1983, Synthetic Substrates in Hemostatic Testing, in: "CRC Critical Review in Laboratory Sciences", CRC Press Inc., Boca Raton.

Gordon, A.H., 1975, in: "Laboratory Techniques in Biochemistry and Molecular Biology", T.W. Work and E. Work, eds., North Holland Publishing Co., Amsterdam.

Hearn, M.T.W., 1983, High Performance Liquid Chromatography of Peptides, in: "HPLC Advances and Perspectives", C. Horvath, ed., Academic Press, New York.

Hearn, M.T.W, Regnier, F.E. and Wehr, C.T., 1983, HPLC of Peptides and Proteins", Academic Press, New York.

Imai, K., Toyo'oka, T. and Miyano, H., 1984, Fluorogenic Reagents for Primary and Secondary Amines and Thiols in High Performance Liquid Chromatography, Analyst, 109:1365.

Jolley, M.E., 1981, Fluorescence Polarization Immunoassay for the Determination of Therapeutic Drug Levels in Human Plasma, J.Anal.Toxicol., 5:236.

Jolley, M.E., Stroupe, S.D., Schwenzer, K.S., Wang, C.J., Lu-Steffes, M., Hill, H.D., Popelka, S.R., Holen, J.T. and Kelso, D.M., 1981b, Fluorescence Polarization Immunoassay III. An Automated System for Therapeutic Drug Determination, Clin.Chem., 27:1575.

Jorgenson, J.W. and Lukacs, K.D., 1983, Capillary Zone Electrophoresis, Science, 222:266.

Jornvall, H., Pohl, G., Bergsdorf, W. and Wallen, P., 1983, Differential Proteolysis and Evidence for a Residue Exchange in Tissue-Plasminogen Activator Suggest Possible Association Between Two Types of Protein Microheterogeneity, FEBS Letters, 156:47.

Kiss, I., Aurell, L., Pozsgay, M. and Elodi, P., 1985, Investigation on the Substrate Specificity of Human Plasmin Using Tripeptidyl p-nitroanilide Substrates, Biochem.Biophys.Res.Commun., 131:928.

Kohler, G. and Milstein, C., 1975, Continuous Cultures of Fused Cells Secreting Antibody of Predefined Specificity, Nature, 256:495.

Liversidge, G., Kinter, L. and Sternson, L., 1986, manuscript in preparation.

Lowry, O.H. and Passonneau, J.V., 1972, "A Flexible System of Enzymatic Analysis, Academic Press, New York.

Lowry, O.H., Rosebrough, N.J., Farr, A.L. and Randall, R.J., 1951, Protein Measurement with the Folin Phenol Reagent, J.Biol.Chem., 193:265.

Lukacs, K.D. and Jorgenson, J.W., 1981, Zone Electrophoresis in Open-Tublar Glass Capillaries: Preliminary Data on Performance, J.High Res.Chrom., 4:230.

Messmore, H.L., Fareed, J., Kniffin, J., Squillaci, G. and Walenga, J.M., 1981, Synthetic Substrate Assays of the Coagulation Enzymes and Their Inhibitors. Comparison with clotting and Immunological Methods for Clinical and Experimental Usage, Ann.N.Y.Acad.Sci., 370:787.

Ohno, Y., Kato, H., Iwanaga, S., Takada, K., Sakakibara, S. and
    Steuflo, J., 1981, A New Fluorogenic Peptide Substrate for Vitamin K
    Dependent Blood Coagulation Factor Bovine Protein C, J.Biochem.,
    90:1387.

Peterson, G., 1979, Review of the Folin Phenol Protein Quantitation
    Method of Lowry, Rosenbrough, Farr and Randall, Anal.Biochem.,
    100:210.

Ranby, M., Bergsdorf, N., Pohl, G. and Wallen, P., 1982, Isolation of Two
    Variants of Native One-Chain Tissue-Plasminogen Activator, FEBS
    Letters, 146:289.

Reghetti, P.G. and Drysdale, J.W., 1975, in: "Laboratory Techniques in
    Biochemistry and Molecular Biology", T.S. Work and E. Work, eds.,
    North Holland Publishing Co., Amsterdam.

Rubenstein, K.E., Schneider, R.S. and Ullman, E.F., 1972, Homogeneous
    Enzyme Immunoassay. A New Immunochemical Technique, Biochem.Biophys
    Res.Commun., 47:846.

Sanger, F., 1945, The Free Amino Groups of Insulin, Biochem.J., 39:507.

Schlabach, T.D., 1984, Post-Column Detection of Serum Proteins with the
    Biuret and Lowry Reactions, Anal.Biochem., 139:309.

Schlabach, T.D. and Wehr, C.T., 1983, Fluorescent Techniques for the
    Selective Detection of Chromatographically Separated Peptides, in:
    "HPLC of Peptides and Proteins", M.T.W. Hearn, F.E. Regnier and
    C.T. Wehr, ed., Academic Press, New York.

Schonherr, O.T. and Houwink, E.H., 1984, Antibody Engineering, a Strategy
    for the Development of Monoclonal Antibodies, Ant.van Leewenhoek,
    50:597.

Schwarz, S., Berger, P. and Wick, G., 1985, Epitope-Selective,
    Monoclonal-Antibody-Based Immunoradiometric Assays of Predictable
    Specificity for Differential Measurement of Choriogonadotropin and
    Its Subunits, Clin.Chem., 31:1322.

Secher, D.S. and Burke, D.C., 1980, A Monoclonal Antibody for Large Scale
    Purification of Human leukocyte Interferon, Nature, 285:446.

Smith, P.K., Krohn, R.I., Hermanson, G.T., Mallia, A.K., Gartner, F.H.,
    Provenzano, M.D., Fujimoto, E.K., Groeke, N.M., Olson, B.J. and
    Klenk, D.C., 1985, Measurement of Protein Using Bicinchoninic Acid,
    Anal.Biochem., 150:76.

Staehelin, T., Durrer, B., Schmidt, J., Takacs, B., Stocker, J.,
    Miggiano, V., Stahli, C., Rubenstein, M., Levy, W.P., Hershberg, R.
    and Pestka, S., 1981, Production of Hybridomas Secreting Monoclonal
    Antibodies to the Human Leukocyte Interferons, Proc.Nat'l.Acad.Sci.
    U.S.A., 78:1848.

Sternson, L.A., Higuchi, T., DeMontigny, P., Repta, A. and Stobaugh, J.,
    1985b, U.S. Patent, "Assaying Method for Primary Amines Using
    Aromatic Dialdehydes", application filed.

Sternson, L.A. and Malefyt, T.R., 1985a, Analytical Aspects of Drug
    Delivery: An Important and Often Overlooked Problem, in: "Directed
    Drug Delivery", Humana Press, Clifton.

Sternson, L.A., Repta, A.J. and Stobaugh, J.F., 1985c, Rational Design and Evaluation of Improved o-phthalaldehyde-like Fluorogenic Reagents, Anal.Biochem., 144:233.

Svendsen, L.G., Fareed, J., Walenga, J.M. and Hoppensteadt, D., 1983, Newer Synthetic Peptide Substrates in Coagulation Testing: Some Practical Considerations for Automated Methods, Seminars in Thrombosis and Hemostasis, 9:250.

Tang, J., Li, S., McGray, P. and Vecchio, A., 1984, Current Status of Activity Assays for Tissue-Plasminogen Activator, Ann.New York Acad.Sci., 434:536.

Wallen, P., Pohl, G., Ranby, M. and Jornvall, H., 1983, Purification and Characterization of a Melanoma Cell Plasminogen Activator, Eur.J.Biochem., 132:681.

Wilson, M.A., Kao, Y. and Miles, L., 1981, Direct Comparison of a Radioimmunoassay and an Immunoradiometric Technique in the Measurement of Human Growth Hormone, Nuc.Med.Commun., 2:68.

Witt, I., Tritschler, W. and Bablok, W., 1981a, Alpha 2-macroglobulin: Values in Serum and Plasma with a Chromogenic Substrate, J.Clin.Chem.Clin.Biochem., 19:887.

Witt, I., 1981b, New Methods for the Analysis of Coagulation Using Chromogenic Substrate, J.Clin.Chem.Clin.Biochem., 19:877.

Yewdell, J.W., Gernard, W. and Bachi, T., 1983, Monoclonal Hemagglutinin Antibodies Direct Irreversible Antigenic Alterations that Coincide with the Acid Activation of Influenza Virus A/PR/834-Mediated Hemolysis, J.Virol., 48:239.

Ying, S.Y., 1981, Radioimmunoassay of Peptide Hormones Using Killed S. Aureus as a Separation Agent, in: "Immunochemical Techniques, Methods in Enzymology", J.J. Langone and H. VanVunakis, eds., Academic Press, New York.

Zimmerman, C.L., Apella, E. and Pisano, J.J., 1977, Rapid Analysis of Amino Acid Phenylthiohydantoins by High Performance Liquid Chromatography, Anal.Biochem., 77:569.

BIOREVERSIBLE DERIVATIZATION OF PEPTIDES

Hans Bundgaard

Royal Danish School of Pharmacy
Department of Pharmaceutical Chemistry AD
2 Universitetsparken, DK-2100 Copenhagen, Denmark

INTRODUCTION

In recent years several biologically active peptides have been discovered, including peptides consisting of only two or three amino acids,
and most certainly, the development of peptide drugs will be a major area
in drug research in the future. The application of peptides as clinically
useful drugs is, however, seriously hampered due to substantial delivery
problems. Peptides are readily degraded by enzymes in the gastrointestinal
system and are absorbed poorly, making the oral route a poor way of administration (Wiedhaup, 1981). Pronounced degradation of peptides does also
occur at routes of administration other than oral, such as the ocular,
nasal, buccal, rectal and vaginal routes (Okada et al., 1982; Kimura, 1984;
Lee et al., 1985; Stratford and Lee, 1986). Another factor contributing to
the poor bioavailability of peptides is most certainly the non-lipophilicity
of peptides. Furthermore, peptides suffer from metabolic lability arising
from hydrolysis by plasma and tissue peptidases and even simple parenteric
administration is problematic, due to the short half-lives of the peptides
once they reach the bloodstream. Several peptides also suffer from systemic
transport problems in that they do not readily penetrate cell membranes to
reach the receptor biophase or cross the blood-brain barrier (Farmer and
Ariëns, 1982; Meisenberg and Simmons, 1983).

A potentially useful approach to solve these delivery problems may be
derivatization of the bioactive peptides to produce prodrugs or transport
forms possessing, with respect to delivery and metabolic stability, enhanced physicochemical properties in comparison to the parent compounds.
Thus, it may be imagined that bioreversible derivatization may protect peptides against degradation by peptidases and other enzymes present at the
mucosal barrier and renders the peptides more lipophilic, resulting in increased bioavailability.

A basic requisite for the application of this approach is the ready
availability of chemical derivative types satisfying the prodrug requirements, the most prominent of these being reconversion to the parent drug
in vivo. In recent years several types of bioreversible derivatives for
the functional groups or chemical entities (such as carboxyl, hydroxyl,
thiol, amino and amido groups) occurring in amino acids and peptides have
been explored. The purpose of the present paper is to review and discuss
various chemical approaches to obtain such prodrug forms. A more extensive

coverage of various types of bioreversible derivatives is published elsewhere (Bundgaard, 1985a).

DERIVATIZATION OF CARBOXYL AND HYDROXYL GROUPS

An obvious way of obtaining bioreversible derivatives of carboxyl and
hydroxyl functions (as well as thiol groups) is ester formation. The popu-
larity of using esters as a prodrug type stems primarily from the fact that
the organism is rich in enzymes capable of hydrolyzing esters. The distribution of esterases is ubiquitous and several types can be found in the
blood, liver and other organs or tissues. In addition, by appropriate esterification of molecules containing a hydroxyl or carboxyl group it is feasible to obtain derivatives with almost any desirable hydrophilicity or
lipophilicity as well as in vivo lability, the latter being dictated by
electronic and steric factors. Accordingly, a great number of alcoholic or
carboxylic acid drugs have been modified for a multitude of reasons using
the ester prodrug approach. Several examples can be found in various reviews (Digenis and Swintosky, 1975; Sinkula and Yalkowsky, 1975; Sinkula,
1975; Roche, 1977; Stella, 1975; Pitman, 1981; Bundgaard, 1982, 1985a,
1985b).

Sometimes, simple aliphatic or aromatic esters may not be sufficiently
labile in vivo to ensure a sufficiently high rate and extent of prodrug
conversion. This is thus the case for penicillin esters. Although various
simple alkyl and aryl esters of the thiazolidine carboxyl groups are rapidly
hydrolyzed to the free penicillin acid in animals, such as rodents, they
proved to be far too stable in man to have any therapeutic potential (Ferres,
1983). This illustrates also - as do many other examples - the occurrence
of marked species differences in the in vivo hydrolysis of ester prodrugs.
A solution to the problem was found in 1965 by Jansen and Russell (1965)
who showed that a special double ester type (acyloxymethyl ester) of benzyl-
penicillin was hydrolyzed rapidly in the blood and tissues of several species including man. The first step in the hydrolysis of such an ester is
enzymatic cleavage of the terminal ester bond with formation of a highly unstable hydroxymethyl ester which rapidly dissociates to the parent penicillin and formaldehyde (Scheme 1). A reason for the different enzymatic stabilities of the acyloxymethyl ester and simple alkyl esters of penicillins
is certainly that the penicillin carboxyl group is highly sterically hindered. The terminal ester in the acyloxymethyl derivative is less hindered
and thus should be more accessible to enzymatic attack.

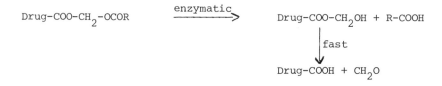

Scheme 1

The principle has been used successfully to improve the oral bioavailability of ampicillin (1), and no fewer than three ampicillin prodrug forms
are now on the market, namely the pivaloyloxymethyl ester (2) (pivampicillin)
(Daehne et al., 1970), the ethoxycarbonyloxyethyl ester (3) (bacampicillin)
(Bodin et al.,1975) and the phthalidyl ester (4) (talampicillin) (Clayton
et al., 1974; Shiobara et al., 1974). The improved oral bioavailability
obtained with these ester prodrugs is primarily due to the increased lipophilicity of the esters achieved by masking the ionized carboxyl group.

50

1 R = H

2 R = CH_2-OOC-C(CH_3)$_3$

3 R = CH-O-C-O-C$_2$H$_5$ / CH$_3$ O

4 R = CH C=O (phthalidyl)

5 R = -H

6 R = -CH-OOC-C(CH$_3$)$_3$ / CH$_3$

7 R = -CH$_2$ (5-methyl-2-oxo-1,3-dioxol-4-yl) CH$_3$

8

9

In more recent years the applicability of this double ester concept in prodrug design has been further expanded. Thus, similar esters have been prepared from cromoglycic acid (Bodor et al., 1980), methyldopa (Saari et al., 1978; Dobrinska et al., 1982; Vickers et al., 1984) and tyrosine (Baldwin et al., 1982). Whereas methyldopa (5) is variably and incompletely absorbed its pivaloyloxyethyl ester (6) is almost completely and more uniformly absorbed in man following oral administration and is rapidly hydrolyzed on the first pass to the parent drug (Dobrinska et al., 1982; Vickers et al., 1984). A different ester type of methyldopa, a (5-methyl-2-oxo-1,3-dioxol-4-yl)methyl derivative (7) was recently reported to be another potentially useful prodrug for improving the oral bioavailability (Saari et al., 1984). A similar ester type of ampicillin has recently been described and shown to be an orally well absorbed prodrug (Sakamoto et al., 1984).

An interesting variant of the acyloxyalkyl double esters is provided in the recent work of Kakeya et al. (1984) on cephalosporins. They have prepared a p-glycyloxybenzoyloxymethyl ester of a cephalosporin. Due to the ionizable amino group in the pro-moiety this prodrug, as a hydrochloride salt, is highly soluble in water but because the pK_a of the glycyl amino group is relatively low the partition coefficient between octanol and water at pH 6.5 (about equal to the pH of the intestine) is sufficient to ensure good absorption. The prodrug contains three ester groupings and depending on the cleavage mechanism (Scheme 2) it may be regarded as a triple prodrug. Phenyl esters of glycine and similar amino acids are known to be rather unstable in neutral aqueous solution and the prodrug may probably undergo an initial cleavage at the glycyl ester grouping before or during the absorption from the gastrointestinal tract.

In recent years simple ethyl esters of various small peptidic angiotensin converting enzyme inhibitors have been exploited for improving the oral bioavailability of the parent drugs by increasing the lipophilicity. Enalapril (8) and pentopril (9) are such ethyl ester prodrugs. The esters are, however, only rather slowly cleaved in the organism to the carboxyl acids (Todd and Heel, 1986; Larmour et al., 1985; Rakhit and Tipnis, 1984; Tipnis and Rakhit, 1985) and especially in the case of pentopril appreci-

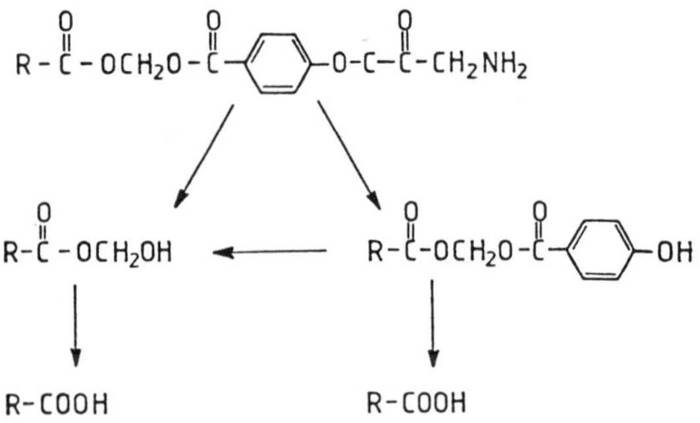

Scheme 2

able quantities of intact prodrug are excreted in intact form in the urine. These examples demonstrate the need for exploring new ester types being more susceptible to undergo enzymatic hydrolysis.

The applicability of acyloxyalkyl esters as biologically reversible transport forms has been extended to include the phosphate group (Farquhar et al., 1983; Srivastva and Farquhar, 1984), phosphinic acids (Jemal et al., 1985) and phenols (Loftsson and Bodor, 1982; Bodor et al., 1983), the derivatives in the latter case being acyloxyalkyl ethers. These ester-ethers are hydrolyzed by a sequential reaction involving the formation of an unstable hemiacetal intermediate (Scheme 3) and they are as susceptible as normal phenol esters to undergo enzymatic hydrolysis by e.g. human plasma enzymes. However, the acyloxyalkyl ethers appear to be more stable against chemical (hydroxide ion-catalyzed) hydrolysis than phenolate esters and this may make them more favorable in prodrug design (Loftsson and Bodor, 1982).

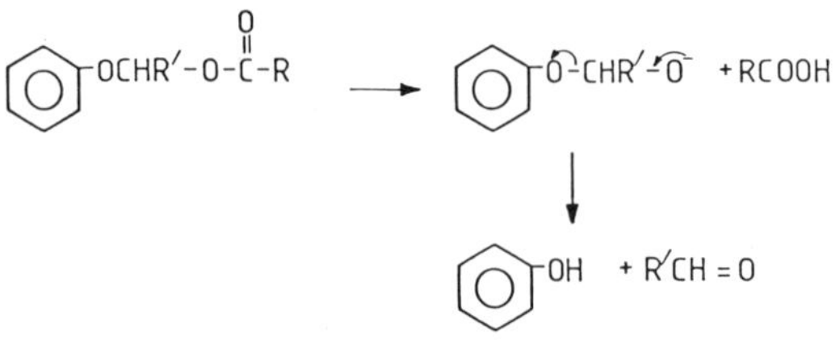

Scheme 3

Carbamate esters may be promising prodrug candidates for phenolic drugs. The enzymatic hydrolytic behaviour of carbamate esters have been examined by Digenis and Swintosky (1975). N-Unsubstituted or N-monosubstituted carbamates derived from phenols showed high lability and strong enzymatic catalysis whereas most N-disubstituted carbamates proved highly stable as did carbamates of aliphatic hydroxy compounds.

Whereas carbamates of alcohols in general appear to be of no value in prodrug design due to their high stability certain activated carbamates may be useful. Imidazole-1-carboxylic acid esters belong to this category and such derivatives have recently been shown to undergo a relatively facile non-enzymatic hydrolysis in aqueous buffer solutions (Klixbüll and Bundgaard, 1983).

DERIVATIZATION OF THE AMINO GROUP

N-Acyl Derivatives

N-Acylation of amines to give amide prodrugs has been used only to a limited extent due to the relative stability of amides in vivo. However, certain activated amides are sufficiently chemically labile and also, certain amides formed with amino acids may be susceptible to undergo enzymatic cleavage in vivo (Bundgaard, 1985a).

Thus, γ-glutamyl derivatives of dopamine, L-Dopa and sulfamethoxazole are readily hydrolyzed by γ-glutamyl transpeptidase in vivo and has been promoted as kidney-specific prodrugs because of their preferential bioactivation in the kidney (Wilk et al., 1978; Orlowski et al., 1979; Kyncl et al., 1979). Similarly, various other amides or dipeptides of L-Dopa including a combined dipeptide-ester structure (10) have been shown to be useful as prodrugs (Bodor et al., 1977). Other enzymatically labile amides include various amino acid derivatives of benzocaine (Zlojkowska et al., 1982). These compounds are highly water-soluble and are cleaved rapidly in the presence of human serum.

Various carbamate derivatives have been assessed as prodrugs for normeperidine, amphetamine, ephedrine and phenethylamine but with limited success (Verbiscar and Abood, 1970; Kupchan and Isenberg, 1967; Baker et al., 1984). Unfortunately, kinetic data on their conversion in aqueous solution and in the presence of plasma or enzymes are not available. As reported by Digenis and Swintosky (1975) carbamate esters of phenol are cleaved very rapidly by plasma enzymes (Scheme 4) and although these authors only classified such structures as possible prodrugs for phenols they can equally well be considered as prodrug candidates for amines. In such a case the phenol would be the transport group. Studies along this line are certainly warranted since there is a paucity of broadly applicable derivatives for the amino group. It is of interest that Sasaki et al.(1983) recently showed that benzyloxycarbonyl derivatives of mitomycin C are susceptible to undergo cleavage by plasma and hepatic enzymes and more so than the corresponding amide derivatives.

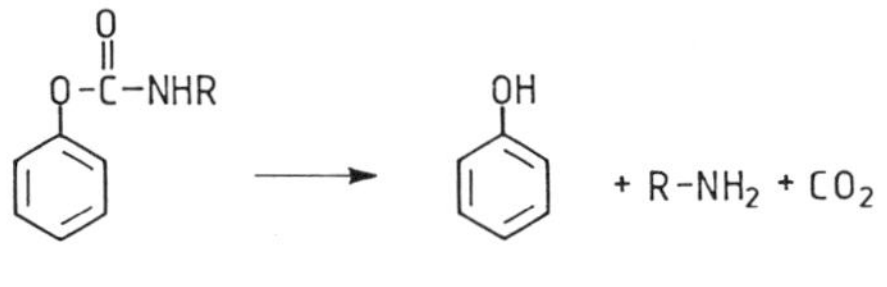

Scheme 4

<u>2-Acyloxymethylbenzamides</u>. A promising approach to obtain an amide pro-
drug capable of releasing the parent amine drug (e.g. a peptide) at physiological conditions of pH and temperature is to make use of intramolecular
chemical catalysis or assistance of the amide hydrolysis. Thus, 2-hydroxy-
methylbenzamides undergo a relatively rapid cyclization in aqueous solution
to give phthalide and free amine (Fig. 1) (Belke et al., 1971; Okuyama and
Schmir, 1972; Chiong et al., 1975; Nielsen and Bundgaard, 1986). A recent
kinetic study (Nielsen and Bundgaard, 1986) has shown that the lactonization
is specific acid- and base-catalyzed as well as subject to buffer catalysis.
The pH-rate profile for the lactonization of N-methyl-2-hydroxymethylbenz-
amide in aqueous solution at 60 $^{\circ}$C is shown in Fig. 2. The rates of cyclization were shown to increase with decreasing steric effects within the alkyl-
amino group of primary amines, the amine basicity being only of minor importance. At pH 7.4 and 37 $^{\circ}$C the cyclization of the 2-hydroxymethylbenzamides
proceeds rather slowly (Nielsen and Bundgaard, 1986) and in order to be a
useful prodrug principle it may be necessary to accelerate the reaction rate,
e.g. by introducing sterically or catalytically accelerating substituents in
the hydroxy-amide moiety. Thus, by substituting the two methylene hydrogen
atoms of 2-hydroxymethylbenzamide with phenyl and methyl groups (<u>11</u>) greatly
increased rates of cyclization have been observed (Chiong et al., 1975).
Further steric acceleration of the lactonization may possibly be achieved by
the introduction of substituents positioned ortho to either the hydroxymethyl
group or the carboxamide group. In fact, the pH-independent cyclization of
3-amino-2-hydroxymethylbenzamide (<u>12</u>) proceeds at a rate 10^3 times greater
than that of unsubstituted 2-hydroxymethylbenzamide (Fife and Benjamin, 1974).
At pH 4-10 and 30 $^{\circ}$C the lactonization of compound <u>12</u> showed a half-life of
only 5-10 min, the large rate enhancement being ascribed to intramolecular
general base catalysis by the 3-amino group. Other possibilities of obtaining steric and catalytic acceleration of the lactonization are presently
being studied in our laboratory

This prodrug principle may become even more attractive by masking the
hydroxyl function in the 2-hydroxymethylbenzamides by acylation to give
stable 2-acyloxymethylbenzamides (Fig. 1) (Nielsen and Bundgaard, 1986; Cain,
1976). In this way the lactonization is blocked and must be preceded by
hydrolysis of the ester grouping, i.e. by the action of esterases in vivo.
Experimental verification of this reaction scheme has recently been provided
(Nielsen and Bundgaard, 1986). It was shown that acetate esters of various

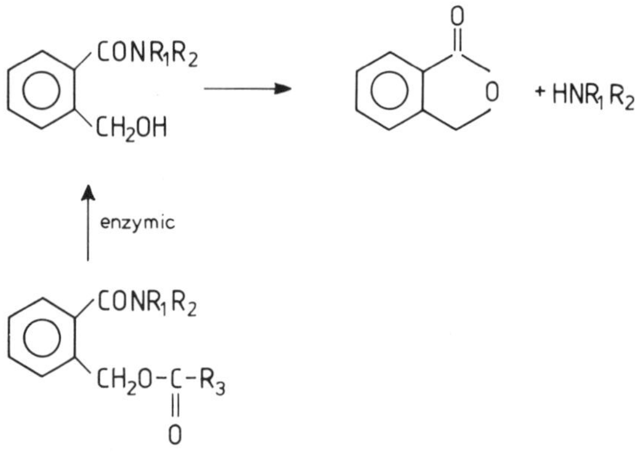

Fig. 1. Principle of the double prodrug
concept: conversion of 2-acyl-
oxymethylbenzamides to 2-hydroxy-
methylbenzamides by enzymic hydrolysis and subsequent cyclization
of these to phthalide with release
of the parent amine drug.

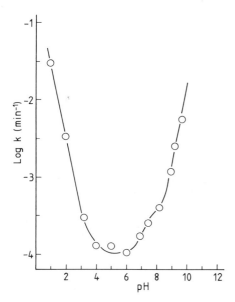

Fig. 2. The pH-rate profile for the degradation of N-methyl-2-hydroxymethylbenzamide in aqueous solution at 60°C.

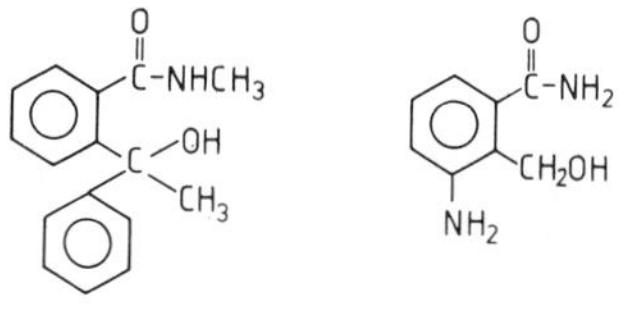

2-hydroxymethylbenzamides are highly stable in aqueous solution but in the presence of human plasma the ester grouping is readily hydrolyzed yielding the parent hydroxy-amide. Thus, such cascade latentiation may be a particularly useful prodrug principle for the amino group affording at the same time adequate in vitro stability and in vivo lability.

N-Mannich Bases

    N-Mannich bases have been proposed as potentially useful prodrug candidates for NH-acidic compounds such as various amides, imides, carbamates and urea derivatives as well as for aliphatic or aromatic amines (Bundgaard, 1982, 1985b; Bundgaard and Johansen, 1980a,b,c, 1981, 1982; Johansen and Bundgaard, 1980, 1982). Such N-Mannich bases were shown to decompose quantitatively to formaldehyde, amine and amide-type compound in aqueous solution at rates being highly dependent on the pH of the solution and on various structural factors.

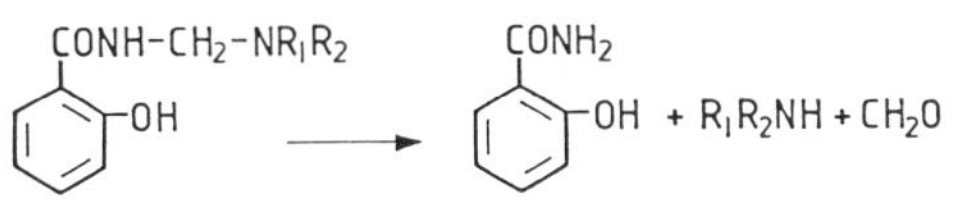

Scheme 5

In considering N-Mannich bases as prodrug forms for primary and secondary amines the amide-type component would act as a transport group. By N-Mannich base formation the pK_a of the amines is lowered by about 3 units (Bundgaard and Johansen, 1980a,b). Therefore, by transforming amino compounds into N-Mannich base transport forms it would be possible to increase the lipophilicity of the parent amines at physiological pH values by depressing their protonation, resulting in enhanced biomembrane-passage properties. This expectation of increased lipophilicity has been confirmed for e.g. the N-Mannich base derived from benzamide and phenylpropanolamine. The partition coefficient of the Mannich base between octanol and phosphate buffer pH 7.4 was found to be almost 100-times greater than than of the parent amine (Johansen and Bundgaard, 1982). By the benzamidomethylation the pK_a of phenylpropanolamine is decreased from 9.4 to 6.15 and the decreased extent of ionization at pH 7.4 is obviously the major contributing factor to the increased lipophilicity of the N-Mannich base derivative.

The selection of biologically acceptable amide-type transport groups affording an appropriate cleavage rate of a Mannich base of a given amine at pH 7.4 is, however, restricted. In a search for generally useful candidates it was observed (Johansen and Bundgaard, 1980b) that N-Mannich bases of salicylamide and different aliphatic amines including amino acids (Scheme 5) showed an unexpectedly high cleavage rate at neutral pH, thus suggesting the utility of salicylamide. As can be seen from Table 1 the half-lives of decomposition of various salicylamide N-Mannich bases at pH 7.4 are of the same order of magnitude and considerably shorter than those of the corresponding benzamide N-Mannich bases.

Although the salicylamide N-Mannich bases are more stable in weakly acidic solutions (pH 2-5) than at pH 7.4 (Johansen and Bundgaard, 1980b) a drawback of this potential prodrug type requiring chemical (non-enzymatic) release of the parent amine drug is the limited in vitro stability, raising some stability-formulation problems. A possible means of improving the stability may be further derivatization of the salicylamide Mannich bases in such a manner that an enzymatic release mechanism is required prior to the spontaneous decomposition of the Mannich bases. Since the hydroxyl group in the salicylamide Mannich base is responsible for the great reactivity of these derivatives (cf. Table 1), possibly by intramolecular catalysis, blocking of this group may be expected to result in derivatives possessing a stability similar to that of benzamide Mannich bases. It has recently been found (Bundgaard et al., 1986) that by performing such blocking through O-acyloxymethylation it is in fact possible to increase the stability in vitro and still obtain a rapid rate of amine release under conditions similar to those encountered in vivo due to the enzymatic lability of the O-acyloxymethyl group introduced. As seen from Fig. 3 the O-acyloxymethyl derivative is considerably more stable than the parent N-Mannich base at pH 2-8, its stability being similar to that of the benzamide Mannich base in this pH-range. In the presence of human plasma the ester grouping is rapidly hydrolyzed by virtue of enzymatic catalysis (Bundgaard et al., 1986), the reaction sequence

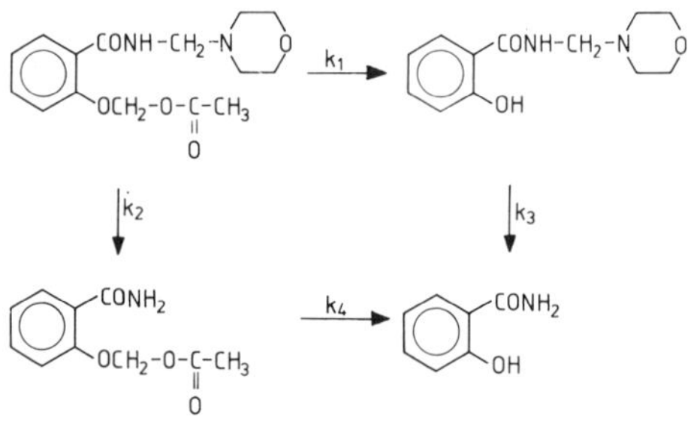

Scheme 6

Table 1. Half-lives of Decomposition of various
N-Mannich Bases Derived From Salicylamide
and Benzamide in Aqueous Solution at 37°C [a]

Compound	$t_{\frac{1}{2}}$ (min)	
	pH 2	pH 7.4
N-(Morpholinomethyl)salicylamide	1.5×10^2	41
N-(Morpholinomethyl)benzamide	1.2×10^3	1400
N-(Piperidinomethyl)salicylamide	4.6×10^3	14
N-(Piperidinomethyl)benzamide	1.7×10^4	47
N-(Methylaminomethyl)salicylamide	-	28
N-(Methylaminomethyl)benzamide	1.7×10^4	600
N-(α-Alanine-methyl)salicylamide	1.2×10^2	17
N-(α-Alanine-methyl)benzamide	3.3×10^2	190
N-(Sarcosin-methyl)salicylamide	73	3
N-(Sarcosin-methyl)benzamide	2.2×10^2	34

[a] From Bundgaard et al. (1986).

being as depicted in Scheme 6. In addition to providing an in vitro stabi-
lizing effect the concept of O-acyloxymethylation makes it possible to obtain prodrug derivatives of a given amine drug with varying physicochemical
properties of importance for drug delivery such as lipophilicity and water
-solubility. This can simply be effected by the selection of an appropriate
acyloxymethyl group.

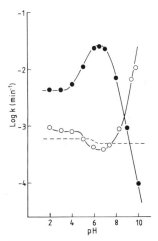

Fig. 3. The pH-rate profiles for
the degradation of O-acetoxy-
methyl-N-(morpholinomethyl)-
salicylamide (o), N-(morpholinomethyl)salicylamide ($\bullet$)
and N-(morpholinomethyl)-
benzamide (---) in aqueous
solution at 37°C.

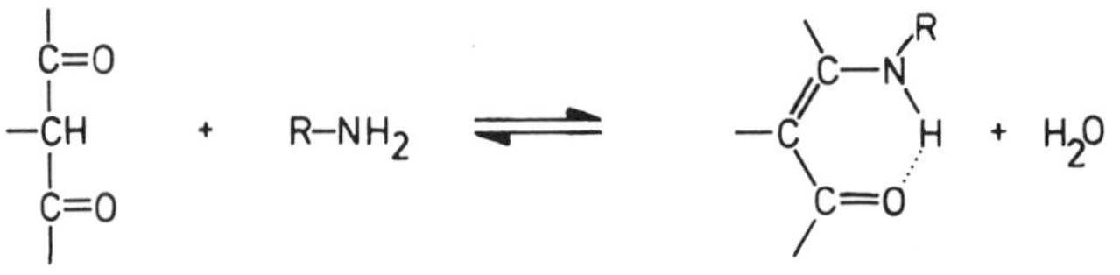

Scheme 7

Enaminones

Enamines, or α,β-unsaturated amines, are, like most Schiff bases, highly unstable in aqueous solution. However, enamines of β-dicarbonyl compounds (enaminones) are stabilized relative to the enamines of monocarbonyl compounds, most probably due to intramolecular hydrogen bonding as depicted in Scheme 7, and such derivatives may be potentially useful prodrugs of amines as originally proposed by Caldwell et al. (1971). They prepared five enaminone derivatives of phenylpropanolamine and showed that the 1,3-dione component had a large influence on the stability at pH 7.4. This was similarly shown by Dixon and Greenhill (1974) in a study of the hydrolysis of various enaminones derived from simple amines and 1,3-diketones and a keto-ester. More recently, the hydrolysis of enaminones derived from ethylacetoacetate and various amino acids or β-lactam antibiotics with a free amino group has been studied at pH 7.4 by a Japanese group (Murakami et al., 1981). The derivatives show promise as prodrugs as their half-lives of hydrolysis at physiological pH are fairly short (from 4 to 98 min at 25°C dependent on the amino compound). In accord with their increased lipophilicity, the enaminones of amino-penicillins and of amino acids such as L- or D-phenylalanine or D-phenylglycine showed markedly improved absorption relative to the parent agents following rectal administration in rabbits or rats (Murakami et al., 1981).

The kinetics of hydrolysis of enaminones derived from various amino acids and 1,3-diketones, keto-esters and keto-amines was recently studied in our laboratory to assess further the suitability of enaminones as prodrugs for amino compounds (Larsen and Bundgaard, 1986). The derivatives studied are shown in Fig. 4. All compounds showed specific acid-catalyzed hydrolysis in the pH-range 4-8 but the stability varied widely as seen from the data in Table 2. The polar effects of the keto, amide or ester groups of the enaminones were found to have a major influence on the reactivity. A potentially useful purpose for transforming amino acids or other amino compounds into enaminone transport forms would be to increase the lipophilicity of the marked amines at physiological pH by depressing their protonation. By enaminone derivatization the pK_a of amines decreases in general by more than 4-5 units (Larsen and Bundgaard, 1986). From a pharmaceutical formulation point of view a definite drawback of enaminones is their high instability in aqueous solutions, making it difficult to prepare solutions with practical shelf-lives. The poor stability in acidic solutions may also preclude oral administration. A possible means of overcoming these problems may be development of enaminones which are stable in vitro but at the same time are susceptible to enzymatic hydrolysis. Enaminones containing two ester groups like compounds XII and XIII fulfill the former condition but

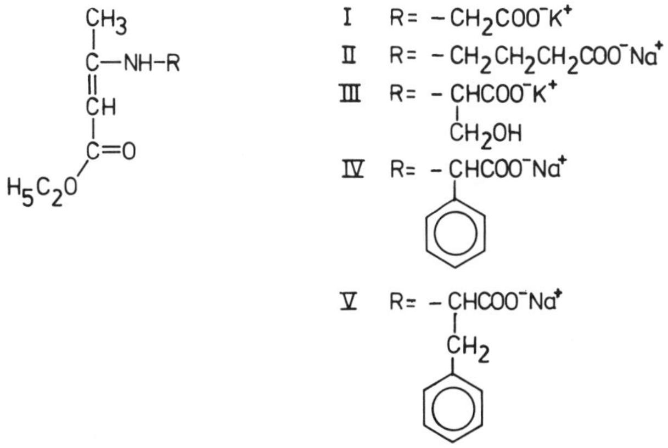
CH3
C—NH-R
CH
C=O
H5C2O
I R= -CH2COO⁻K⁺
II R= -CH2CH2CH2COO⁻Na⁺
III R= -CHCOO⁻K⁺
CH2OH
IV R= -CHCOO⁻Na⁺
V R= -CHCOO⁻Na⁺
CH2

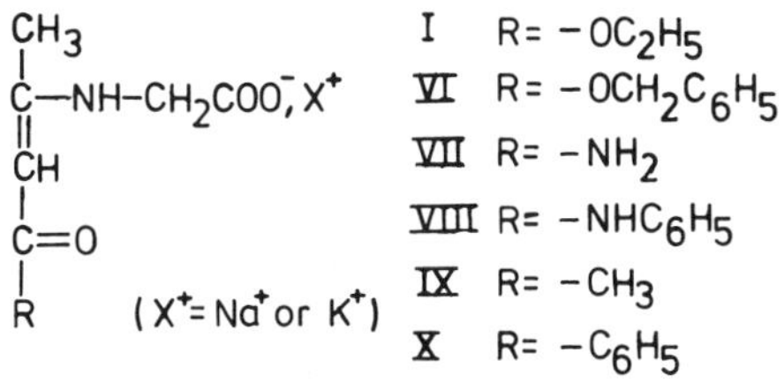
CH3
C—NH-CH2COO⁻, X⁺
CH
C=O
R
(X⁺= Na⁺ or K⁺)
I R= -OC2H5
VI R= -OCH2C6H5
VII R= -NH2
VIII R= -NHC6H5
IX R= -CH3
X R= -C6H5

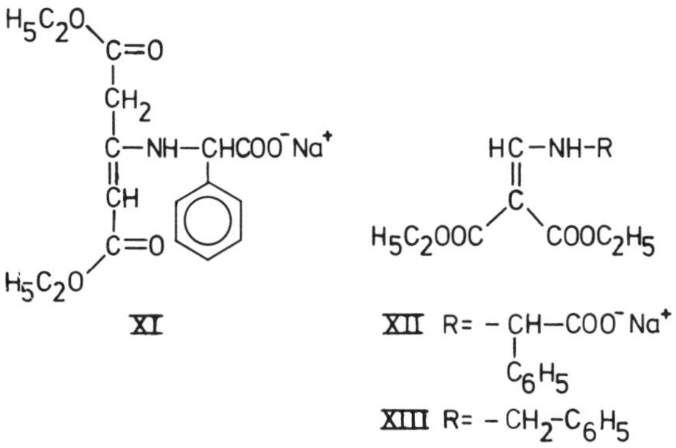
H5C2O
C=O
CH2
C—NH—CHCOO⁻Na⁺
CH
C=O
H5C2O
XI
HC-NH-R
C
H5C2OOC
COOC2H5
XII R= -CH—COO⁻Na⁺
C6H5
XIII R= -CH2-C6H5

Fig. 4. Chemical structures of various enaminones.

Table 2. Rate data for the hydrolysis of various
enaminones in aqueous solution ($\mu = 0.5$)
at 37°C [a]

Compound	$\dfrac{k_H}{(M^{-1}\ min^{-1}}$	$t_{\frac{1}{2}}$ (min) pH 5.0	pH 7.4
I	5.9×10^6	0.01	3
II	2.1×10^6	0.03	9
III	3.2×10^6	0.02	6
IV	1.3×10^6	0.05	16
V	2.5×10^6	0.03	9
VI	4.5×10^6	0.02	5
VII	8.9×10^7	0.008	0.2
VIII	5.4×10^7	0.001	0.4
IX	1.0×10^5	0.7	180
X	1.1×10^4	6	1660
XI	2.1×10^4	3	1020
XII	6.3	183 h	4.6×10^4 h

[a] From Larsen and Bundgaard (1986).

not the latter. The observed resistance of the esters to undergo enzymatic
hydrolysis may most likely be ascribed to the large steric hindrance within
the acyl moieties (Larsen and Bundgaard, 1986). Studies are in progress to
find other enaminones of the ester type with the desired characteristics.

Other Bioreversible Derivatives for Amines

As stated above the utility of carbamates as prodrug derivatives for
amines is limited due to the resistance of carbamates in general to undergo
enzymatic cleavage in vivo. By introducing an enzymatically hydrolyzable
ester function in the carbamate structure it may, however, be possible to
circumvent this problem. As recently described in a patent application
(Alexander, 1985) (acyloxyalkoxy)carbonyl derivatives of primary or secondary amines may be readily transformed to the parent amines in vivo. Enzymatic hydrolysis of the ester moiety in such derivatives would lead to a
(hydroxyalkoxy)carbonyl derivative which is assumed to spontaneously de-
compose into the parent amine via an unstable carbamic acid (Scheme 8).

$$Drug-NH-COOCR_1R_2OOCR_3 \xrightarrow{enzymic} Drug-NH-COOCR_1R_2OH + R_3COOH$$

$$Drug-NH_2 + CO_2 \longleftarrow Drug-NH-COOH + R_1R_2C = O$$

Scheme 8

Such carbamate esters may indeed be promising prodrug derivatives for amino
groups in drugs including peptides since they are neutral compounds and
should combine a high in vitro stability with an appropriate in vivo lability.
Studies on their stability and enzymatic hydrolysis are certainly warranted.

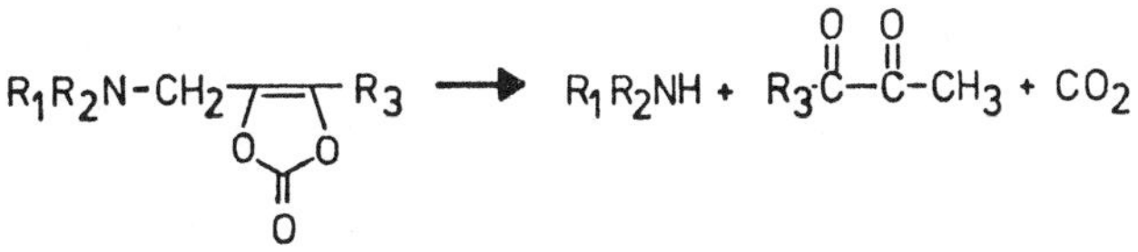

$$R_1R_2N-CH_2 \overline{} R_3 \longrightarrow R_1R_2NH + R_3\overset{O}{\overset{\|}{C}}-\overset{O}{\overset{\|}{C}}-CH_3 + CO_2$$

$$\underline{13}$$

Another potentially useful prodrug type for amines is N-(5-substituted 2-oxo-1,3-dioxol-4-yl)methyl derivatives (13). Sakamoto et al. (1985) have shown that such derivatives formed with the secondary amino group of the piperazinyl moiety of norfloxacin are readily hydrolyzed in mouse blood in vitro and at the same time being relatively stable in acidic and neutral aqueous solutions. The mechanism of liberation of the parent amine from such derivatives has not been elucidated but the enzymatic cleavage may certainly involve hydrolysis of the cyclic carbonate ester moiety. As described above similar derivatives have been proposed as prodrugs for carboxylic acid agents (cf. structure 7).

4-IMIDAZOLIDINONES AS PRODRUGS FOR THE α-AMINOAMIDE MOIETY

The α-aminoamide moiety is found in almost all peptides and a potentially useful and broadly applicable prodrug type for this group may be 4-imidazolidinones (Scheme 9) as recently suggested by Klixbüll and Bundgaard (1984). These authors studied the hydrolysis kinetics of five 4-imidazolidinones derived from acetone and the dipeptides Ala-Gly, Ala-Ala, Phe-Leu, Leu-Gly and Asp-Phe methyl ester (Fig. 5). The imidazolidinyl peptides which may be regarded as cyclic N-Mannich bases were shown to undergo a complete hydrolysis in the pH range 1-10 at 37°C and most of them showed a sigmoidal pH-rate profile with maximum rates at pH > 4 (Fig. 6). The stability of the derivatives varied widely, the following half-lives being obtained at pH 7.40 and 37°C: 0.8 h (Asp-Phe methyl ester), 3.4 h (Phe-Leu), 24.6 h (Ala-Ala), 410 h (Ala-Gly) and 530 h (Leu-Gly). These rates might not be expected to change much in vivo (Klixbüll and Bundgaard, 1984). The major structural factor influencing the stability appears to be the steric properties within the C-terminal amino acid residue. For the further evaluation of 4-imidazolidinones as a prodrug type for peptides it is, however, of importance to establish the effect of the carbonyl component on the reactivity of the

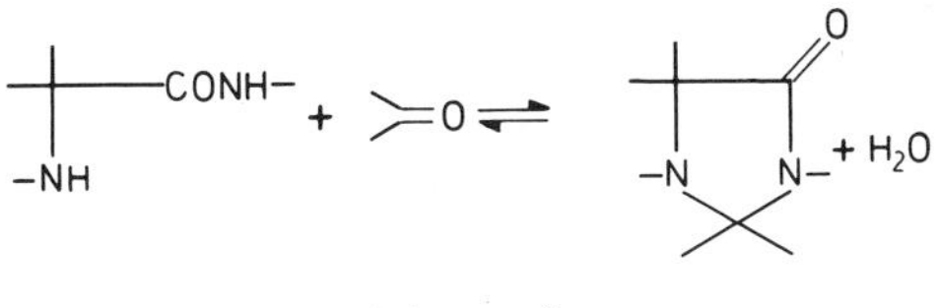

Scheme 9

61

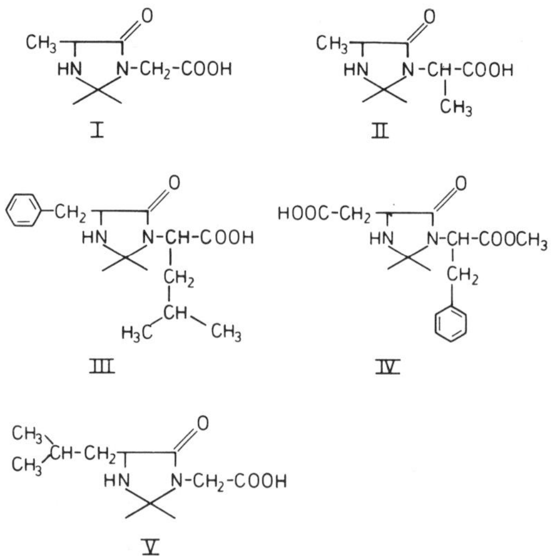

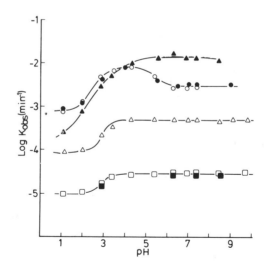

Fig. 5. Chemical structures of 4-imidazolidinones
derived from acetone and the following
dipeptides: I (ala-Gly), II (Ala-Ala),
III (Phe-Leu), IV (Asp-Phe methyl ester)
and V (Leu-Gly).

Fig. 6. The pH-rate profiles for the
hydrolysis of the 4-imidazoli-
dinones I (□), II (Δ), III
(o, ●), IV (▲) and V (■)
at 37°C.

derivatives. In the case of 4-imidazolidinones derived from ampicillin which may be regarded as a model of a peptide containing an α-aminoamide moiety, the rate of 4-imidazolidinone hydrolysis shows only a small dependence on the carbonyl component (aldehyde or ketone) (Klixbüll and Bundgaard, 1985) but this does not necessarily apply to other imidazolidinyl peptides.

In considering 4-imidazolidinones as a potential prodrug type for peptides the large decrease obtained in basicity of the reacting N-terminal amino group should be appreciated. The 4-imidazolidinones mentioned above are much weaker bases (pK_a about 3.1) than the parent dipeptides and such depression of amino protonation brings about an increase in the lipophilicity of the N-terminal amino acid part at physiological pH as confirmed by partition experiments in octanol-aqueous buffer systems (Klixbüll and Bundgaard, 1984). The increased lipophilicity attained which obviously will be further influenced by the lipophilicity of the substituents of the carbonyl component, may be of value in situations where delivery problems of peptide drugs are due to low lipophilicity.

It is interesting to note that several 4-imidazolidinones have been prepared from peptides although their stability or delivery behaviour have not been examined or considered. Thus, 4-imidazolidinones were reported to be formed by condensation of acetaldehyde with various oligopeptides (Cardinaux and Brenner, 1974), by reaction of acetone with the tripeptide L-protyl-L-leucyl-glycineamide (Hruby et al., 1968) and oxytocin (Hruby et al., 1968; Yamashiro et al., 1965) and by reaction of acetaldehyde with various enkephalins and β-endorphin (Summers et al., 1980; Summers and Lightman, 1981). There is, however, already one 4-imidazolidinone prodrug derivative in clinical use, namely hetacillin, formed by condensation of ampicillin with acetone (Hardcastle et al., 1966). It is readily hydrolyzed to the active ampicillin in aqueous solution, the half-life being 17 min at pH 7.4 and 37°C (Klixbüll and Bundgaard, 1985) and about 11 min in vivo as determined after intravenous administration in man (Jusko and Lewis, 1973). An advantage of hetacillin is its higher stability in concentrated aqueous solutions (Schwartz and Hayton, 1972) compared with ampicillin sodium which undergoes a facile intermolecular aminolysis by attack of the side-chain amino group in one molecule on the β-lactam moiety of a second molecule (Bundgaard, 1976).

CONCLUSION

Theoretically, the prodrug concept may be highly useful to improve the delivery of peptides. Thus, by derivatization of a functional group in a peptide it may be possible to obtain a derivative which is resistant to degradation by peptidases in e.g. the gastro-intestinal tract. This should especially hold true for small peptides containing 2-5 amino acid residues. In addition, the passage of peptides through the mucosal and cellular barriers may be improved by administering the peptide agents in the form of more lipophilic transport forms. The types of bioreversible derivatives being applicable to peptides have increased greatly during the past few years and there are now a number of possibilities for performing bioreversible derivatization of the various functional groups of peptides. Studies on the effect of derivatization on the susceptibility of peptides towards various kinds of peptidases are almost lacking but are highly needed in order to explore the potential utility of the prodrug concept in peptide delivery.

REFERENCES

Alexander, J. 1985, (Acyloxyalkoxy)carbonyl derivatives as bioreversible
   prodrug moieties for primary and secondary amine functions in drugs,
   their preparation and pharmaceutical compositions containing said
   derivatives, Eur. Pat. Appl., No. 130, 119.
Baker, G.B., Coutts, R.T., Nazarali, A.J., Danielson, T.J., and Rubens,
   M., 1984, Carbamate prodrugs of phenylethylamines: A neurochemical
   investigation, Proc. West. Pharmacol. Soc. 27:523.
Baldwin, J.J., Denny, G. H., Ponticello, G.S., Sweet, C.S. and Stone,
   C.A., 1982, Tyrosine progenitors as antihypertensive agents, Eur. J.
   Med. Chem., 17:297.
Belke, C.J., Su, S.C.K., and Shafer, J.A., 1971, Imidazole-catalyzed
   displacement of an amine from an amide by a neighboring hydroxyl
   group. A model for the acylation of chymotrypsin, J. Am. Chem. Soc.
   93:4552.
Bodin, N.O., Ekström, B., Forsgren, U., Jalar, L.P., Magni, L. Ramsey,
   C.H., and Sjöberg B., 1975, Bacampicillin: A new orally well-absorbed
   derivative of ampicillin, Antimicrob. Agents. Chemother. 8:518.
Bodor, N., Sloan, K.B., Higuchi, T, and Sasahara, K., 1977, Improved
   delivery through biological membranes. 4. Prodrugs of L-Dopa, J. Med.
   Chem. 20:1435.
Bodor, N., Zupan, J., and Selk, S., 1980, Improved delivery through bio-
   logical membranes VII. Dermal delivery of chromoglycic acid
   (cromolyn) via its prodrugs, Int. J. Pharm. 7:64.
Bodor, N., Sloan, K.B., Kminski,J.J., Shih, C., and Pogani, S., 1983, A
   convenient synthesis of (acyloxy)alkyl α-ethers of phenols, J. Org.
   Chem. 48:5280.
Bundgaard, H., 1976, Polymerization of penicillins: kinetics and mechanisms of di- and polymerization of ampicillin in aqueous solution,
   Acta Pharm. Suec. 13:9.
Bundgaard, H., 1982, Novel bioreversible derivatives of amides, imides,
   ureides, amines and other chemical entities not readily derivatiz-
   able, in: "Optimization of drug delivery", H. Bundgaard, A.B. Hansen
   and H. Kofod eds., Munksgaard, Copenhagen.
Bundgaard, H., 1985a, Design of prodrugs: Bioreversible derivatives for
   various functional groups and chemical entities, in: "Design of prodrugs", H. Bundgaard ed., Elsevier Biomedical Press, Amsterdam.
Bundgaard, H., 1985b, The formation of prodrugs of amines, amides,
   ureides and imides. Methods in Enzymology 112:347.
Bundgaard, H. and Johansen, M., 1980a, Pro-drugs as drug delivery systems. IV. N-Mannich bases as potential novel pro-drugs for amides,
   ureides, amines, and other NH-acidic compounds, J. Pharm. Sci.
   69:44.
Bundgaard, H. and Johansen, M., 1980b, Pro-drugs as drug delivery systems. X. N-Mannich bases as novel pro-drug candidates for amides,
   imides, urea derivatives, amines and other NH-acidic compounds. Kinetics and mechanisms of decomposition and structure-reactivity relationships, Arch. Pharm. Chem., Sci. Ed. 8:29.
Bundgaard, H. and Johansen, M., 1980c, Pro-drugs as drug delivery systems. XV. Bioreversible derivatization of phenytoin, acetazolamide,
   chlorzoxazone and various other NH-acidic compounds by N-aminome-
   thylation to effect enhanced dissolution rates, Int. J. Pharm.
   7:129.
Bundgaard, H. and Johansen, M. 1981, Hydrolysis of N-Mannich bases and
   its consequences for the biological testing of such agents, Int. J.
   Pharm. 9:7.
Bundgaard, H. and Johansen, M., 1981, Pro-drugs as drug delivery systems.
   XVIII. Bioreversible derivatization of allopurinol by N-aminomethy-
   lation to effect enhanced dissolution rates, Acta Pharm. Suec.
   18:129.

Bundgaard, H. and Johansen, M., 1982, Prodrugs as drug delivery systems. XIX. Bioreversible derivatization of aromatic amines by formation of N-Mannich bases with succinimide, Int. J. Pharm. 8:183.

Bundgaard, H., Klixbüll, U., and Falch, E., 1986, Prodrugs as drug delivery systems. 43. O-Acyloxymethyl salicylamide N-Mannich bases as double prodrug forms for amines, Int. J. Pharm. 29:19.

Cain, B.F., 1976, 2-Acyloxymethylbenzoic acids. Novel amine protective functions providing amides with the lability of esters, J. Org. Chem. 41:2029.

Caldwell, H.C., Adams, H.J., Jones, R.G., Mann, W.A., Dittert, L.W., Chong, C.W., and Swintosky, J.V., 1971, Enamine prodrugs J. Pharm. Sci. 60:1810.

Cardinaux, F. and Brenner, M., 1973, N,N'-Alkylidenpeptide: Peptidsynthese-Nebenprodukte bei Einwirkung von Carbonylverbindungen, Helv. Chim. Acta 56:339.

Chiong, K.N.G., Lewis, S.D., and Shafer, J.A., 1975, Rationalization of the rate of the acylation step in chymotrypsin-catalyzed hydrolysis of amides, J. Am. Chem. Soc. 97:418.

Clayton, J.P., Cole, M., Elson, S.W., and Ferres, H., 1974, BRL.8988 (talampicillin), a well-absorbed oral form of ampicillin. Antimicrob. Agents Chemother. 5:670.

Daehne, W.v., Frederiksen, E., Gundersen, E., Lund, F., Mørch, P., Petersen, H.J., Roholt, K., Tybring, L., and Godtfredsen, W.O., 1970, acyloxymethyl esters of ampicillin, J. Med. Chem. 13:607.

Digenis, G.A. and Swintosky, J.V., 1975, Drug latentiation, Handbook of Experimental Pharmacology, 28/3:86.

Dixon, K. and Greenhill, J.V., 1974, A study of the rates of hydrolysis of certain enaminones, J. Chem. Soc. Perkin II, 164.

Dobrinska, M.R., Kukovetz, W., Beubler, E., Leidy, H.L., Gomez, H.J., Demetriades, J., and Bolognese, J.A., 1982, Pharmacokinetics of the pivaloyloxyethyl (POE) ester of methyldopa, a new prodrug of methyldopa, J. Pharmacokin. Biopharm. 10:587.

Farmer, P.S. and Ariëns, E.J., 1982, Speculations on the design on non-peptidic peptidomimetics, Trends Pharm. Sci. 3:362.

Farquhar, D., Srivastva, D.N., Kuttesch, N.J., and Saunders, P.P., 1983, Biologically reversible phosphate-protective groups, J. Pharm. Sci. 72:324.

Fife, T.H. and Benjamin, B.M., 1974, Intramolecular general base-catalyzed alcoholysis of amides, J. Chem. Soc., Chem. Comm. 525.

Ferres, H., 1983, Pro-drugs of β-lactam antibiotics, Drugs of Today 19:499.

Hardcastle, G.A., Johnson, D.A., Panetta, C.A., Scott, A.I., and Sutherland, S.A., 1966, The preparation and structure of hetacillin, J. Org. Chem. 31:897.

Hruby, V.H., Yamashiro, D., Vigneaud, V. du, 1968, The structure of acetone-oxytocin with studies on the reaction of acetone with various peptides. J. Am. Chem. Soc. 90:7106.

Jansen, A.B.A. and Russell, T.J., 1965, Some novel penicillin derivatives, J. Chem. Soc. 2127.

Jemal, M., Ivashkiv, E., Ribick, M., and Cohen, A.I., 1985, Determination of SQ 27,519, The active phosphinic acid-carboxylic acid of the prodrug SQ 28,555, in human serum by capillary gas chromatography with nitrogen-phosphorus detection after a two-step derivatization, J. Chromatogr. 345:299.

Jusko,W.J. and Lewis, G.P., 1973, Comparison of ampicillin and hetacillin pharmacokinetics in man, J. Pharm. Sci. 62:69.

Johansen, M. and Bundgaard, H., 1980a, Pro-drugs as drug delivery system. XII. Solubility, dissolution and partitioning behaviour of N-Mannich bases and N-hydroxymethyl derivatives, Arch. Pharm. Chem., Sci. Ed. 8:141.

Johansen, M. and Bundgaard, H., 1980b, Pro-drugs as drug delivery systems. XIII. Kinetics of decomposition of N-Mannich bases of salicylamide and assessment of their suitability as possible pro-drugs for amines, Int. J. Pharm. 7:119.

Johansen, M. and Bundgaard, H., 1982, Pro-drugs as drug delivery systems. XXIV. N-Mannich bases as bioreversible lipophilic transport forms of ephedrine, phenethylamine and other amines, Arch. Pharm. Chem., Sci. Ed. 10:111.

Kakeya, N., Nishimura, K.-I., Yoshimi, A., Nakamura, S., Nishizawa, S., Tamaki, S., Matsui, H., Kawamura, T., Kasai, M., and Kitae, K., 1984, Studies of prodrugs of cephalosporins. I. Synthesis of biological properties of glycyloxybenzoyloxymethyl and glycylaminobenzoyloxymethyl esters of 7 β-[2-(2-aminothiazol-4-yl)-(Z)-2-methoxyimino-acetamido]-3-methyl-3-cephem-4-carboxylic acid, Chem. Pharm. Bull. 32:692.

Kimura, T., 1984, Transmucosal absorption of small peptide drugs, Pharm. Int. 5:75.

Klixbüll, U. and Bundgaard, H., 1983, Prodrugs as drug delivery systems. XXIX. Imidazole-1-carboxylic acid esters of hydrocortisone and testosterone, Arch. Pharm. Chem., Sci. Ed. 11:101.

Klixbüll, U. and Bundgaard, H., Prodrugs as drug delivery systems. XXX. 4-Imidazolidinones as potential bioreversible derivatives for the α-aminoamide moiety in peptides, Int. J. Pharm. 20:273.

Klixbüll, U. and Bundgaard, H., 1985, Kinetics of reversible reactions of ampicillin with various aldehydes and ketones with formation of 4-Imidazolidinones, Int. J. Pharm. 23:163.

Kupchan, S.M. and Isenberg, A.C., 1967, Drug latentiation. III. Labile amide derivatives of normeperidine, J. Med. Chem. 10:960.

Kyncl, J.J., Minard, F.N., and Jones, P.H., 1979, L-α-Glutamyl dopamine, an oral dopamine prodrug with renal selectivity, Adv. Biosci. 20:369.

Larmour, I., Jackson, B., Cubela, R. and Johnston, C.I., 1985, Enalapril (MK421) activation in man: importance of liver status, Br. J. Clin. Pharmacol. 19:701.

Larsen, J.D. and Bundgaard, H., 1986, Prodrugs as drug delivery systems. 49. Hydrolysis kinetics of enaminones derived from various amino acids and 1,3-diketones, keto-esters and keto-amides, Arch. Pharm. Chem., Sci. Ed. 14:52.

Lee, V.H.L., Stratfors, R.E., Carson, L.W., and Kashi, S.D., 1985, Effect of ocular aminopeptidases on ocular absorption of enkephalins, Invest. Ophthalmol. Vis. Sci. Suppl. 26:106.

Loftsson, T. and Bodor, N., 1982, Synthesis and hydrolysis of some pivaloyloxymethyl and pivaloyl derivatives of phenolic compounds, Arch. Pharm. Chem., Sci. Ed. 10:104.

Meisenberg, G. and Simmons, W.H., 1983, Peptides and the blood-brain barrier, Life Sci. 32:2611.

Murakami, T., Tamauchi, H., Yamazaki, M., Kubo, K., Kamada, A., and Yata, N., 1981, Biopharmaceutical study on the oral and rectal administrations of enamine prodrugs of amino acid-like β-lactam antibiotics in rabbits, Chem. Pharm. Bull. 29:1986.

Murakami, T., Yata, N., Tamauchi. H., Nakai, J., Yamazaki, M., and Kamada, A., 1981, Studies on absorption promotors for rectal delivery preparations. I. Promoting efficacy of enamine derivatives of amino acids for the rectal absorption of β-lactam antibiotics in rabbits, Chem. Pharm. Bull. 29:1998.

Nielsen, N.M., and Bundgaard, H., 1986, Prodrugs as drug delivery systems. Part. 42. 2-Hydroxymethylbenzamides and 2-acyloxymethylbenzamides as potential prodrug forms for amines, Int. J. Pharm. 29:9.

Okada, H., Yamazaki, I., Ogawa, Y., Hirai, S., Yoshiki, T., and Mima, H.J., 1982, Vaginal absorption of a potent luteinizing hormone-releasing hormone analog (Leuprolide) in rats I: Absorption by various routes and absorption enhancement, J. Pharm. Sci. 71:1367.

Okuyama, T. and Schmir, G.L., 1972, Hydrolysis of 1-benzylimino-1,3-dihydroisobenzofuran. Implications for the mechanism of lactonization of 2-hydroxymethylbenzamides, J. Am. Chem. Soc. 94:8805.

Orlowski, M., Mizoguchi, H., and Wilk, S., 1979, N-Acyl-γ-glutamyl derivatives of sulfamethoxazole as models of kidney-selective prodrugs, J. Pharmacol. Exp. Ther. 212:167.

Pitman, I.H., 1981, Prodrugs of amides, imides and amines, Med. Res. Rev. 1:189.

Rakhit, A. and Tipnis, V., 1984, Liquid-chromatographic determination of an angiotensin converting enzyme inhibitor, CGS 13945, and its active metabolite (CGS 13934) in plasma, Clin. Chem. 30:1237.

Roche, E.B., ed., 1977, "Design of biopharmaceutical properties through prodrugs and analogs", Washington, D.C., American Pharmaceutical Association.

Saari, W.S., Freedman, M.B., Hartman, R.D., King, S.W., Raab, A.W., Randall, W.C., Engelhardt, E.L., Hirschman, R., Rosegay, A., Ludden, C.T., and Scriabine, A., 1978, Synthesis and antihypertensive activity of some ester progenitors of methyldopa, J. Med. Chem. 21:746.

Saari, W.S., Halczenko, W., Cochran, D.W., Dobrinska, M.R., Vincek, W.C., Titus, D.C., Gaul, S.L., and Sweet, C.S., 1984, 3-Hydroxy-α-methyltyrosine progenitors: Synthesis and evaluation of some (2-oxo-1,3-dioxol-4-yl)methylesters, J. Med. Chem. 27:713.

Sakamoto, F., Ikeda, S., and Tsukamoto, G., 1984, Studies on prodrugs. II. Preparation and characterization of (5-substituted 2-oxo-1,3-dioxolen-4-yl)methyl esters of ampicillin, Chem. Pharm. Bull. 32:2241.

Sakamoto, F., Ikeda, S., Kondo, H., and Tsukamoto, G., 1985, Studies on prodrugs. IV. Preparation and characterization of N-(5-substituted 2-oxo-1,3-dioxol-4-yl)methyl norfloxacin, Chem. Pharm. Bull. 33:4870.

Sasaki, H., Mukai, E., Hashida, M., Kimura, T., and Sezaki, H., 1983, Development of lipophilic prodrugs of mitomycin C. I. Synthesis and antitumor activity of 1a-N-substituted derivatives with aromatic pro-moiety, Int. J. Pharm. 15:49.

Sasaki, H., Mukai, E., Hashida, M., Kimura, T., and Sezaki, H., 1983, Development of lipophilic prodrugs of mitomycin C. II. Stability and bioactivation of 1a-N-substituted derivatives with aromatic pro-moiety, Int. J. Pharm. 15:61.

Sasaki, H., Fukumoto, M. Hashida, M., Kimura, T., and Sezaki, H., 1983, Development of lipophilic prodrugs of mitomycin C. III. Physicochemical and biological properties of newly synthesized alkoxycarbonyl derivatives, Chem. Pharm. Bull. 31:4083.

Schwartz, M.A. and Hayton, W.L., 1972, Relative stability of hetacillin and ampicillin in solution, J. Pharm. Sci. 61:906.

Shiobara, Y., Tachibana, A., Sasaki, H., Watanabe, T., and Sado, T., 1974, Phthalidyl D-α-aminobenzylpenicillinate hydrochloride (PC-183), a new orally active ampicillin ester. J. Antibiot. 27:665.

Sinkula, A.A., 1975, Prodrug approach in drug design, Annual Reports in Medicinal Chemistry, 10:306.

Sinkula, A.A. and Yalkowsky, S.H., 1975, Rationale for design of biologically reversible drug derivatives: Prodrugs, J. Pharm. Sci. 64:181.

Srivastva, D.N. and Farquhar, D., 1984, Bioreversible phosphate protective groups: Synthesis and stability of model acyloxymethyl phosphates, Bioorg. Chem. 12:118.

Stella, V., 1975, Pro-drugs: An overview and definition, in: "Pro-drugs as novel drug delivery systems", T. Higuchi and V. Stella, eds., American Chemical Society, Washington, D.C.

Stratford, R.E. and Lee, V.H.L., 1986, Aminopeptidase activity in homogenates of various absorptive mucosae in the albino rabbit: implications in peptide delivery, Int. J. Pharm. 30:73.

Summers, M.C., Gidley, M.J., and Sanders, J.K., 1980, "Acetaldehyde-enkephalins": elucidation of the structure of the acetaldehyde adducts of methionine-enkephalin and leucine-enkephalin, FEBS Lett. 111:307.

Summers, M.C. and Lightman, S.L., 1981, A reaction of acetaldehyde with enkephalins and related peptides, Biochem. Pharmacol. 30:1621.

Tipnis, V. and Rakhit, A., 1985, Determination of pentopril, an angiotensin converting enzyme inhibitor, and its active metabolite in urine, J. Chromatogr. 345:396.

Todd, P.A. and Heel, R.C., 1986, Enalapril. A review of its pharmacodynamic and pharmacokinetic properties, and therapeutic use in hypertension and congestive heart failure, Drugs, 31:198.

Verbiscar, A.J. and Abood, L.G., 1970, Carbamate ester latentiation of physiologically active amines, J. Med. Chem. 13:176.

Vickers, S., Duncan, C.A.H., Ramjit, H.G., Dobrinska, M.R., Dollery, C.T., Gomez, H.J., Leidy, H.L., and Vincek, W.C., 1984, Metabolism of methyldopa in man after oral administration of the pivaloyloxyethyl ester, Drug Metab. Disp. 12:242.

Wiedhaup, K., 1981, The stability of small peptides in the gastrointestinal tract, in: "Topics in Pharmaceutical Sciences", D.D. Breimer and P. Speiser, eds., Elsevier/North-Holland Biomedical Press, Amsterdam.

Wilk, S., Mizoguchi, H., and Orlowski, M., 1978, γ-Glutamyl Dopa: A kidney-specific dopamine precursor, J. Pharmacol. Exp. Ther. 206:227.

Yamashiro, D., Aanning, H.L., and Vigneaud, V. du, 1965, Inactivation of oxytocin by acetone, Proc. Natl. Acad. Sci. U.S.A., 54:166.

Zlojkowska, Z., Krasuka, H.J., and Pachecka, J., 1982, Enzymatic hydrolysis of amino acid derivatives of benzocaine, Xenobiotica 12:359.

AN APPROACH TO TARGETED THERAPY: SYNTHESIS AND BIOLOGICAL ACTIVITY OF

HYDROPHOBIC AND HYDROPHILIC ENKEPHALIN ANALOGUES

José M. García-Antón, Francesca Reig and Gregorio Valencia

Laboratory of Peptides
Biological Organic Chemistry Department C.S.I.C.
Jorge Girona Salgado 18-26
08034 Barcelona, Spain

INTRODUCTION

The mechanisms whereby opioid peptides (naturally occuring peptides with opiate - like biological properties) activate processes on their target receptors are still at an early stage of exploration. The aim of receptor research is to purify and isolate receptor glycoproteins or glycolipids in order to further implement the knowledge of the physicochemical aspects involved in the interaction of opioids with their receptor.

Opioid peptides like other neuroactive peptides, are derived from large molecular weight proteins and are synthesized with ribosomal participation. To date, it is now clear that there are at least three different families of endogenous opioid peptides : the enkephalins, the endorphins and the dynorphins, that may act as neurotransmitters or neurohormones. It is also well stablished that these various opioid peptides are derived from three biosynthetic precursors: the Proenkephalin-A, that contains 6 copies of [Met]- enkephalin and one copy of [Leu]- enkephalin; the Pro-opiomelanocortin, that contains the sequence of the β - endorphin; and the Prodynorphin that includes the sequences of the dynorphins. The primary structures of these precursors have been deduced by the use of recombinant DNA techniques. It is possible to isolate and purify the pro-hormone mRNA from hormone rich tissues. DNAs complementary to the mRNAs encoding these precursors have been cloned and the determination of their nucleotide sequences has lead to the elucidation of the amino acid sequences of the precursor proteins.

The physiological action of these peptides is mediated by Opioid Receptors. Such receptors consist of both a recognition site, to which the peptide binds ,and a nervous device that translates the binding into biochemical events that lead to a biological response. Three different subtypes of opioid receptors : (μ, δ and k) have been characterized so far.Each of them are supposed to mediate different physiological effects. Thus, μ receptors appear to be involved in analgesia and more precisely in heat mediated nociception. They are supposed to mediate the respiratory depressant effects of opiates as well as the inhibition of

69

intestinal motility. The development of physical dependence seems to be mediated by the μ binding sites; δ - receptors seem to be involved in respiratory depression and circulatory shock. It is still not clear whether δ - receptors are involved in analgesia; k receptors,on the contrary, seem to mediate analgesia and, particularly, pressure nociception. They are also involved in diuresis and feeding behaviour.

The concept of multiple Opioid Receptor subtypes offers a new strategy for the development of targeted therapy if specific "in vivo" effects can be undoubtely associated with the occupancy of specific receptors.

Design of opioids with analgesic efficacies dissociated from respiratory depression or the development of physical dependence is obviously of the utmost importance. In this regard, there is evidence that the administration of a δ -selective antagonist, reversed hypotension associated with endotoxin shock,without altering the levels of analgesia induced by morphine, which is supposed to interact with the μ.- subtype (Holaday et al. 1982).

To go further in this objective of " targeted therapy " it is of great importance to obtain information on the chemical requirements of each binding - site. To date the best way to obtain information concerning the chemical structure of the opioid receptors is to conduct investigations based on physicochemical principles that would help in the isolation of the binding sites. Such studies should be complementary to those dealing with the in situ properties within the membrane.

As far as the isolation of the opioid receptors is concerned it is worth remembering that many efforts have been made in this direction by either the two major approaches to the isolation of surface receptors. In the first a labeled ligand is bound to the receptor, and the ligand binding site complex is solubilized and isolated; in the other, the binding sites are solubilized and isolated in the absence of opioids . However, nearly all attempts have failed and the studies on the isolation of the opioid binding sites are still at an early stage.

One of the most interesting studies to date in this respect is that by Gioannini et al. 1984, who found that opioid binding sites solubilized from bovine striatum were specifically retained by affinity chromatography on a wheat germ agglutinin agarose column. Although wheat germ agglutinin not only recognizes N-acetyl glucosamine residues and also sialoproteins, further studies with specific lectins for sialic acid did not retain any of the solubilized binding sites. These results suggested that the extracted material might be a glycoprotein containing N-acetyl glucosamine residues.

On the other hand, in our laboratory, the present authors could demonstrate, by an indirect approach, using monolayer techniques and studying the profiles of the different isotherms, that gangliosides, a group of sialic acid containing glycosphingolipids, were involved in the chemical structure of the opioid receptors. By monolayer techniques one can easily examine the interactions between neuronal membrane lipids and opioid agonists and antagonists. Lipid monolayers may be arranged at an air-water interface using a Langmuir balance (Albretch, 1983). The interactions between the monolayer components and solutes included in the aqueous subphase may be examined through measurement of the lateral compresibility of the monolayer (Phillips et al., 1968). Mixed monolayers, of various lipids prepared from the stock solution and spread over a range of surface concentrations, yield isotherms which are dependent upon the molar fraction of each lipid. When examined at low pressures in the case of mixed monolayers of soybean lecithin and gangliosides, as it is shown in Fig 1, the area per molecule does not exhibit ideal behaviour and consistently falls to very low values at 0.9 molar fraction of lecithin. However the inclusion of morphine or naloxone results in monolayer expansion for nearly every mixture which contains

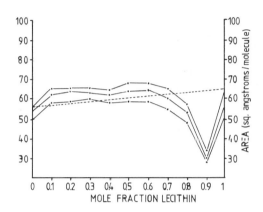

Figure 1. The mean area per molecule in mixed monolayers of lecithin and gangliosides to the molecular proportions of the two components at three different surface pressures: 3 dyn/cm (solid line), 6 dyn/cm (-o-) and 9 dyn/cm (-●-) on a twice-distilled water subphase. Pure lecithin on the right, pure gangliosides on the left. The dotted line is the expected plot for ideal mixtures.

gangliosides as can be observed in Fig. 2 . In general the effect is greatest for morphine. These effects occur even at the lowest levels of ganglioside tested (0.1 mole fraction), but do not increase in a simple manner with increasing mole fraction. The specificity of lipid expansion for gangliosides over lecithins may localize the opioid-lipid interabctions to nervous tissues in vivo.

This type of investigation has been extended to other lipids (phosphatidylserine, phosphatidylinositol) as well as to other opiates such as buprenorphine, methadone, meperidine, ethylmorphine, codeine, dextrometorphan, etc. In this regard, a set of studies has been carried out in our laboratory comparing the interaction of buprenorphine, a partial agonist, and naloxone, a typical antagonist, with phosphatidylinositol monolayers. For reference purposes we worked also, in a similar way, with phosphatidylcholine in order to differentiate non-specific interactions from the specific ones. Moreover, as the affinity of opioid molecules, in biochemical assays, is greatly modified by ions we have also studied the influence of Na^+, Ca^{2+} and Mn^{2+} in these physicochemical interactions.

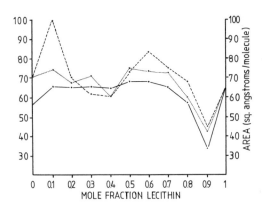

Figure 2. The mean area per molecule in mixed monolayers of lecithin and gangliosides to the molar proportion of the two components at the following subphases: twice-distilled water (solid line), 1.4×10^{-5}M morphine hydrochloride solution (dashed line) and 1.4×10^{-5}M naloxone hydrochloride solution (dotted line) at a surface pressure of 3 dyn/cm.

Figure 3 shows an important interaction between buprenorphine and phosphatidylinositol, larger than the one existing with naloxone. This interaction is highly dependent on the ionic content of the subphase in the case of buprenorphine but not for naloxone. This fact could be related to Zajac's (1985) observations concerning the changes induced by sodium on the allosteric conformation of the opioid receptor promoting a decrease in agonist affinity, leaving on the contrary the antagonist affinity unchanged (sodium index of naloxone being equal to 1).

These striking differences can not be attributed to differences in hydrophobicity because they are not found with phosphatidylcholine monolayers taken as reference.

Besides, the interaction between phosphatidylserine and morphine or naloxone were studied and also in this system the influence of ions was checked. By measuring the area occupied per molecule of phosphatidylserine in films spread on subphases containing the different opioid molecules and ions, it could be acertained that the highest variability with regard to the ionic content is found in morphine containing subphases (agonist).

The results obtained are, thus, in general similar to the ones previously reported with phosphatidylinositol and buprenorphine or naloxone. They suggest that it is possible to establish a similar mechanism of interaction between opioid agonists and some acidic phospholipids involved in the opioid receptor, different from the type of interaction the same phospholipids have with opioid antagonists.

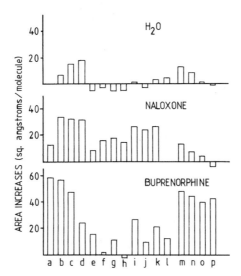

Figure 3. Area increases experienced by Phosphatidylinositol monolayers when spread on the following subphases:
a) water; b), c), d) NaCl 10^{-3}M, 10^{-2}M, 10^{-1}M; e), f) CaCl$_2$ 10^{-3}M, 10^{-2}M; g), h) MnCl$_2$ 10^{-3}M, 10^{-2}M; i), j) NaCl 10^{-1}M + CaCl$_2$ 10^{-3}M, 10^{-2}M; k), l) NaCl 10^{-1}M + MnCl$_2$ 10^{-3}M, 10^{-2}M; m) TRIS; n), o), p) TRIS + NaCl 10^{-1}M, or CaCl$_2$ 10^{-2}M or MnCl$_2$ 10^{-2}M.

This simple membrane model (monolayers), has proved to be very useful for the selection of the phospholipids that could be a part of the opioid receptor. By comparing the affinities or selectivities of the opioid molecules for the different opioid receptors, with the degree of interaction of the same molecule with phospholipids it could be possible to obtain knowledge of the chemical constituents of the opioid receptor subtypes.

HYDROPHOBIC ENKEPHALIN DERIVATIVES

Once the involvement of certain lipids, as constituents of the opioid receptors had been established, and bearing in mind that the interaction between opioid peptides and the membrane lipids, probably depends on the formation of specific hydrophobic bonds between the non – polar parts of both ligands and receptors, we decided to prepare a series of hydrophobic enkephalin analogues . Furthermore, hydrophobicity is a basic property that enables opioids to cross the blood – brain barrier allowing them to exhibit higher levels of potency. Thus, it is not difficult to predict that by means of hydrophobic modifications of a parent enkephalin, one could, in principle, improve both affinity and transport properties.

With this in mind and as a first approach we decided to synthesize a series of hydrophobic enkephalin amides:

Tyr-D.Met-Gly-Phe-Pro-X

being $X = NH-[CH_2]_n-CH_3$; $n = 5,7,9,11$ and 13. Where the parent compound ($[D.Met^2, Pro-NH_2^5]$ enkephalin), is generally accepted as a μ-selective ligand.

All the analogues were synthesized by solution phase procedures with isolation and characterization of intermediate and final products (Garcia Anton et al., 1985). The synthetic route is outlined in Fig. 4. A considerable decrease in the last coupling step (d), was observed in the case of the C_{12} and C_{14} derivatives, probably due to steric hindrance of the aliphatic chain in the C - terminal position.

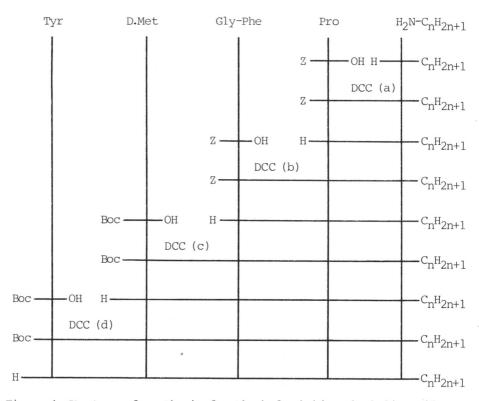

Figure 4. Strategy of synthesis for the hydrophobic enkephalin amides.

Purification of final peptides was carried out by semipreparative reversed phase HPLC on a μ -Bondapack C_{18}, 10 µm with a 1.1 ml loop. The homogeneity of the peptides was checked by TLC and reversed phase HPLC on a C_{18}, 5 µm column using a solvent system $CH_3CN/H_2O-0.05$ % TFA and gradient elution from 9 to 100% of CH_3CN, with a linear rate of 3.5%/min.

Biological Activity

The compounds were tested in vitro on the guinea pig ileum (GPI) preparation . They proved to be more potent than the parent compound and a direct relation between hydrophobicity and opioid activity was observed, the IC_{50} values for the C_6, C_{10} and C_{14} respectively : $4.3x10^{-7}$M, $8.0x10^{-10}$M and $5.0 \cdot 10^{-11}$M. An increasing affinity for the guinea pig ileum preparation was observed as the hydrophobicity increased such that the C_{14} derivative was very sligthly displaced from the ileum by naloxone or repeated washings.

The in vivo tests were performed on male albino Sprague Dawley rats, body weight 250 - 300 gr. which were kept before and during the experiment in the animal room under normal conditions. All the in vivo tests were carried out with the operator unaware of which analogue he was testing. The readings from animals which showed control responses greater than 75% of the chosen cut - off value were discarded.

Hot plate and tail flick tests provided different results for the same derivative depending on the mode of administration. Thus, for instance, in the case of the C_{10} derivative by parenteral injection, analgesia was not detected in the tail flick test, whereas hyperalgesia was observed in the hot plate test. Moreover, when the same analogue was injected intrathecally, a pronounced activity in both tests, was observed (Reig, et al.,1986).

As the derivatives are completely resistant to enzymatic hydrolysis, are homogeneous as determined by HPLC, are correctely characterized and each value is the mean of six experiments one has to assume that this anomalous pharmacological behaviour could be due to a shift in the affinity towards different opioid receptors. Further experiments are required to elucidate such a possibility. Nevertheless, an answer to the question of " what are we really measuring in the hot plate and tail flick tests ?", seems to be of the utmost importance.

In this regard, Dickenson (1986) has also found, studying the antinociceptive properties of peptidase inhibitors, that bestatin, thiorphan and kelatorphan, induce analgesia in the vocalization and hot plate jumping tests, whereas the tail flick test is not sensitive to the inhibitors.

SACCHARIDE RECEPTOR MEDIATED DRUG DELIVERY

The presence of glycolipidic material in mammalian surface receptors has been evidenced by many authors in the last few years (Ashwell et al., 1982; Sly et al., 1982; Behnam et al. 1984),and it has became widely accepted that exposed sugar residues on glycolipids or glycoproteins serve as determinants for receptor recognition. Moreover, mammalian hepatic receptors are known to be specific for terminal D - galactose, whereas in avian liver, the receptors recognize terminal D - glucose . On the other hand macrophages and Kupffer-cells have been shown to bind D - mannose residues.

In this respect one interesting approach could be the use of synthetic specific glycomaterial as ligands for the delivery of pharmaceuticals to target tissues.

Being aware of such a possibility one can easily assume that the incorporation of sugar moieties in the enkephalin sequence, could improve the affinity of the molecule for its receptor,exhibiting as a consequence a higher biological response. Thus,we decided to synthesize two glycopeptides:

β-D-glucopiranosylamide   (I)

Tyr-D-Met-Gly-Phe-Pro
                                    β-D-galactopiranosylamide (II)

with the sugar moiety bonded to the C-terminal carboxyl group of the
parent peptide by means of the amide bond. For comparative purposes we
selected the same parent peptide as in the hydrophobic series refered to
before.

SYNTHESIS OF GLYCOPEPTIDES

Glycopeptides (I) and (II) were obtained by the liquid phase
procedure. Three different strategies have been attempted for the
incorporation of the saccharide moiety into the peptide. The one
providing better yields for both derivatives is outlined in Fig. 5.

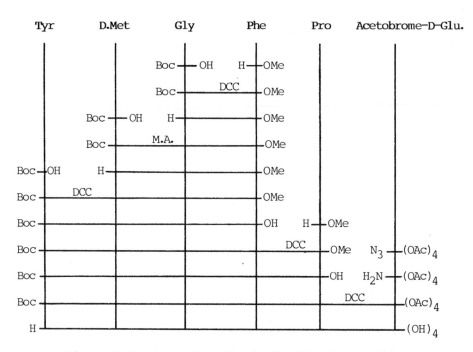

Figure 5. Strategy of synthesis for the glycopeptides.

Final glycolipids were purified by semipreparative reversed phase
HPLC. Characterization of both peptides was ascertained by elemental
analysis,amino acid composition, n.m.r. and FAB-MS.

Biological activity

In vitro GPI test.

Compounds (I),(II),(D-Met,ProNH$_2$) enkephalin and morphine were
subjected to the GPI test according to the Kosterlitz description.

In vivo analgesia

Antinociceptive activity after intraperitoneal injection of morphine sulphate and glycopeptides (I) and (II), was obtained for the tail inmersion test both in rats and mice (Rodriguez, et al., 1986) Table 1 shows the ED_{50} (95% confidence limits) of the antinociceptive activity produced by morphine sulphate and glycopeptide (I).

Table 1. Antinociceptive activity results.

Compound	RATS		MICE	
	ED_{50}	n. animals	ED_{50}	n. animals
(I)	1.2 (0.75-1.92)	10	5.0 (2.7-9.2)	12
Morph. sulfate	2.66 (2.05-3.46)	6	900 (801-1007)	7

ED_{50} (µg/animal); 95% confidence limits for tail inmersion; intraperitoneal injections.

No significant differences were observed between compounds (I) and(II). The results obtained show that the antinociceptive activity by intraperitoneal administration of the glycopeptides is 2000 times higher in rats than that observed with morphine. In addition, the same experiments in mice show that glycopeptides are nearly 200 times more potent than morphine.

However , in the GPI test, the IC_{50} of compound (I) was:64.9 nM, whereas the corresponding IC_{50} for (II) was:117.3 nM, showing a slight difference between the derivatives. The IC_{50} for the parent compound under the same conditions was 10.8 nM, which accounts for a slight decrease in the affinity for the µ-subtype as a consequence of the saccharide incorporation.

In order to further investigate the above findings, other routes of administration and different antinociceptive tests, as well as binding measurements to elucidate receptor selectivity, are under study.

ACKNOWLEDGEMENTS

The biological activity of the enkephalin analogues was carried out by Raquel E.Rodriguez in the University of Salamanca,to whom the authors are grateful for her guidance and expert cooperation.

REFERENCES

Albrecht, O., 1983, The Construction of a Microprocessor-controlled Film Balance for Precision Measurement of Isotherms and Isobars. The Thin Films, 99:227.
Ashwell, G. and Harford, J., 1982, Carbohydrate-specific Receptors of the Liver. Ann. Rev. Biochem., 51:531.

Behnam, B. A. and Deber, C. M., 1984, Evidence for a Folded Conformation of Methionine- and Leucine-Enkephalin in a Membrane Environment, J. Biol. Chem., 259:14.935.

Dickenson, A. H., 1986, Enkephalins: A new Approach to Pain Relief? Nature, 320:681.

Garcia-Anton, J. M., Sole, N., and Reig, F., 1985, Synthesis of Hydrophobic Enkephalin amides, Int. J. Peptide Protein Res., 26:591.

Gioannini, T. L., Howard, A., Hiller, J. M. and Simon, E. J., 1984, Affinity Chromatography of Solubilized Opioid Binding Sites using CH-Sepharose modified with a new Naltrexone Derivative, Biochem. Biophys. Res. Commun., 119:624.

Holaday, J. W., Ruvio, B. A., Robles, L. E., Johnson, C. E., and D'Amato, R. J., 1982, M 154,129, A Putative delta Antagonist reverses Endotoxic Shock Without altering Morphine Analgesia, Life Sci., 31:2209.

Phillips, M. C. and Chapman, D., 1968, Monolayer Characteristics of Saturated 1,2- diacyl Phosphatidylcholines (lecithins) and Phosphatidylethanolamines of the Air-water Interphase, Biochim. Biophys. Acta, 163:301.

Rodriguez, R. E., Sole, N., Reig, F., 1986, Analgesic Effects of (D-Met^2-Pro^5-NH$_2$) - Enkephalin Analogues in Rats, Life Sci., (in press).

Sly, W. S. and Fisher, H. D., 1982, The Phosphomannosyl Recognition System for Intracellular Pools of Receptor and their Roles in Receptor Recycling, J. Cellular Biochim., 18:67.

Zajac, J. M., and Roques, B. P., 1985, Differences in Binding Properties of mµ and delta Opioid Receptor Subtypes from Rat Brain: Kinetic Analysis and Effects of Ions and Nucleotides, J. of Neurochem., 44:1605.

TEMPORAL AND PHARMACOKINETIC ASPECTS

IN DELIVERY OF PEPTIDES AND PROTEINS

Leslie Z. Benet and Robert A. Baughman, Jr.

School of Pharmacy, University of California
San Francisco, CA and
Genentech, Inc., South San Francisco, CA

The rational administration of any drug to a patient requires some knowledge of the anticipated efficacy and toxicity for a particular dose of
that drug. When an understanding of how an individual patient will
absorb and eliminate a drug is coupled together with knowledge of the
pharmacologic effects of a given amount of the drug, a particular dose
can be selected that will result in clinical efficacy and minimal toxicity. Such considerations have been defined adequately for many classical
drugs; however, this approach has not been used as yet for the new peptide and protein therapeutic agents. Thus, today we are interested in
gaining an understanding of the pharmacokinetics and pharmacodynamics of
peptide and protein drugs. Pharmacokinetics may be simply described as
the mathematical relationship that exists between the dose of a drug and
the measureable concentration in a readily accessible site in the body
(e.g., plasma or blood). Pharmacodynamics extends this relationship to a
correlation between measured concentrations of drug and the pharmacologic
effect. As a simple description, pharmacokinetics describes what the
body does to the drug, as opposed to pharmacodynamics which describes
what the drug does to the body. There are two major uses for pharmacokinetics. First, as a tool in therapeutics to help the clinician choose
the right dosage regimen for a particular drug in a specific patient.
Second, pharmacokinetics may be used as a tool in defining drug disposition. As indicated above, up to the present time the therapeutic use of
pharmacokinetics for proteins and peptide drug compounds has not been
realized. However, regulatory agencies do require information concerning
drug disposition which can be best described using pharmacokinetic principles, i.e., the use of pharmacokinetics as a tool in defining drug
disposition.

A large number of pharmacokinetic parameters may be determined in
defining a new drug substance. However, certain critical parameters are
of primary importance (Benet, 1984). The first of these is clearance, a
measure of the body's ability to eliminate the drug. In therapeutic
terms, clearance defines the dosing rate since the product of total body
clearance and the desired steady state drug concentration in the body is
equal to the appropriate dosing rate. In defining the drug substance,
regulatory agencies will also want to know how clearance is divided into
its component parts. For example, what fraction of the total body clearance results from metabolic pathways? In addition, for classical drugs,
regulatory agencies will want information related to the specific meta-

bolic processes involved and an understanding of the pattern of metabolism. It is generally necessary to define the fraction of the clearance due to renal mechanisms. Since pharmacokinetic parameters are often determined using plasma concentration measurements, knowledge of the blood to plasma ratio is necessary if one wishes to relate clearance as a fraction of the blood flow to any particular eliminating organ.

The second fundamental kinetic parameter useful in discussing drug disposition is volume. The volume of distribution relates the amount of drug in the body to the concentration of drug in the blood or plasma, depending upon the fluid measured. When pharmacokinetics is used as a tool in therapeutics, an understanding of the volume of distribution is of only minor consequence. However when kinetics is used as a tool in defining drug disposition, the volume of distribution describes the space available in the body into which the drug may distribute. Since the clearing organs can only remove drug from the blood flowing through them, a drug that distributes into a large volume of distribution (i.e., out of the plasma) will not be available for rapid elimination. As may be expected the volume of distribution can be strongly influenced by protein binding. A drug which has a high degree of binding to plasma proteins will generally exhibit a small volume of distribution and a change in protein binding may result in an increase in the distribution space.

The third fundamental pharmacokinetic parameter is half-life, an expression of the relationship between volume and clearance. Since the organs of elimination can only clear drug from the blood or plasma in direct contact with the organ, the time course of drug in the body will depend upon both the volume of distribution and the clearance:

$$t_{1/2} = 0.693 \ V/CL$$

where V is the volume of distribution and CL is total body clearance. Half-life is an extremely useful kinetic parameter in terms of therapeutics, since this parameter defines the dosing interval at which drugs should be administered. Half-life also dictates the time required to attain steady-state or to decay from steady-state conditions after a change in the dosing regimen (i.e., starting or stopping a particular rate of drug administration). However, as an indication of either drug elimination or distribution, half-life has little value. Early studies of drug pharmacokinetics in disease states were compromised by reliance on drug half-life as the sole measure of alterations in drug disposition. Disease states can affect both of the physiologically related parameters, volume of distribution and clearance; thus, the derived parameter, $t_{1/2}$, will not necessarily reflect expected changes in drug elimination.

The fourth major pharmacokinetic parameter of interest, and of particular interest to the topic of this text, is bioavailability. Bioavailability is defined as the fraction of the unchanged drug reaching the site of drug action, or more usually the systemic circulation, following administration by any route. For an intravenous dose of the drug, bioavailability is defined as unity. For a drug administered orally, bioavailability may be less than one due to several causes: the drug may be incompletely absorbed; it may be metabolized in the gut, the gut wall, the portal blood or the liver prior to entry into the systemic circulation; or it may undergo enterohepatic cycling with incomplete absorption following elimination in the bile. Although bioavailability is most often described following oral dosing, the processes related to absorption and first pass metabolism can occur when drugs are administered via other routes of administration. For the therapeutic use of pharmacokinetics, bioavailability defines the adjustment which must be made in the dosing rate due to loss of the drug via various processes prior to entry into the systemic circulation.

Bioavailability, as described above, refers to the extent of availability to the systemic circulation. A bioavailability parameter related to the rate of availability is also desired when drugs are given other than by the intravenous route. For many classical drugs, such rate information may be expressed in terms of the peak time and the peak concentration of a drug following dosing. In addition, sophisticated mathematical analyses may be carried out to define the actual rate processes involved in drug absorption.

The above parameters are those generally desired by regulatory agencies when any new drug is presented for registration. That is, clearance and the various pathways by which clearance occurs, volume of distribution, half-life, the extent of protein binding, and the extent and the rate of availability. However, since drugs are usually dosed in a repetitive manner, it is also required that information be provided as to dose and time "stability" of these parameters. That is, is there proportionality over the range of doses which might be expected to be administered to a patient? Nonlinearities can occur due to saturable metabolic and renal processes, saturable protein binding and changes in membrane permeability which can affect all of the parameters listed above. In addition with prolonged dosing, the drug substance may cause stimulation or inhibition of various processes. These potential nonlinearities must also be investigated.

To describe drug kinetics, either for therapeutic uses or for a basic understanding of drug disposition, one presupposes the ability to measure the "active drug" substance in various biological fluids. Almost all pharmacokinetic work with peptide and protein drugs up to the early 1980's was based on bioassay methods. The variability inherent in such methodology probably restricts our ability to adequately describe the disposition of these compounds. Specifically, interferon (IFN) bioassays most often employ the detection of antiviral activity. As such, these assays require cell death as the assay endpoint. In this bioassay, target cells are seeded in a 96-well plate. Biological fluid containing interferon is serially diluted across the plate. The IFN concentration is determined by the first well with cell killing. As such, the variation can be as great as ± one well, equating to a potential two-fold variability in the reported concentration.

The recent implementation of more sensitive analytical methodology such as the ELISA and IRMA procedures may alleviate this variability problem. This is evident from the initial work with the interferons. The "sandwich" binding assay could measure significantly lower IFN concentrations than could be detected by the bioassay, resulting in very poor correlations between the two methods. These newer methods, as utilized to analyze peptide and protein drugs, are based on immunological recognition of a specific site(s) on the "drug" molecule. Thus, even when the protein has been "clipped" it is possible for the ELISA method to yield a measurement. However, under these conditions, we may in fact have reduced activity as measured by the bioassay.

The concern with specificity leads us directly to a problem generally recognized for classical drugs, but little investigated for proteins and peptides. That is, are metabolites being measured, and/or should they be measured? For example, consider the one chain versus the two chain forms recombinant tissue plasminogen activator (rtPA). Should we characterize the concentration of both forms or is the ELISA which measures the sum adequate? Rijken et al. (1982) showed that naturally

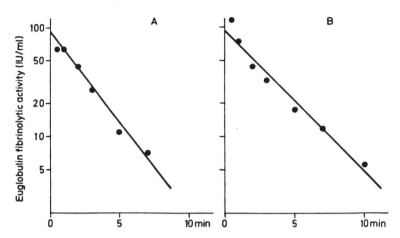

Fig. 1.   Plasma tPA concentrations as measured by euglo-
          bulin fibrinolytic activity in two 3 kg
          rabbits, one receiving 20,000 IU of two chain
          tPA (Panel A) and the second receiving the same
          dose of one chain (Panel B). Reproduced with
          permission.

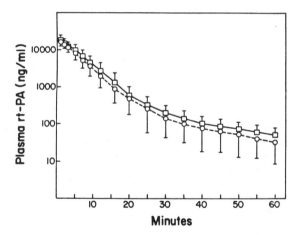

Fig. 2.   Mean plasma rtPA concentrations in two groups
          of 6 rhesus monkeys receiving 1 mg/kg bolus
          intravenous injections of one chain (circles)
          and two chain (squares) rtPA. The two chain
          rtPA was derived from the same lot of one chain
          rtPA by limited plasmin proteolysis. Bars
          indicate standard deviations.

derived tissue-type plasminogen activator exists in both the one-chain and two-chain forms. These workers showed that both forms had the same fibrinolytic properties. Korninger et al. (1981) attempted to determine whether both forms had exhibited the same pharmacokinetics in rabbits. As depicted in Fig. 1, they found that the disappearance rate of the two forms, as measured by the fibrinolytic activity in the euglobulin fraction of rabbit plasma, was similar for the two forms. The half-lives were approximately 2 and 3 minutes for the two-chain and one-chain forms, respectively. We have calculated the apparent one-compartment volume of distribution to be approximately 70 ml/kg for both forms in the rabbit.

Hotchkiss et al. (1986) using an ELISA assay further investigated this phenomena. One chain rtPA and two chain rtPA were administered to rhesus monkeys. As can be seen in Fig. 2, no significant differences in the pharmacokinetics were observed. This study has several advantages compared to previous work addressing this question. First, a sensitive, accurate and precise immunochemical assay was used. This allowed plasma rtPA to be measured over an hour following dosing vs. the 10 minutes of measureable concentrations (30 minute sampling) observed by Korninger et al. (1981) as seen in Fig. 1. This increased sensitivity allowed Hotchkiss et al. (1986) to define the two characteristics of rtPA. The 2 compartment characteristics are somewhat apparent in the rabbit data (Fig. 1), although the half-lives were determined assuming a one compartment model.

Another area of consideration in which peptide and protein drugs differ from classical compounds is the test population in which kinetics are determined. It is highly unlikely that "drugs" such as tumor necrosis factors (TNF), luteinizing hormone-releasing hormone (LHRH), and high dose interferons could be given to normal volunteers. For example, most human pharmacokinetic studies with rIFNs were carried out in various populations of cancer patients (Foon et al., 1985; Van der Burg et al., 1985; Kurzrock et al., 1985; Vadhan-Raj et al., 1986) although Wills et al. (1984) did define the pharmacokinetics of rIFN-αA in 3 groups of 6 healthy men. Thus, under these conditions the pharmacokinetics which are determined may be perturbed from that which might be expected to be found in other populations. This, in itself, is not a disqualification for these types of studies. However, variability is inherent in a patient population at a significantly higher level than that found in a well controlled normal subject panel in which many classical drugs are initially tested. This patient population variability due to the heterogeneity of the disease state together with the variability found in many of the analytical methods used previously to define the kinetics of peptides and proteins may obviate our ability to obtain accurate kinetic measures for such compounds.

When analytical methods are sufficiently sensitive, most protein and peptide drug show multicompartment pharmacokinetics, as do classical drugs. Figure 3 depicts the serum concentrations of rIFN-αA after a 40 min intravenous infusion and after intramuscular and subcutaneous injections (Wills et al., 1984). Since these proteins are naturally occurring at much lower concentrations, must we be concerned with the tissue contributions of these agents at therapeutic doses as reflected by the multicompartment kinetics, and more specifically must we measure the accummulation of these substances at particular tissue sites? If the answer to this question is yes, then we face the even more difficult problem of convincing ourselves and the regulatory agencies, that studies in animals may yield meaningful results that can be extrapolated to man. This question is made more difficult when we attempt to carry out such studies with human specific proteins in animals, or extrapolate data from animal specific proteins to humans. (See Bocci, 1985 for a discussion of this point with respect to IFN.)

At the present there is only limited temporal and kinetic data available for proteins and peptides. Such studies have been carried out with recombinant derived insulin, hGH, LHRH analogs, interferons, interleukins and TNFs. For example, the studies depicted in Fig. 3 describe the pharmacokinetics of rIFN-αA in patients following three different routes of administration. Wills and co-worker (1984) determined the primary pharmacokinetic parameters: clearance, volume of distribution steady-state, and terminal half-life from the intravenous data. They determined that the bioavailability was 83% for the intramuscular dose and 90% for the subcutaneous dose. Numerous pharmacokinetic studies have been carried out with insulin (e.g. Owen et al., 1981 and Waldhäusl et al., 1983). The pharmacokinetics of synthetic long acting LHRH analogs has been recently reviewed by Nestor et al. (1984). Modification of the time course of LHRH agonists and antagonists has been accomplished both by chemical modification and by dosage form and route of administration modifications. Probably the most studied peptide drug in terms of altered delivery is insulin (Binder et al., 1984). Here again chemical, dosage form and route of administration modifications have been utilized.

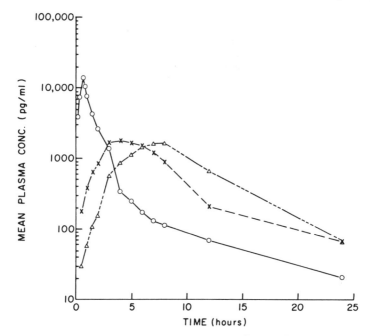

Fig. 3. Mean serum rIFN-αA concentrations after a single 36 x 10^6 U dose as an intravenous infusion (circles) or an intramuscular (x) or subcutaneous injection (triangles) in three groups of 6 healthy men. Reproduced with permission.

Only limited data on the pharmacokinetics of peptide and protein drugs has been published. The main reason for this lack of information is related to the variability and nonspecificity of the analytical measurements previously available. Up to the present time, where pharmacokinetic measurements have been reported this information has been utilized only to describe the disposition of specific protein and peptide drugs. As yet, little correlation of pharmacodynamic measurements with pharmacokinetics has been made. Thus, at present pharmacokinetics is limited to the elucidation of parameter values which can be given to regulatory agencies to satisfy a specific criteria related to the understanding of drug disposition and the linearity of drug kinetics. Hopefully, in the future, when more experience has been obtained with such compounds, the therapeutic use of pharmacokinetics may be invoked in the development of rationale drug dosing regimens.

REFERENCES

Benet, L.Z., 1984, Pharmacokinetic parameters; which are necessary to define a drug substance? Eur. J. Resp. Dis., 65(Suppl 134):45-61.

Binder, C., Lauritzen, T., Faber, O. and Pramming, S., 1984, Insulin pharmacokinetics, Diabetes Care, 7:188-199.

Bocci, V., 1985, Distribution, catabolism and pharmacokinetics of interferons, in: "Interferon, Vol.4," Finter, N.B. and Oldham, R., eds., Elsevier, Amsterdam.

Foon, K.A. Sherwin, S.A., Abrams, P.G., Stevenson, H.C., Holmes, P., Maluish, A.E., Oldham, R.K. and Herberman, R.B., 1985, A phase I trial of recombinant gamma interferon in patients with cancer, Cancer Immunol. Immunother., 20:193-197.

Hotchkiss, A., Ross, M., Refino, C., Chen, S., Fuller, G. and Baughman, R.A., 1987, Circulation, submitted for publication.

Korninger, C., Stassen, J.M., and Collen, D., 1981, Turnover of human extrinsic (tissue-type) plasminogen activator, Thromb. Haemostas. (Stuttgart), 46:658-661.

Kurzrock, R., Rosenblum, M.G., Sherwin, S.A., Rios, A. Talpaz, M. Quesada, J.R., and Gutterman, J.U., 1985, Pharmacokinetics, single-dose tolerance, and biological activity of recombinant α-interferon in cancer patinets, Cancer Res., 45:2866-2872.

Nestor, J.J., Ho, T.L., Tahilrami, R., McRae, G.I., and Vickery, B.H., 1984, Long acting LH-RH agonists and antagonists, Int. Cong. Ser.- Excerpta Med., 656:24-35.

Owens, D.R., Hayes, T.M., Alberti, K.G.M.M., Jones, M.K., Heding, L.G., Home, P.D., and Burrin, J.M., 1981, Comparative study of subcutaneous, intramuscular, and intravenous administration of human insulin, Lancet 1:118-122.

Rijken, D.C., Hoylaerts, M., and Collen, D., 1982, Fibrinolytic properties of one-chain and two-chain human extrinsic (tissue-type) plasminogen activator, J. Biol. Chem., 257:2920-2925.

Vadhan-Raj, S., Al-Katib, A., Bhalla, R., Pelus, L., Nathan, C.F., Sherwin, S.A., Oettgen, H,.F., and Krown, S.E., 1986, Phase I trial of recombinant interferon gamma in cancer patients, J. Clin. Oncol., 4:137-146.

Van der Burg, M., Edelstein, M., Gerlis, L., Liang, C-M., Hirschi, M., and Dawson, A., 1985, Recombinant interferon-γ (Immuneron): Results of a phase I trial in patients with cancer, J. Biol Response Modifiers, 4:264-272.

Waldhäusl, W.K. Bratush-Marrain, P.R. Vierhapper, H., and Nowotny, P., 1983, Insulin pharmacokinetics following continuous infusion and bolus injection of regular porcine and human insulin in healthy man. Metabolism, 32:478-486.

Wills, R.J., Dennis, S., Spiegel, H.E., Gibson, D.M., and Nadler, P.I., 1984, Interferon kinetics and adverse reactions after intravenous, intramuscular, and subcutaneous injection, Clin. Pharmacol. Ther., 35:722.

ENZYMATIC BARRIERS TO PEPTIDE AND PROTEIN ABSORPTION AND THE USE OF
PENETRATION ENHANCERS TO MODIFY ABSORPTION

Vincent H.L. Lee

University of Southern California
School of Pharmacy
Los Angeles, California 90033 U.S.A.

INTRODUCTION

The mammalian body possesses several extremely efficient mechanisms
to restrict the entry of macromolecules. These include the presence of
various epithelia that are poorly absorptive, the presence of significant
levels of enzymatic activity at various locations between the point of
entry into the systemic circulation and the target site of a peptide or
protein, the availability of multiple enzymes to degrade peptides and
proteins at a given location, and varying levels of immunoglobulins to
neutralize peptides and proteins both before and after they are absorbed.
The inevitable result is that the bioavailability of peptides and proteins is likely to be much less than that for small drug molecules, a
factor that must be kept in mind in designing realistic strategies to
optimize peptide and protein absorption. These strategies include the co-
administration of penetration enhancers to alter membrane permeability,
coadministration of inhibitors to restrain the activity of proteolytic
enzymes primarily at the absorption site, and the design of analogs that
are metabolically stable and which, at the same time, may be more readily
absorbed.

This review will be in two parts. The first part will be on the
efficiency of various enzymatic barriers in degrading peptides and proteins, including various sites of administration, the liver and the
kidneys. The second part will be on various aspects of penetration enhancers, including (1) types and possible mechanisms, (2) efficacy in promoting peptide and protein absorption from various sites of administration as well as factors influencing their efficacy, and (3) potential
toxicities.

ENZYMATIC BARRIERS TO PEPTIDE AND PROTEIN ABSORPTION

In order to circumvent the enzymatic barriers thereby optimizing
peptide and protein absorption, the nature of these barriers must be
understood.   Unlike most small drug molecules that are currently in use,
peptides and proteins are usually susceptible to degradation not only in
the liver, but also at the site of administration, in the blood, in the
kidney, and while crossing the vascular endothelia en route to their site

of action. This suggests that protection of peptides and proteins against degradation in more than one anatomical site is necessary in order to maximize their bioavailability. Moreover, as illustrated in Table 1 for substance P (Bunnett et al., 1985), a given peptide or protein is usually susceptible to degradation at more than one linkage within the molecule, each locus of hydrolysis being mediated by a certain peptidase. This observation, plus the fact that almost all of the relevant enzymes are usually present in a given anatomical site where the peptide or protein is located (Najdovski et al., 1985; Palmieri et al., 1985; Palmieri and Ward, 1983; Ward, 1984), indicates that protecting a peptide or protein from degradation by one enzyme may not necessarily lead to marked increases in its stability or in the amount of peptide or protein reaching its site of action (Dodda Kashi and Lee, 1986; Lee et al., 1986).

The plasma half-life of peptides and proteins is relatively short, on the order of 15 minutes or less. This is due in part to the rapid clearance of these substances by the liver and kidney (Bocci et al., 1982; Johnson and Maack, 1977; Pimstone et al., 1977; Temperley et al., 1971), as illustrated in Fig. 1 for growth hormone. The kidneys play a key role in clearing peptides and proteins with a molecular weight of less than 50,000 by glomerular filtration followed by digestion of the reabsorbed peptide or protein in the epithelial cells comprising the proximal tubule (Carone and Peterson, 1980; Johnson and Maack, 1977; Maack, 1975). To date, there has been no deliberate attempt to curtail renal clearance such as by encouraging binding of the administered peptide or protein to plasma proteins including albumin and globulin.

The clearance of peptides and proteins by the liver has been found to occur in both parenchymal and non-parenchymal cells, both of which are capable of degrading peptides and proteins (Gardner et al., 1985; Segre et al., 1981). Gardner et al. (1985) demonstrated that vasoactive intestinal peptide was taken up primarily by the non-parenchymal cells, whereas insulin was taken up primarily by parenchymal cells (Fig. 2) - a finding which has yet to be exploited in terms of redirecting a peptide or protein away from the cell type that favors its degradation. However, there is preliminary evidence that peptide and protein degradation in the liver can be altered through chemical modifications of these substances. Strunz et al. (1978), for instance, discovered that modifying the molecular size of gastrin significantly altered its stability in the liver.

Table 1. Enzymes Involved in the Hydrolysis of Substance P (Bunnett et al., 1985)

Arg-Pro-Lys-Pro-Gln-Gln-Phe-Phe-Gly-Leu-MetNH$_2$

1   2   3   4   5   6   7   8   9   10 11

Enzymes Involved	Bonds Cleaved
Endopeptidase-24.11	6-7, 7-8, 9-10
Angiotensin converting enzyme	8-9, 9-10
Dipeptidylpeptidase IV	2-3, 3-4
Substance Pase	6-7, 7-8, 8-9
Prolyl endopeptidase	4-5

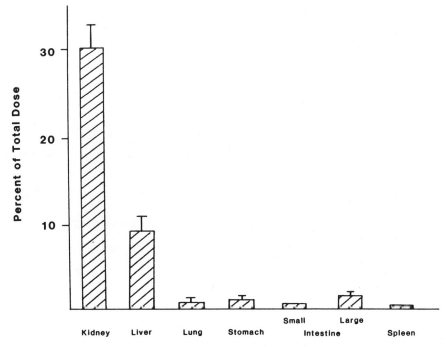

Fig. 1. Relative distribution of recombinant growth hormone in various organs of the rat at 10 min after intravenous administration. Values are means $\pm$ SEM expressed as percentage of total administered dose (Johnson and Maack, 1977).

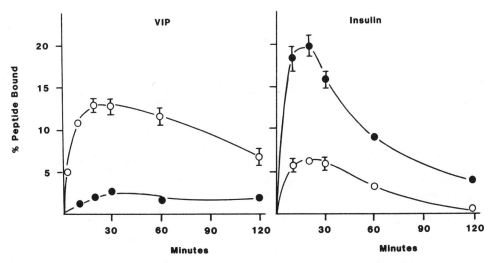

Fig. 2. Time course of binding of vasoactive intestinal peptide (VIP) and insulin to hepatocytes (●) and nonparenchymal cells (○) at 37° (Gardner et al., 1985)

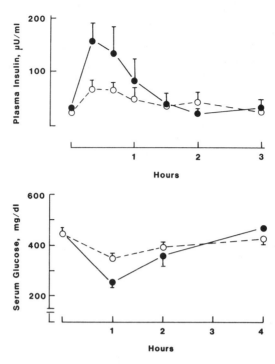

Fig. 3. Effect of Boc–Gly–Pro–Leu–Gly on the absorption of subcutaneously administered insulin and on the lowering of serum glucose in rats. Error bars represent standard error of the mean. Key: ○ , control; ● , coadministration with inhibitor (Hori et al., 1983).

In addition to the liver and kidney, peptides and proteins can also be degraded at the site of administration. Hori et al. (1983) found that insulin was degraded in the subcutaneous tissues of the rat with a half-life of about 60 minutes. However, this small protein was 16 times less susceptible to hydrolysis in the presence of a synthetic peptidase inhibitor (Boc–Gly–Pro–Leu–Gly), resulting in a doubling of its amount absorbed with a corresponding lowering in blood glucose (Fig. 3).

By far the site that has received the most attention is the gastrointestinal tract because of a persistent desire to deliver peptides and proteins orally. Unfortunately, the gastrointestinal tract is well equipped with digestive enzymes which collectively can remove orally administered peptides and proteins within 10 minutes of administration (Bunnett et al., 1985; Laskowski et al., 1958). This leads to the investigation of alternative routes such as the nasal, buccal, rectal and vaginal routes for peptide and protein delivery. For the limited number of peptides and proteins studied thus far, their delivery via the alternative routes, while a considerable improvement over the oral route, still lags behind the parenteral route in the fraction of intact peptide absorbed (Anik et al., 1984; Ishida et al., 1981; Moses et al., 1983; Nishihata et al., 1983; Okada et al., 1982; Su et al., 1985; Yoshioka et al., 1982). This is partly due to the possible existence of a sub-stantial enzymatic barrier in the epithelial cells constituting a given mucosal route of administration (Hussain et al., 1985). Indeed, Lee and his co-workers (Stratford and Lee, 1986; Dodda Kashi and Lee, 1986) demonstrated that the activity of aminopeptidases in homogenates of mucosal tissues in the albino rabbit was comparable to that in the ileum. At a protein concentration of 10 mg/ml, the half-life of degradation of methionine enkephalin, a pentapeptide, in homogenates of the nasal, buccal, rectal, and vaginal mucosae of the albino rabbit ranged from 11 to 22 minutes, as compared with a half-life of 15 minutes in ileal homogenates (Table 2). This indicates that the same enzymatic barrier as exisiting in the oral route is also present in the alternate routes of peptide and protein delivery. Nonetheless, the alternate routes still favor peptide and protein absorption when compared with the oral route. There are four possible reasons for this improvement, as follows.

First, compared with the oral route, there is a deficiency of lumi-nal enzymes in the alternate route of delivery. Second, the alternative routes may be "leaker" than the oral route in membrane permeability (Hayashi et al., 1985), thereby minimizing contact of peptides and pro-teins with the resident enzymes. Third, peptides and proteins when delivered via the alternative routes may be exposed to a smaller surface area, hence a smaller fraction of the total enzymes present, when com-pared with the oral route. Fourth, peptides and proteins are subjected to less dilution in the alternative routes since the resident fluid volume is less, thereby maximizing the concentration gradient for peptide and protein absorption.

In summary, various peptidases participate in the degradation of peptides and proteins from the moment of administration to their arrival at their sites of action. The impracticality associated with controlling the activity of all of these enzymes in every site where they exist indicates that peptides and proteins will be subjected to varying extents of degradation while in the body. It is speculated that the misconcep-tion that non-oral routes of delivery are deficient in peptidases may be responsible for the scarce information on the extent to which peptidase inhibitors may promote peptide and protein absorption from these routes. Indeed, work has only begun to circumvent this enzymatic barrier either with peptidase inhibitors or by designing metabolically stable analogs that retain the pharmacological activity of the natural peptides and proteins.

Table 2. Half-life of Methionine Enkephalin Hydrolysis in Homogenates of Various Mucosal Tissues of the Albino Rabbit (Dodda Kashi and Lee, 1986)

Mucosal Tissue	Half-Life (Minutes)
Nasal	16.3 ± 1.4
Buccal	12.0 ± 1.1
Rectal	11.3 ± 1.6
Vaginal	22.2 ± 2.1
Ileal	15.1 ± 2.0

Penetration enhancers are compounds, generally of low molecular weight, that facilitate the absorption of solutes across biological membranes. With few exceptions and regardless of the non-parenteral route of administration, penetration enhancers are required for the absorption of peptides and proteins in pharmacologically active amounts. In principle, penetration enhancers should work synergistically with peptidase inhibitors in optimizing peptide and protein absorption. This is indeed the case for the coadministration of deoxycholate, a penetration enhancer, with soybean trypsin inhibitor, a peptidase inhibitor, in improving the absorption of insulin from the ileum of the rat (Fig. 4, Kidron et al., 1982).

Types and Mechanisms of Action of Penetration Enhancers

Penetration enhancers are of four major types. They are: (1) chelators, such as EDTA, citric acid, salicylates, N-acyl derivatives of collagen, and enamines (N-amino acyl derivatives of β-diketones), (2) surfactants, such as sodium lauryl sulfate, polyoxyethylene-9-lauryl ether, and polyoxyethylene-20-cetyl ether, (3) bile salts, such as sodium deoxycholate, sodium glycocholate, and sodium taurocholate, and (4) fatty acids, such as oleic acid and monoolein.

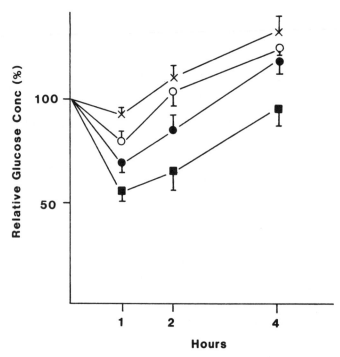

Fig. 4. Effects of 3 mg soybean trypsin inhibitor (STI) and 2 mg sodium deoxycholate (DOC) on the absorption of 12 U insulin administered in the ileum of the rat. Each point represents mean ± SEM for 6 animals. Key: X , control; O , DOC alone; ● , STI alone; ■ , combination of DOC and STI (Kidron et al., 1982).

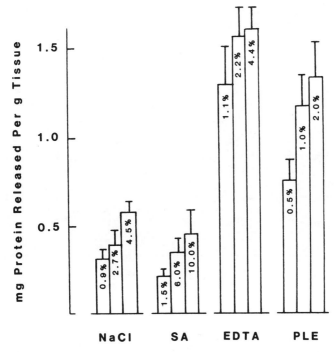

Fig. 5. Effects of various concentrations of sodium
chloride (NaCl), sodium salicylate (SA),
disodium EDTA (EDTA) and polyoxyethylene–
23–lauryl ether (PLE) on protein release
from the rat rectal sac following 1 hour of
incubation at 30°C. Error bars represent
standard deviations with n ⩾ 4 (Nishihata
et al., 1985).

Generally, penetration enhancers improve peptide and protein absorption by one or combinations of several mechanisms. Bile salts have been
shown to reduce the viscosity of the mucus layer adhering to all mucosal
surfaces, thereby facilitating peptide and protein diffusion towards the
membrane surface (Martin et al., 1978). Chelators (Kamada et al., 1981;
Nishihata et al., 1983; Nishihata et al., 1985a; Okada et al., 1983;
Yamashita et al., 1985) and, to a certain extent, polyoxyethylated
nonionc surfactants (Sakai et al., 1986), interfere with the ability of
calcium ions to maintain the dimension of the intercellular space, thereby permitting the paracellular transport of peptides and proteins which
otherwise will be excluded from this pathway. Interestingly, all of the
penetration enhancers are capable of increasing membrane fluidity either
by creating disorder in the phospholipid domain in the membrane, as is
the case for salicylates, oleic acid and monoolein (Kajii et al., 1985;
Muranushi et al., 1980, 1981), or by facilitating the leaching of proteins from the membrane, as is the case for surfactants and EDTA (Nishihata et al., 1985b). As illustrated in Fig. 5, polyoxyethylene–9–
lauryl ether and EDTA were equally effective in releasing proteins from
the rectal sac of the rat in a dose-dependent manner. In the case of
surfactants, Hirai et al. (1981b) demonstrated that the extent of lowering of blood glucose following nasal administration of insulin in the rat
correlated well with the extent of protein release (Table 3). On the

Table 3.   Correlation of Decrement in Blood Glucose with Extent of Protein Released and Inhibition of Leucine Aminopeptidase Activity Following Nasal Administration of Insulin in the Rat (Hirai et al., 1981a)

Surfactant	Protein Released (µg/min/g body wt)	Inhibition of LAP Activity (%)	Decrement in blood glucose (%)
Saline	0.11 ± 0.02[a]		
POE 9 lauryl ether	0.83 ± 0.13	22.7 (19.6–28.2)[b]	60.9 ± 2.9
POE 10 monostearate	0.09 ± 0.01	20.1 (15.7–28.3)	16.6 ± 3.2
Na lauryl sulfate	1.99 ± 0.07	98.3 (97.4–100.0)	52.9 ± 1.4
Na taurocholate	0.29 ± 0.00	87.4 (80.7–96.3)	56.7 ± 3.3
Na cholate	0.36 ± 0.03	84.9 (79.2–89.2)	53.1 ± 4.8
Na glycocholate	0.21 ± 0.02	87.2 (80.5–93.2)	53.1 ± 2.7
Saponin	0.77 ± 0.01	36.9 (28.6–42.7)	53.9 ± 2.5

[a] Mean ± standard error of the mean for 4 experiments.
[b] Figure within parentheses represents range for 3 experiments.

other hand, the equal effectiveness of bile salts (sodium taurocholate, sodium cholate, and sodium glycocholate) in enhancing nasal insulin absorption as surfactants, despite their lower efficiency in eluting proteins from membranes, was attributed to their ability to inhibit peptidases responsible for the degradation of insulin (Table 3, Hirai et al., 1981b).

Recent studies by Fix et al. (1983) and Shiga et al. (1985) indicate that sodium ion transport and the associated water flux are a component of the penetration enhancing mechanism of salicylate, taurocholate, and EDTA. This suggests that other compounds which interfere with these transport processes may also affect peptide and protein absorption. Indeed, Cooper et al. (1978) observed an enhancement in the intestinal uptake of horseradish peroxidase (M.W. 40,000) upon exposing a jejunal segment of the rat to hyperosmotic solutions for 60 minutes, even though water flux was in the opposite direction to solute movement. Similarly, the ability of polyacrylic acid gel to enhance the rectal and vaginal absorption of insulin was also attributed to its effect on water flux (Morimoto et al., 1982, 1983).

Efficiency of Penetration Enhancers in Promoting Peptide and Protein Absorption and Factors Influencing Their Efficacy

Each of the four types of penetration enhancers mentioned earlier has been used to promote peptide and protein absorption from the oral, rectal, and vaginal routes, whereas only the bile salts and surfactants have been used to promote nasal absorption of peptides and proteins. The preferred enhancer appears to be sodium glycocholate for the nasal and buccal routes, salicylates for the rectal route, citric acid for the vaginal route, and oleic acid-monoolein mixed micelles for the oral route. With one or two exceptions, the bioavailability of a limited number of peptides and proteins is no more than 40%, as shown in Table 4.

The efficacy of penetration enhancers depends on several factors, including peptide type, physicochemical properties of the delivery system as relate to peptide and protein release, lipophilicity of the enhancer, intrinsic ability of the enhancer to perturb membrane permeability, site of application of enhancer, and animal species used.

Table 4. Efficiency of Peptide and Protein Absorption From Various Routes of Administration in the Presence of Various Types of Penetration Enhancers (Adjuvants).

Adjuvant	Route	Peptide	% Absorbed	Ref.
Chelators	Nasal	None	--	
	Rectal	Insulin	14-28	Kim et al., 1983; Yagi et al., 1983
		Gastrin	18	Yashioka et al., 1982
		Pentagastrin	33	Yashioka et al., 1982
	Vaginal	Leuprolide	13-39	Okada et al., 1982; Okada et al., 1983a
	Oral	Insulin	10	Nishihata et al., 1981
Surfactants	Nasal	Insulin	30	Hirai et al., 1981a
		Leuprolide	2	Okada et al., 1982
	Rectal	Insulin	3-50	Bar-On et al., 1981; Ichikawa et al., 1980; Touitou et al., 1978
	Vaginal	Leuprolide	4	Okada et al., 1982
	Oral	Insulin	?	Touitou et al., 1980
Bile Salts	Nasal	Insulin	10-30	Hirai et al., 1981a; Moses et al., 1983; Pontiroli et al., 1982
		Leuprolide	3	Okada et al., 1982
		DADLE	94	Su et al., 1985
	Rectal	Interferon	2	Bocci et al., 1985
	Vaginal	Leuprolide	7	Okada et al., 1982
	Oral	Leuprolide	0.054	Okada et al., 1982
Oleic Acid/ Monoolein	Nasal	None		
	Rectal	Heparin	12-15x	Taniguchi et al., 1980
	Vaginal	Leuprolide	3	Okada et al., 1982
	Oral	Leuprolide	0.054	Okada et al., 1982

Table 5. Effect of 1% Sodium Glycocholate on Nasal Peptide Absorption in
the Rat.

Peptide	% Bioavalability		Factor	Ref.
	(−)	(+)		
Leuprolide	0.11	3.0	27.3	Okada et al., 1982
Insulin	5	30	6	Hirai et al., 1981a
DADLE[a]	59	94	1.6	Su et al., 1985
Metkephamid	91	91	1	Su et al., 1985

[a] Tyr–D–Ala–Gly–Phe–D–Leu

Peptide Type.   The intrinsic ability of peptides to cross biological membranes is anticipated to be a complex function of their physicochemical properties.   From Table 5 it is clear that the bioavailability
of peptides following nasal administration varies with their primary
structure, although the precise relationship between permeation and physicochemical properties is as yet unknown.   As expected, the co–administration of peptides with 1% Na glycocholate brings about the greatest
increase in the absorption of a poorly absorbed peptide, namely, leuprolide, while having no effect on the absorption of a relatively well
absorbed peptide, namely, metkephamid.   Interestingly, even in the presence of adjuvants, the bioavailability of leuprolide and insulin is far
from complete.

Delivery System.   The selection of a delivery system for a peptide
and its penetration enhancer must take into account the vast differences
in physicochemical properties that may exist between these two substances, because of which their release rates from this system may be
very different.   For a penetration enhancer to be effective, it must be
released either simultaneously with the peptide or shortly before the
peptide itself is released.   This requirement is supported by the findings of Nishihata et al. (1985a), in that the bioavailability of insulin
following rectal administration in the rat was reduced from 30.2% to
12.8% when the release of DL–phenylalanyl ethylacetoacetate, the adjuvant, from the suppository was delayed from 17.5 to 30 minutes prior to
the administration of insulin.   Okada et al. (1982) attributed the enhanced interaction between leuprolide and polyethylene glycol as being
responsible for the lack of effectiveness of 5% citric acid in enhancing
the vaginal absorption of leuprolide in the rat upon incorporation into a
polyethylene glycol–based jelly as opposed to a starch–based jelly, since
peptide and adjuvant release was now desynchronized.   On the other hand,
the enhanced effectiveness of 10% citric acid in promoting vaginal absorption of leuprolide in the rat upon incorporation in a tablet consisting of lactose, corn starch, hydroxypropylcellulose and magnesium stear-
ate, relative to incorporation in an aqueous solution, was due to the
formation of a highly concentrated adjuvant solution locally at the
absorptive surface as the adjuvant was released from the tablet.

Nature of Enhancer.   Generally, a penetration enhancer must be able
to penetrate the membrane and, at the same time, achieve a high enough
concentration to perturb membrane structure (Nishihata et al., 1984a).
Kim et al. (1983), for instance, found that the phenylalanyl derivative

of ethylacetoacetate was 4 times more effective than its less lipophilic glycyl counterpart in enhancing the rectal absorption of insulin in the rabbit. Similarly, Hirai et al. (1981b) determined that somewhat lipophilic ester and ether type non-ionic surfactants with HLB values of 10-14 appeared to optimize the nasal absorption of insulin in the rat when compared with extremely hydrophilic or lipophilic derivatives. Interestingly, weak adjuvants which are so by virtue of their inability to penetrate membranes, such as tripolyphosphate and phytate, have been found to improve upon their potency significantly in the presence of an intrinsically potent enhancer, in this instance, α-glycerophosphate (Nishihata et al., 1984b), as shown in Table 6. The coadministration of monoolein and bile salt has also been found to bring about a synergistic effect in enhancing the oral absorption of heparin in the rat (Table 7), presumably due to facilitation of membrane penetration of the bile salt by monoolein (Taniguchi et al., 1980). In spite of its attractiveness in optimizing the efficiency of adjuvants, the approach of using co-adjuvants that operate by different mechanisms has not been carefully explored.

The potency of an enhancer is another factor that determines the magnitude of absorption enhancement. As reported by Kamada et al. (1981), in a series of phenylalanyl enamine type enhancers, which act by chela-

Table 6. Effect of Co-Adjuvants on Rectal Absorption of Cefoxitin (Nishihata et al., 1984b)

mmoles/body			% Bioavailability
α-Glycerophosphate	Tripolyphosphate	Phytate	
0	0	0	3.6
0	0.135	0	5.3
1.03	0.054	0	30.6
0	0	0.065	6.5
1.03	0	0.026	35.9
1.03	0	0	19.0

Table 7. Effect of Bile Salts and Monoolein on the Plasma Clearing Factor Activity Following Administration of Heparin to the Small and Large Intestine (Taniguchi et al., 1980)

Condition	Plasma Clearing Factor	
	Small	Large
Control	0.020	0.009
10 mM Taurocholate	–	0.017
10 mM Taurocholate + 10 mM Monoolein	0.035	0.214
40 mM Glycocholate	0.049	–
40 mM Glycocholate + 40 mM Monoolein	0.231	–
40 mM Taurocholate + 40 mM Monoolein	0.229	0.349
Trioctanoin emulsion	0.068	0.011

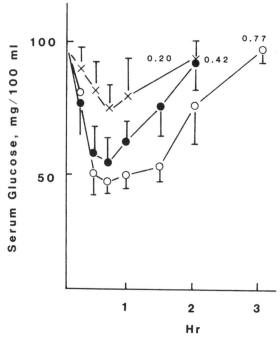

Fig. 6. Correlation of chelating ability
of enamine derivatives on absorption efficiency of rectally administered insulin in the rabbits. Figures represent g of
Ca^{2+} ions chelated per mole of
compound. Error bars represent
standard deviation. The derivatives were sodium phenylglycin-
ates of ethoxyethyl acetoacetate
(✗), ethyl acetoacetate (●),
and diethyl ethoxymethylene ma-
lonate (○) (Kamada et al., 1981).

ting Ca^{2+}, the extent of hypoglycemia in rabbits following rectal
administration of insulin was most pronounced for the most potent chela-
tor in the series (Fig. 6).

Site of Administration. Because each mucosal site differs in permeability characteristics (Hayashi et al., 1985), a given type of adjuvant may affect the absorption of a certain peptide differently depending
on the site of administration. As evidence, Okada et al. (1982) observed that polyoxyethylene-9-lauryl ether (PLE) and sodium glycocholate
were far more effective in promoting the nasal absorption of leuprolide
than vaginal absorption (Table 8), not a surprising finding in light of
the fact that the nasal epithelium is comprised of columnar cells whereas
the vaginal epithelium is comprised of stratified squamous cells (Bloom
and Fawcett, 1968). In addition, Taniguchi et al. (1980) demonstrated
that the large intestine of the rat was far more sensitive than the small
intestine to the adjuvant action of taurocholate-monoolein mixed micelles
(Fig. 7), possibly due to differences in microvilli length and density
(Carr and Toner, 1984).

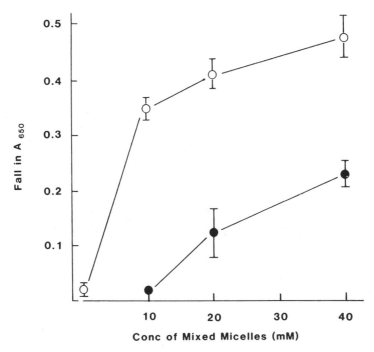

Fig. 7. Effect of concentration of monoolein–Na taurocholate mixed micelles on plasma clearing factor activity following administration of heparin in the small (●) and large intestines (○) of the rat (Taniguchi et al., 1980).

Table 8. Influence of Adjuvants on the Efficacy of Leuprolide Following Nasal and Vaginal Administration in the Rat (Okada et al., 1982)

Adjuvant (10%)	ED_{50} (µg/kg)	
	Nasal	Vaginal
Control	33.4	270
PLE	2.08	254
Na Glycocholate	1.28	151
Citric acid	–	56

Animal Model. The animal model that reliably mimics peptide and protein absorption in human, both in the presence and absence of penetration enhancers, has yet to be established. Preliminary evidence, collected in Table 9, suggests that, at least in the case of nasal absorption of insulin, the extent of enhancement may be a function of the animal model chosen.

Table 9. Effect of 1% Na Glycocholate on Percent of Dose Absorbed
Following Nasal Administration of Insulin in Various
Animal Species.

Species	(−)	(+)	Ref.
Rat	5	30	Hirai et al., 1981
Dog	25	25−30	Hirai et al., 1981
Human	< 5	12.5	Pontiroli et al., 1982
		10−20[a]	Moses et al., 1983

[a] 1% Na Deoxycholate

Potential Toxicities of Penetration Enhancers

Because all penetration enhancers promote peptide and protein absorption by perturbing membrane integrity, it is inevitable that varying
extents of insult would occur to the mucosal tissues which are in intimate contact with the enhancer. To date, only a few studies have been
undertaken to determine the nature of potentially exaggerated effects or
toxicities of various types of penetration enhancers (Hirai et al.,
1981a; Kajii et al., 1986; Nishihata et al., 1983; Okada et al., 1983;
Sithigorngul et al., 1983; Stanzani et al., 1981; Yagi et al., 1983).
Overall, non-surfactant type enhancers appear to cause less severe and
more readily reversible morphological changes than their surfactant counterparts when used on an acute basis. Moreover, they tend to cause no
long-lasting morphological changes in the mucosal tissues even when used
on a chronic basis, i.e., 7-60 days. Sithigorngul et al. (1983) reported that the exposure of rectal columnar cells to 2% salicylate for 10-20
minutes resulted in a 2-3 fold reduction in the microvilli length and a
shift of the distribution of microvilli towards the sparse and bare
arrangement.

Aside from morphological changes, however, there is virtually no
information on (1) the biochemical changes that may occur locally or (2)
the systemic toxicity which may result from the absorption of the penetration enhancers themselves and from the absorption of toxins at the
mucosal surface that otherwise would be excluded from the systemic circulation. This information must be available before penetration enhancers
can be used on a routine basis.

CONCLUSION

The key to promoting peptide and protein absorption from any route
of administration is to recognize that there is an upper limit to the
percent of an applied dose of peptide or protein which can be absorbed,
due primarily to the synergistic effects of enzymatic and transport
barriers both at and beyond a given site of administration. To some
extent, both of these barriers can be circumvented by using penetration
enhancers and peptidase inhibitors, respectively, but the extent to which
these barriers can be altered safely and transiently is as yet unknown.

Future work on circumventing the enzymatic barrier must be directed
towards understanding the type, distribution, and properties of pepti-

dases principally at the anatomical sites where peptides and proteins are most vulnerable to degradation. Eventually, it will be necessary to understand the tissue and cellular trafficking of peptides and proteins, so as to design strategies to channel these substances away from the primary areas of peptide and protein degradation.

Insofar as circumventing the transport barrier is concerned, future work must be focused on, initially, comparative studies on the mechanisms, effectiveness, and toxicities of different classes of penetration enhancers, thereby permitting the selection of penetration enhancers that are both relatively safe and effective. On the long term, it will be necessary to determine the characteristics that render an absorptive surface, including the blood brain barrier, relatively impermeable, information which should be useful in guiding the design of novel penetration enhancers on a rational basis. Studies should also be conducted to design delivery systems which would carry both an enhancer and a peptide or protein to the vicinity of the latter's target site, where transient modification of the vascular endothelia that isolate the target site from the systemic circulation could occur.

REFERENCES

Anik , S.T., McRae, G., Nerenberg, C., Worden, A., Foreman, J., Hwang, J., Kushinsky, S., Jones, R.E., and Vickery, B., 1984, Nasal absorption of nafarelin in rhesus monkeys, J. Pharm. Sci., 73: 684.

Bar-On, H., Berry, E.M., Eldor, A., Kidron, M., Lichtenberg, D., and Ziv, E., 1981, Enteral administration of insulin in the rat, Br. J. Pharmac., 73: 21.

Bloom, W. and Fawcett, D.W., 1968, "A Textbook of Histology," W.B. Saunders Co., Philadelphia.

Bocci, V., Naldini, A., Corradeschi, F., and Lencioni, E., 1985, Colorectal administration of human interferon-α, Int. J. Pharm., 24: 109.

Bocci, V., Pacini, A., Bandinelli, L., Pessina, G.P., Muscettola, M., and Paulesu, L., The role of liver in the catabolism of α- and β-interferon, J. Gen. Virol., 60: 397.

Bunnett, N.W., Orloff, M.S., and Turner, A.J., 1985, Catabolism of substance P in the stomach wall of the rat, Life Sci., 37: 599.

Carone, F.A. and Peterson, D.R., 1980, Hydrolysis and transport of small peptides by the proximal tubule, Am. J. Physiol., 238: F151.

Carr, K.E. and Toner, P.G., 1984, Morphology of the intestinal mucosa, in: "Pharmacology of Intestinal Permeation I," Csaky, T.Z., ed., Springer-Verlag, Berlin.

Cooper, M., Teichberg, S., and Lifshitz, F., 1978, Alterations in rat jejunal permeability to a macromolecular tracer during a hyperosmotic load, Lab. Invest., 38: 447.

Dodda Kashi, S. and Lee, V.H.L., 1986, Enkephalin hydrolysis in homogenates of various absorptive mucosae of the albino rabbit: similarities in rates and involvement of aminopeptidases, Life Sci., 38: 2019.

Gardner, D.F., Kilberg, M.S., Wolfe, M.M., McGuigan, J.E., and Misbin, R.I., 1985, Preferential binding of vasoactive intestinal peptide to hepatic nonparenchymal cells, Am. J. Physiol., 248: G663.

Fix, J.A., Leppert, P.S., Porter, P.A., and Caldwell, L.J., 1983, Influence of ionic strength on rectal absorption of gentamicin sulfate in the presence and absence of sodium salicylate, J. Pharm. Sci., 72: 1134.

Hayashi, M., Hirasawa, T., Muraoka, T., Shiga, M., and Awazu, S., 1985, Comparison of water influx and sieving coefficient in rat jejunal, rectal and nasal absorption of antipyrine, Chem. Pharm. Bull., 33: 2149.

Hirai, S., Yashiki, T., and Mima, H., 1981a, Effect of surfactants on the nasal absorption of insulin in rats, Int. J. Pharm., 9: 165.

Hirai, S., Yashiki, T., and Mima, H., 1981b, Mechanisms for the enhancement of the nasal absorption of insulin by surfactants, Int. J. Pharm., 9: 173.

Hori, R., Komada, F., Okumura, K., 1983, Pharmaceutical approach to subcutaneous dosage forms of insulin, J. Pharm. Sci., 72: 435.

Hussain, A., Faraj, J., Aramaki, Y., and Truelove, J.E., 1985, Hydrolysis of leucine enkephalin in the nasal cavity of the rat — a possible factor in the low bioavailability of nasally administered peptides, Biochem. Biophys. Res. Commun., 133: 923.

Ichikawa, K., Ohata, I., Mitomi, M., Kawamura, S., Maeno, H., and Kawata, H., 1980, Rectal absorption of insulin suppositories in rabbits, J. Pharm. Pharmacol., 32: 314.

Ishida, M., Machida, Y., Nambu, N., and Nagai, T., 1981, New mucosal dosage form of insulin, Chem. Pharm. Bull., 29, 810–816, 1981.

Johnson, V. and Maack, T., 1977, Renal extraction, filtration, absorption, and catabolism of growth hormone, Am. J. Physiol., 233: F185.

Kajii, H., Horie, T., Hayashi, M., and Awazu, S., 1985, Fluorescence study on the interaction of salicylate with rat small intestinal epithelial cells: possible mechanism for the promoting effects of salicylate on drug absorption in vivo, Life Sci., 37: 523.

Kamada, A., Nishihata, T., Kim, S., Yamamoto, M., and Yata, N., 1981, Study of enamine derivatives of phenylglycine as adjuvants for the rectal absorption of insulin, Chem. Pharm. Bull., 29: 2012.

Kidron, M., Bar-On, H., Berry, E.M., and Ziv, E., 1982, The absorption of insulin from various regions of the rat intestine, Life Sci., 31: 2837.

Kim, S., Kamada, A., Higuchi, T., and Nishihata, T., 1983, Effect of enamine derivatives on the rectal absorption of insulin in dogs and rabbits, J. Pharm. Pharmacol., 35: 100.

Laskowski, M., Haessler, H.A., Miech, R.P., Peanasky, R.J., and Laskowski, M., 1958, Effect of trypsin inhibitor on passage of insulin across the intestinal barrier, Science, 127: 1115.

Lee, V.H.L., Carson, L.W., Dodda Kashi, S., and Stratford, R.E., 1986, Barriers to the ocular absorption of topically applied enkephalins, in preparation.

Maack, T., 1975, Renal handling of low molecular weight proteins, Am. J. Med., 58: 57.

Martin, G.P., Marriott, C., and Kellaway, I.W., 1978, Direct effect of bile salts and phospholipids on the physical properties of mucus, Gut, 19: 103.

Morimoto, K., Kamiya, E., Takeeda, T., Nakamoto, Y., and Morisaka, K., 1983, Enhancement of rectal absorption of insulin in polyacrylic acid aqueous gel bases containing long chain fatty acid in rats, Int. J. Pharm., 14: 149.

Morimoto, K., Takeeda, T., Nakamoto, Y., and Morisaka, K., 1982, Effective vaginal absorption of insulin in diabetic rats and rabbits using polyacrylic acid aqueous gel bases, Int. J. Pharm., 12: 107.

Moses, A.C., Gordon, G.S., Carey, M.C., and Flier, J.S., 1983, Insulin administered intranasally as an insulin-bile salt aerosol: effectiveness and reproducibility in normal and diabetic subjects. Diabetes, 32: 1040.

Muranishi, S., Tokunaga, Y., Taniguchi, K., and Sezaki, H., 1977, Potential absorption of heparin from the small intestine and the large intestine in the presence of monoolein mixed micelles, Chem. Pharm. Bull., 25: 1159.

Muranushi, N., Nakajima, Y., Kinugawa, M., Muranishi, S., Sezaki, H.,

1980, Mechanism for the inducement of the intestinal absorption of poorly absorbed drugs by mixed micelles II. Effect of the incorporation of various lipids on the permeability of liposomal membranes. Int. J. Pharm., 4: 281.

Muranushi, N., Takagi, N., Muranishi, S., and Sezaki, H., 1981, Effect of fatty acids and monoglycerides on permeability of lipid bilayer. Chem. Phys. Lipids, 28: 269.

Najdovski, T., Collette, N., and Deschodt-Lanckman, M., 1985, Hydrolysis of the C-terminal octapeptide of cholecystokinin by rat kidney membranes: characterization of the cleavage by solubilized endopeptidase-24.11, Life Sci., 37: 827.

Nishihata, T., Higuchi, T., and Kamada, A., 1984a, Salicylate-promoted permeation of cefoxitin, insulin and phenylalanine across red cell membrane. Possible mechanism, Life Sci., 34: 437.

Nishihata, T., Kim, S., Morishita, S., Kamada, A., Yata, N., and Higuchi, T., 1983, Adjuvant effects of glyceryl esters of acetoacetic acid on rectal absorption of insulin and inulin in rabbits, J. Pharm. Sci., 72: 280.

Nishihata, T., Lee, C.S., Nghiem, B.T., and Higuchi, T., 1984b, Possible mechanism behind the adjuvant action of phosphate derivatives on rectal absorption of cefoxitin in rats and dogs, J. Pharm. Sci., 73: 1523.

Nishihata, T., Okamura, Y., Kamada, A., Higuchi, T., Yagi, T., Kawamori, R., and Shichiri, M., 1985a, Enhanced bioavailability of insulin after rectal administration with enamine as adjuvant in depancreatized dogs. J. Pharm. Pharmacol., 37: 22.

Nishihata, T., Rytting, J.H., Kamada, A., and Higuchi, T., 1981, Enhanced intestinal absorption of insulin in rats in the presence of sodium 5-methoxysalicylate, Diabetes, 30: 1065.

Nishihata, T., Tomida, H., Frederick, G., Rytting, J.H., and Higuchi, T., 1985b, Comparison of the effects of sodium salicylate, disodium ethylenediaminetetraacetic acid and polyoxyethylene-23-lauryl ether as adjuvants for the rectal absorption of sodium cefoxitin, J. Pharm. Sci., 37: 159.

Okada, H., Yamazaki, I., Ogawa, Y., Hirai, S., Yashiki, T., and Mima, H.J., Vaginal absorption of a potent luteinizing hormone-releasing hormone analog (leuprolide) in rats. I. Absorption by various routes and absorption enhancement, J. Pharm. Sci., 71: 1367.

Okada, H., Yamazaki, I., Ogawa, Y., Hirai, S., Yashiki, T., and Mima, H.J., Vaginal absorption of a potent luteinizing hormone-releasing hormone analog (leuprolide) in rats. II. Mechanism of absorption enhancement with organic acids, J. Pharm. Sci., 72: 75.

Palmieri, F.E., Petrelli, J.J., and Ward, P.E., 1985, Vascular, plasma membrane aminopeptidase M. Metabolism of vasoactive peptides, Biochem. Pharmacol., 34: 2309.

Palmieri, F.E. and Ward, P.E., 1983, Mesentery vascular metabolism of substance P, Biochim. Biophys. Acta, 755: 522.

Pimstone, B., Epstein, S., Hamilton, S.M., LeRoith, D., and Hendricks, S., Metabolic clearance and plasma half disappearance time of exogenous gonadotropin releasing hormone in normal subjects and in patients with liver disease and chronic renal failure, J. Clin. Endocrinol. Metab., 44: 356.

Pontiroli, A.E., Alberetto, M., Secchi, A., Dossi, G., Bosi, I., and Pozza, G., 1982, Insulin given intranasally induces hypoglycaemia in normal and diabetic subjects, Brit. Med. J., 284: 303.

Sakai, K., Kutsuna, T.M., Nishino, T., Fujihara, Y., and Yata, N., 1986, Contribution of calcium ion sequestration by polyoxyethylated nonionic surfactants to the enhanced colonic absorption of p-aminobenzoic acid, J. Pharm. Sci., 75: 387.

Segre, G.V., Perkins, A.S., Witters, L.A., and Potts, J.T., Metabolism of parathyroid hormone by isolated rat Kupffer cells and hepatocytes. J. Clin. Invest., 67: 449.

Shiga, M., Muraoka, T., Hirasawa, T., Hayashi, M., and Awazu, S., 1985, The promotion of drug rectal absorption by water absorption, J. Pharm. Pharmacol., 37: 446.

Sithigorngul, P., Burton, P., Nishihata, T., and Caldwell, L., 1983, Effects of sodium salicylate on epithelial cells of the rectal mucosa of the rat: a light and electron microscopic study, Life Sci., 33: 1025.

Stanzani, L., Mascellani, G., Corbelli, G.P., and Bianchini, P., 1981, Rectal absorption of some glycosaminoglycan sulphates and heparin in rats, J. Pharm. Pharmacol., 33: 783.

Stratford, R.E. and Lee, V.H.L., 1986, Aminopeptidase activity in homogenates of various absorptive mucosae in the albino rabbit: implications in peptide delivery, Int. J. Pharm, 30: 73.

Strunz, U.T., Thompson, M.R., Elashoff, J., and Grossman, M.I., 1978, Hepatic inactivation of gastrins of various chain lengths in dogs, Gastroenterology, 74: 550.

Su, K.S.E., Campanale, K.M., Mendelsohn, L.G., Kerchner, G.A., and Gries, C.L., 1985, Nasal delivery of polypeptides I: Nasal absorption of enkephalins in rats, J. Pharm. Sci., 74: 394.

Taniguchi, K., Muranishi, S., and Sezaki, H., 1980, Enhanced intestinal permeability to macromolecules II. Improvment of the large intestinal absorption of heparin by lipid-surfactant mixed micelles in rat. Int. J. Pharm., 4: 219.

Temperley, J.M., Stagg, B.H., and Wyllie, J.H., 1971, Disappearance of gastrin and pentagastrin in the portal circulation, Gut, 12: 372.

Touitou, E., Donbrow, M., and Azaz, E., 1978, New hydrophilic vehicle enabling rectal and vaginal absorption of insulin, heparin, phenol red, and gentamicin, J. Pharm. Pharmacol., 30: 662.

Touitou, E., Donbrow, M., and Rubinstein, A., 1980, Effective intestinal absorption of insulin in diabetic rats using a new formulation approach, J. Pharm. Pharmacol., 32: 108.

Ward, P.E., 1984, Immunoelectrophoretic analysis of vascular, membrane-bound angiotensin I converting enzyme, aminopeptidase M, and dipeptidyl(amino)peptidase IV, Biochem. Pharmacol., 33: 3183.

Yagi, T., Hakui, N., Yamasaki, Y., Kawamori, R., Shichiri, M., Abe, H., Kim, S., Miyake, M., Kamikawa, K., Nishihata, T., and Kamada, A., Insulin suppository: enhanced rectal absorption of insulin using an enamine derivative as a new promoter, J. Pharm. Pharmacol., 35: 177.

Yamashita, S., Saitoh, H., Nakanishi, K., Masada, M., Nadai, T., and Kimura, T., 1985, Characterization of enhanced intestinal permeability; electrophysiological study on the effects of diclofenac and ethylenediaminetetraacetic acid, J. Pharm. Pharmacol., 37: 512.

Yoshioka, S., Caldwell, L., and Higuchi, T., 1982, Enhanced rectal bioavailability of polypeptides using sodium 5-methoxysalicylate as an absorption promoter, J. Pharm. Sci., 71: 593.

INTRACELLULAR SORTING OF PROTEINS

Claudia Bibus

Biocenter, University of Basel
Klingelbergstrasse 70
CH-4056 Basel / Switzerland

INTRODUCTION

Compartmentalization is an essential requirement for cellular function and growth. Each compartment contains a unique set of proteins
designed to perform specialized functions, such as oxidative phosphory-
lation within the mitochondria or ribosome assembly within the nuc-
leolus. How do cells generate and maintain such an asymmetric, highly
organized distribution of their proteins? Five major targets of protein
transport have been studied in detail: (1) the eukaryotic secretory
system; (2) the nucleus; (3) the mitochondria; (4) the chloroplasts; (5)
the bacterial secretory system. The scope of this review does not allow
in-depth treatment of all important aspects of protein sorting. For
detailed reviews see Schekman (1985), Garoff (1985), Farquhar (1985) and
Benson et al. (1985).

EUKARYOTIC SECRETORY SYSTEM

The proteins populating compartments as diverse as the extracellular space, the periplasm, the plasma membrane, the secretory vesicles,
the vacuole, the lysosome, the Golgi apparatus and the endoplasmic reticulum (ER) all share at least the first step of their localization pathway: They are synthesized on ribosomes bound to the ER membrane and are
transported into or across the ER membrane (Palade, 1975). The early in
vitro translocation experiments (Milstein et al., 1972; Blobel and Dobberstein, 1975) showed that newly synthesized precursor proteins contain
an N-terminal signal peptide which is (in most cases) removed during
translocation. Many signal peptides have been identified and sequenced.
They contain a stretch of hydrophobic amino acids flanked by a few basic
residues on either side. They are quite variable in length and amino
acid composition. A series of classical experiments (reviewed by Walter
et al., 1984) showed that, as the signal peptide emerges from the ribosome, it interacts with a ribonucleoprotein particle called the signal
recognition particle (SRP). The SRP then directs the nascent polypeptide
to the ER membrane by binding to the "docking protein" or SRP receptor
which is an integral ER membrane protein. Both the SRP as well as its
receptor have been purified. In addition, the purification of the signal
peptidase has been reported recently (Evans et al., 1986). In a process
called core-glycosylation almost all proteins destined for the Golgi

stack receive an oligosaccharide chain consisting of 14 sugar units attached to an asparginine residue. Quickly, while the protein is still in the ER, 4 sugar units are removed. As the core-glycosylated protein travels through the Golgi stack the oligosaccharide chain is further modified (Rothman, 1985). In addition to proteolytic processing and glycosylation, secretory proteins may be phosphorylated, sulfated or acylated. Proteins secreted into the ER may become soluble in the ER lumen or become anchored in the membrane. The topology with respect to the membrane depends on the number, length and distribution of hydrophobic amino acid stretches within the protein. Wickner and Lodish (1985) present models on how proteins with various topologies may be inserted into the lipid bilayer. In vivo, protein synthesis and translocation into the ER appear to be at least temporally coupled since proteolytic modification and glycosylation on the luminal side of the ER membrane occur on nascent polypeptides. In vitro studies using mammalian ER suggested a mechanistic coupling between translation and translocation since translocation occurred only if the ER membrane vesicles (microsomes) were present during translation (reviewed by Walter et al., 1984). Recently, however, two novel in vitro systems were developed in which translocation could be uncoupled from translation. On the one hand, Hansen et al., Rothblatt and Meyer, and Waters and Blobel (all 1986) independently developed homologous yeast in vitro translation / translocation systems in which the yeast mating factor and/or invertase can be post-translationally transported across the ER membrane. The process was shown to be dependent on ATP hydrolysis and independent of an electrochemical potential across the ER membrane. In an alternative approach, Perara et al. (1986) uncoupled translation from translocation in vitro by studying translocation of almost full-length precursor polypeptide chains which were still attached to the ribosome. When these nascent chains were added to mammalian microsomal membranes under conditions where further protein synthesis was inhibited with an antibiotic (such as cycloheximide or emetine), the nascent chains were translocated across the ER membrane in a process that was independent of chain elongation, but dependent on attachment of the polypeptide chain to the ribosome. Thus, obligate co-translational transport can no longer serve as a feature which mechanistically distinguishes protein transport across the ER membrane from that across all other membrane systems although temporal coupling of translation to translocation is observed in vivo.

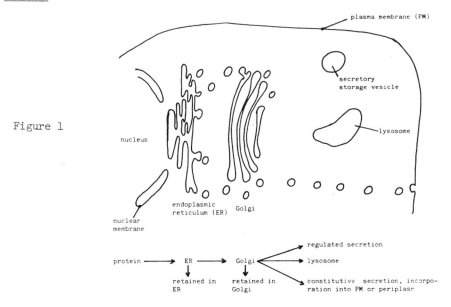

Figure 1

While much is known about the signal and the mechanism for protein translocation across the ER membrane, there is still very little under-standing of how the sorting of proteins along the pathway outlined in Figure 1 is accomplished. Although it is generally accepted that protein traffic between these compartments is mediated by vesicle flow, it is, for example, not yet known whether the travelling proteins contain specific retention signals if they are to be retained in a certain com-partment (such as a Golgi cisterna) without which they would be secreted to the plasma membrane or the extracellular space.

There are some examples in which a specific sorting signal on proteins transported by vesicular membrane flow has been identified. One of them diverts lysosomal enzymes from the secretory pathway to the lysosome. Another one initiates the first step in the receptor-mediated endocytosis pathway, namely the clustering of a receptor in coated pits. Incidentally, these two examples discussed below were discovered by studying mutations causing a human genetic disease.

Lysosomal enzymes (as reviewed by Farquhar, 1985; Garoff, 1985) are first secreted into the ER where they are core-glycosylated. They then migrate to a cis-cisterna of the Golgi complex, where, in contrast to other glycoproteins containing N-linked sugar branches, they receive mannose-6-phosphate (man-6-P) residues added to their oligosaccharide chains. A man-6-P receptor has been identified in the cis-cisternae of the Golgi which diverts the lysosomal enzymes from the secretory pathway and directs them to the lysosome via vesicular transport. The man-6-P receptor can be trapped in the endosomal compartment (see below) by reagents which raise the intracellular pH such as chloroquine (Gonzales-Noriega et al., 1980), because the increased endosomal pH prevents receptor ligand dissociation and receptor recycling. Intere-stingly, such trapping of the man-6-P receptor causes lysosmal enzymes to be mistargeted and secreted.

Low density lipoprotein (LDL) is internalized via receptor-mediated endocytosis. The LDL receptor cycles between the plasma membrane and the endosome. As reviewed by Brown and Goldstein (1986), the LDL receptor present on the plasma membrane clusters in coated pits independent of ligand binding. Upon binding LDL it is internalized in coated vesicles which, after uncoating, fuse to form an endosome. As the endosomal pH falls below 5.5, LDL dissociates from the receptor and the receptor cycles back to the plasma membrane. The LDL receptor contains a large exoplasmic domain which includes the LDL binding domain, a transmembrane segment of 22 amino acids and a cytosolic domain of 50 amino acids. There are mutated forms of the LDL receptor which still bind LDL but no longer cluster into coated pits. Three of such mutant receptors have been analyzed at the molecular level and all three are due to an altera-tion in the cytoplasmic tail. It will be interesting to identify this signal within the cytoplasmic domain and to learn how it mediates clustering of the receptor into coated pits. Roth et al. (1986) were able to induce clustering into coated pits of influenza virus hemagglu-tinin (which physiologically has a very long life span on the cell sur-face and is not internalized through coated pits) by fusing it to the transmembrane segment and cytoplasmic domain of two viral glycoproteins which are endocytosed in a fashion resembling cell surface receptors.

TARGETING OF PROTEINS TO THE NUCLEUS

Proteins destined for the nuclear matrix are synthesized on free cytoplasmic ribosomes and transported to the nucleus post-translational-ly. The large size of the pores in the nuclear membrane which in prin-ciple would allow passage of proteins up to 70 kd poses the still unresolved question of how the nucleus maintains its identity. Interestingly, proteins isolated from the nucleus, when injected into the cytoplasm of an oocyte can be relocalized efficiently to the nucleus. This is in marked contrast to the localization of proteins to all other compartments.

Targeting of proteins to the nucleus, too, seems to involve discrete signal sequences which may be N-terminal, internal, or C-terminal. By limited proteolysis of nucleoplasmin, Dingwall et al. (1982) found a polypeptide domain which specifies migration of nucleoplasmin into the nucleus. In more recent studies using both deletion analysis and gene fusion, Kalderon et al. (1984) identified the nuclear targeting signal of the SV40 T-antigen to be the peptide Pro(126)-Lys-Lys-Lys-Arg-Lys-Val(132). By fusing this peptide to the N-terminus of pyruvate kinase and β-galactosidase they targeted both proteins to the nucleus. Interestingly, this nuclear targeting peptide functions both in its physiological internal location and in the artificial N-terminal position of the two hybrid proteins, suggesting that it is structurally autonomous. In addition, it appears that multiple nuclear targeting sequences in one protein may exert a cooperative effect as indicated by studies on polyoma virus large-T nuclear localization (Richardson et al., 1986). Targeting signals for other nuclear proteins including the influenza virus nuclear protein (Davey et al., 1985) and the α2-protein of yeast were identified (Hall et al., 1984). The former is internal, the latter N-terminal. All of them contain basic residues and some contain a hydrophobic core. Nuclear targeting signals are not proteolytically removed after transport into the nuclear matrix.

IMPORT OF PROTEINS INTO MITOCHONDRIA AND CHLOROPLASTS

General Remarks

Mitochondria and chloroplasts both contain their own genome which codes for only a few of the organellar polypeptides. The vast majority of the hundreds of distinct mitochondrial and chloroplast proteins are encoded in the nucleus and synthesized on soluble ribosomes as precursor molecules; most of these contain a transient N-terminal presequence. Again with a few exceptions, they are translocated across 1 to 3 membranes in an energy-dependent fashion and have their signal sequence proteolytically removed. The resulting mature polypeptide may be further covalently modified or assembled into protein complexes (see Hay et al., 1984 and Ellis, 1981 for detailed reviews).

One difference between mitochondrial and chloroplast import is that the energy requirement of the mitochondrial system is met by an electrochemical gradient across the inner mitochondrial membrane (Schleyer et al., 1982, Gasser et al., 1982) whereas chloroplast import is driven by ATP hydrolysis (Grossmann et al., 1980). Since translocation across the ER, too, requires ATP hydrolysis whereas bacterial secretion requires an electrochemical potential, these different energy requirements might point to some basic mechanistic variation. However, chloroplast and mitochondrial import are very similar and particularly so the mitochondrial and chloroplast presequences. For example, the 31 N-terminal amino acids of the small subunit of ribulose-1,5-bisphosphate carboxylase can direct an attached protein into yeast mitochondria (Hurt et al., 1986).

Recent Results in the Analysis of Mitochondrial Import

Advances in mitochondrial import studies during the past few years stem from gene fusion experiments, biochemcial analysis and classical genetic methods. Gene fusion studies were instrumental for understanding the targeting mechanism of mitochondrial prepieces. It was shown that the cleavable signal sequence of a mitochondrial precursor protein when fused in front of a cytosolic protein (which otherwise would not cross a membrane) was sufficient to efficiently direct the resulting fusion protein into the mitochondria, both in vivo and in vitro. In fact, the fusion protein was localized to the correct submitochondrial space. Subsequently, signal sequences from proteins of each of the four submitochondrial compartments (outer membrane, intermembrane space, inner membrane, matrix) were attached to cytosolic proteins and in all cases the signal sequence alone specifically targeted the protein to the correct intramitochondrial location. Experiments in which only portions of such signal sequences were fused to a cytosolic protein led to the current model in which the most N-terminal part of the signal directs the protein to the mitochondria and, in fact, into the matrix space. Further domains in the signal may cause transport to stop at an earlier point such that the protein ends up for example in the outer membrane or the intermembrane space. For a review and references see Hurt and van Loon (1986). Allison and Schatz (manuscript in preparation) engineered totally artificial presequences (via chemically synthesized oligonucleotides) composed of only three different amino acids (lys, leu, ser) which are able to specify mitochondrial location in vivo and in vitro.

Mitochondrial protein import has been studied in a cell-free in vitro system (Hay et al., 1984). The longstanding goal of reconstituting the import process with purified components is being approached by the identification and purification of individual components. Purification of the matrix-localized protease has been reported (Böhni et al., 1983; McAda and Douglas, 1982; Miura et al., 1982). There is evidence for one or more cytosolic factors involved in the import mechanism. However, none of the factors described has been purified yet (Ohta and Schatz, 1984; Argan et al., 1983; Miura et al., 1983). Several precursor molecules have been purified (Argan and Shore, 1986; Ohta and Schatz, 1984). The question of whether or not these precursors unfold during import could be tackled with the purified proteins. Eilers and Schatz (1986) purified an artificial mitochondrial precursor from E. coli transformed with a fusion gene encoding the mitochondrial targeting sequence of cytochrome c oxidase subunit IV (COX IV; 22 N-terminal amino acids) and the entire mouse dihydrofolate reductase (DHFR). This artificial precursor resembles authentic precursors in all criteria applied to mitochondrial import. For example, it is imported into isolated mitochondria in an energy-dependent fashion. However, two different folate antagonists block import of this precursor into mitochondria. Since the only known effect of these antifolates on the artificial COX IV-DHFR precursor or on isolated mitochondria is their tight binding to (and stabilization of) the DHFR moiety, their inhibitory effect on import implies that the precursor has to at least partially unfold in order to translocate across the mitochondrial membranes.

A recent very elegant study carried out by Schleyer and Neupert (1985) with isolated Neurospora mitochondria provided the first biochemical indication that proteins are transported through contact sites between the inner and outer mitochondrial membrane. By lowering the incubation temperature in an in vitro import reaction or by binding antibodies specific for the mature part of a precursor polypeptide, a transport intermediate was isolated which had its targeting signal removed by the matrix protease but which was still sensitive to externally added protease. Thus, this translocation intermediate had to span both outer and inner membrane, presumably at a point where both membranes were in close apposition.

Experiments have also been performed with chemically synthesized mitochondrial signal peptides (Ito et al., 1985; Gillespie et al., 1985; Roise et al., 1986). Roise et al. (1986) showed that various lengths of the presequence of cytochrome c oxidase subunit IV can spontaneously insert into lipid monolayers, lyse liposomes and can uncouple mitochondria. The amino acid sequences of more than 20 mitochondrial targeting peptides can be deduced from the nucleotide sequences of the corresponding genes. Comparison reveals no extensive sequence homology; in general, these peptides lack acidic amino acids, are rich in the hydroxylated amino acids serine and threonine and in the basic amino acids lysine and arginine. Many of these peptides can form an amphiphilic α—helix (Roise et al., 1986; von Heijne, 1986). However, experiments with artificial presequences argue that an amphiphilic α-helix is not an obligate prerequisite for a functional mitochondrial targeting sequence (Allison, manuscript in preparation).

In a microorganism such as S. cerevisiae, classical genetic methods can be applied towards the understanding of the mechanism of mitochondrial protein import. Two mutants which are defective in mitochondrial assembly (termed mas 1 and mas 2) were isolated in a screen identifying strains which accumulate mitochondrial precursors at an elevated temperature. These strains are temperature-sensitive lethals since mitochondrial import is a process vital to the cell. Biochemical analysis of mas 1 yielded strong evidence that this mutant carries a defective gene required for the matrix-localized protease activity (Yaffe et al., 1984, 1985). For both mas 1 and mas 2, the corresponding wild-type alleles have been cloned and sequenced and their function is being analyzed in more detail. Presently, methods are being developed to select more mutants since their analysis may well lead to the identification of additional components essential for mitochondrial import and to a better understanding of the molecular mechanism by which proteins are imported into mitochondria.

BACTERIAL SECRETORY SYSTEM

While some features of bacterial secretion resemble translocation across the eukaryotic ER, others are more similar to mitochondrial import. As mentioned above, both bacterial export and mitochondrial import share the requirement of an electrochemical potential for translocation. On the other hand, bacterial leader sequences resemble eukaryotic signal sequences with which they can be functionally exchanged. For example, if the N-terminal leader sequence of bacterial β-lactamase (28 amino acids) is fused to α-globin, it directs the hybrid protein into mammalian microsomes (Lingappa et al., 1984). The specificities of bacterial leader peptidase and of ER signal peptidase are closely similar, if not identical. Translocation of many bacterial precursor proteins can be entirely post-translational whereas others are translocated while still nascent but after at least 80% of the protein has been synthesized (Randall, 1983). Bacterial leader sequences appear to be necessary but not sufficient for secretion. Thus, the mature protein may contain some additional discrete regions directing export (Benson and Silhavy, 1983). Genetically, various gene products have been identified (reviewed by Benson et al., 1985) which block export of some proteins but not of others, suggesting that there exist multiple export pathways. Many of the export mutants appear to contain an altered protein synthesizing system, which makes it difficult to interpret their phenotype in molecular terms. However, the existence of these mutants suggests that there is an interaction between the ribosome and components of the translocation machinery. Furthermore, the development of an in vitro translocation system of bacterial proteins across inverted E. coli plasma membrane vesicles (Müller and Blobel, 1984) should contribute to the biochemical identification of these genetically defined components.

Acknowledgment

I would like to thank Professor G. Schatz and my colleagues in the Schatz laboratory who commented on the manuscript and Michèle Probst for typing the manuscript.

References

Argan, C., Lusty, C.J. and Shore, G.C., 1983, Membrane and cytosolic components affecting transport of the precursor for ornithine carbamyl transferase into mitochondria, J. Biol. Chem., 258:6667.

Argan, C. and Shore, G.C., 1986, The precursor to ornithine carbamyl transferase is transported to mitochondria as a 5S complex containing an import factor, in press.

Benson, S.A. and Silhavy, T.J., 1983, Information within the mature lamB protein necessary for localization to the otuer membrane of E. coli K12, Cell, 32:1325.

Benson, S.A., Hall, M.N. and Silhavy, T.J., 1985, Genetic analysis of protein export in Escherichia coli K12, Ann. Rev. Biochem., 54:101.

Blobel, G. and Dobberstein, B., 1975, Transfer of proteins across membranes. II. Reconstitution of functional rough microsomes from heterologous components, J. Cell Biol., 67:852.

Böhni, P.C., Daum, G., Schatz, G., 1983, Import of proteins into mitochondria: partial purification of a matrix-located protease involved in cleavage of mitochondrial precursors, J. Biol. Chem., 258:4937.

Brown, M.S. and Goldstein, J.L., 1986, A receptor-mediated pathway for cholesterol homeostasis, Science, 232:34.

Davey, J., Dimmock, N.J. and Colman, A., 1985, Identification of the sequence responsible for the nuclear accumulation of the influenza virus nucleoprotein in Xenopus oocytes, Cell, 40:667.

Eilers, M. and Schatz, G., 1986, Binding of a specific ligand inhibits import of a purified precursor protein into mitochondria, Nature, in press.

Ellis, R.J., 1981, Chloroplast proteins: synthesis, transport and assembly, Ann. Rev. Plant Physiol., 32:111.

Evans, E.A., Gilmore, R. and Blobel, G., 1986, Purification of microsomal signal peptidase as a complex, Proc. Natl. Acad. Sci. USA, 83:581.

Farquhar, M.G., 1985, Progress in unravelling pathways of Golgi traffic, Ann. Rev. Cell Biol., 1:447.

Garoff, H., 1985, Using recombinant DNA techniques to study protein targeting in the eukaryotic cell, Ann. Rev. Cell Biol., 1:403.

Gasser, S.M., Daum, G. and Schatz, G., 1982, Import of proteins into mitochondria: energy-dependent uptake of precursors by isolated mitochondria, J. Biol. Chem., 257:13034.

Gillespie, L.L., Argan, C., Taneja, A.T., Hodges, R.S., Freeman, K.B. and Shore, G.C., 1985, A synthetic signal peptide blocks import of precursor proteins destined for the mitochondrial inner membrane or matrix, J. Biol. Chem., 260:16045.

Gonzales-Noriega, A., Gruto, J.H., Talkad, V. and Sly, W.S., 1980, Chloroquine inhibits lysosomal enzyme pinocytosis and enhances lysosomal enzyme secretion by impairing receptor recycling, J. Cell. Biol., 85:839.

Grossmann, A., Bartlett, S. and Chua, N.H., 1980, Energy-dependent uptake of cytoplasmically synthesized polypeptides by chloroplasts, Nature, 285:625.

Hall, M.N., Hereford, L. and Herskowitz, I., 1984, Targeting of E. coli β-galactosidase to the nucleus in yeast, Cell, 36:1057.

Hansen, W., Garcia, P.D. and Walter, P., 1986, In vitro protein translocation across the endoplasmic reticulum of Saccharomyces cerevisiae: Post-translational translocation and glycosylation of
the precursor to α-factor, Cell, in press.

Hay, R., Böhni, P. and Gasser, S., 1984, How mitochondria import proteins, Biochim. Biophys. Acta, 779:65.

Hurt, E.C. and van Loon, A.P.G.M., 1986, How proteins find mitochondria
and intramitochondrial compartments, Trends Biochem. Sci.,
11:204.

Hurt, E.C., Soltanifar, N., Goldschmidt-Clérmont, M., Rochaix, J.D. and
Schatz, G., 1986, The cleavable presequence of an imported
chloroplast protein directs attached polypeptides into yeast
mitochondria, EMBO J., June issue.

Ito, A., Ogishima, T., Ou, W., Omura, T., Aoyagi, H., Lee, S., Mihara,
H. and Izumiya, N., 1985, Effects of synthetic model peptides
resembling to the extension peptides of mitochondrial enzyme
precursors on import of the precursors into mitochondria, J.
Biochem. (Tokyo), 98:1571.

Kalderon, D., Roberts, B.L., Richardson, W.D. and Smith, A.E., 1984, A
short amino acid sequence able to specifiy nuclear localization,
Cell, 39:499.

Lingappa, V.R., Chaidez, J., Yost, C.S. and Hedgpeth, J., 1984, Determinants for protein localization: β-lactamase signal sequence
directs globin across microsomal membranes, Proc. Natl. Acad.
Sci., 81:456.

McAda, P.C. and Douglas, M.G., 1982, A neutral metalloendoprotease
involved in the processing of an F_1ATPase subunit precursor in
mitochondria, J. Biol. Chem., 257:3177.

Milstein, C., Brownlee, G., Harrison, T. and Mathews, M.B., 1972, A
possible precursor of immunoglobulin light chains, Nature New
Biol., 239:117.

Miura, S., Mori, M., Amaya, Y. and Tatibana, M., 1982, A mitochondrial
protease that cleaves the precursor of ornithine carbamoyl
transferase, Eur. J. Biochem., 122:641.

Miura, S., Mori, M., Tatibana, M., 1983, Transport of ornithine carba-
moyltransferase precursor into mitochondria: Stimulation by
potassium ion, magnesium ion and a reticulocyte cytosolic pro-
tein(s), J. Biol. Chem., 258:6671.

Müller, M. and Blobel, G., 1984, In vitro translocation of bacterial
proteins across the plasma membrane of E. coli, Proc. Natl.
Acad. Sci. USA, 81:7421.

Ohta, S. and Schatz, G., 1984, A purified precursor polypeptide requires
a cytosolic protein fraction for import into mitochondria, EMBO
J., 3:651.

Palade, G., 1975, Intracellular aspects of the process of protein secretion, Science, 189:347.

Perara, E., Rothman, R.E. and Lingappa, V.R., 1986, Uncoupling translocation from translation: Implications for transport of proteins across membranes, Science, 232:348.

Randall, L.L., 1983, Translocation of domains of nascent periplasmic
proteins across the cytoplasmic membrane is independent of elongation, Cell, 33:231.

Richardson, W.D., Roberts, B.L. and Smith, A.E., 1986, Nuclear location
signals in polyoma virus large-T., Cell, 44:77.

Roise, D., Horvath, S.J., Tomich, J.M., Richards, J.H. and Schatz, G.,
1986, A chemically synthesized presequence of an imported mitochondrial protein can form an amphiphilic helix and perturb
natural and artificial phospholipid bilayers, EMBO J., June
issue.

Roth, M.G., Doyle, C., Sambrook, J. and Gething, M.J., 1986, Heterologous transmembrane and cytoplasmic domains direct functional
chimeric influenza virus hemagglutinins into the endocytic pathway, J. Cell Biol., 102:1271.

Rothblatt, J.A. and Meyer, D.I., 1986, Secretion in yeast: Reconstitution of the translocation and glycosylation of α-factor and invertase in a homologous cell-free system, Cell, 44:619.

Rothman, J.E., 1985, The compartmental organization of the Golgi apparatus, Sci. Am., 253:74.

Schekman, R., 1985, Protein localization and membrane traffic in yeast, Ann. Rev. Cell. Biol., 1:115.

Schleyer, M., Schmidt, B. and Neupert, W., 1982, Requirement of a membrane potential for post-translational transfer of proteins into mitochondria, Eur. J. Biochem., 125:109.

Schleyer, M. and Neupert, W., 1985, Transport of proteins into mitochondria: translocational intermediates spanning contact sites between outer and inner membranes, Cell, 43:339.

Von Heijne, G., 1986, Mitochondrial targeting sequences may form amphiphilic helixes, EMBO J., June issue.

Walter, P., Gilmore, R. and Blobel, G., 1984, Protein translocation across the endoplasmic reticulum, Cell, 38:5.

Waters, M.G. and Blobel, G., 1986, Secretory protein translocation in a yeast cell-free system can occur post-translationally and requires ATP hydrolysis, J. Cell Biol., 102:1543.

Wickner, W.T., and Lodish, H.F., 1985, Multiple mechanisms of protein insertion into and across membranes, Science, 239:400.

Yaffe, M.P. and Schatz, G., 1984, Two nuclear mutations that block mitochondrial protein import in yeast, Proc. Natl. Acad. Sci. USA, 81:4819.

Yaffe, M.P., Ohta, S. and Schatz, G., 1985, A yeast mutant temperature-sensitive for mitochondrial assembly is deficient in a mitochondrial protease activity that cleaves imported precursor polypeptides, EMBO J., 4:2069.

BIODEGRADABLE POLYMERS FOR SUSTAINED RELEASE OF POLYPEPTIDES

F. G. Hutchinson and B. J. A. Furr

Pharmaceutical Department and Research Department

Imperial Chemical Industries PLC, Pharmaceuticals Division
Mereside, Alderley Park
Macclesfield, Cheshire SK10 4TG, U.K.

INTRODUCTION

Recent years have seen major advances in genetic engineering and consequent bacterial production of many interesting and pharmacologically active polypeptides as well as improvements in techniques leading to total chemical synthesis of lower molecular weight peptides such as 'Zoladex' (ICI 118630; D—Ser (But)^6—Azgly^{10}—LHRH; 'Zoladex' is a trade mark, the property of Imperial Chemical Industries PLC). However the therapeutic and commercial potential of polypeptide drugs will only be realised if these advances are accompanied by dosage form design leading to practical and effective formulations.

The use of polypeptides in human and animal diseases is fraught with problems. These macromolecular drugs are usually ineffective by the oral route as they are rapidly degraded and deactivated by proteolytic enzymes in the alimentary tract. Even if stable to enzymatic digestion their molecular weights are too high for absorption through the intestinal wall to occur. Consequently they are usually administered parenterally but since such drugs often have very short half—lives frequent injections are required to produce an effective therapy. The most appropriate dosage form for peptide hormones using the parenteral route would therefore be one which would release drug continuously at a controlled rate over a period of weeks or even months. Preferably the formulation should be biodegradable and so disappear from the site of administration. Long experience with homopolymers and copolymers of lactic and glycolic acids has shown these to be non—toxic and biocompatible. Consequently these polymers are invariably the preferred materials of use in initial design of parenteral sustained delivery systems using a biodegradable carrier, particularly when release over many weeks is required. We have adopted this approach and evaluated polylactides [Fig 1] as carriers for delivery of peptides and proteins with particular emphasis on design of delivery systems for 'Zoladex'.

RATIONALE

The advent of many clinically useful peptides such as 'Zoladex' has provided renewed impetus for development of sustained—release biodegradable delivery systems. However this objective can only be achieved by recognition and resolution of a number of major problems posed by these

115

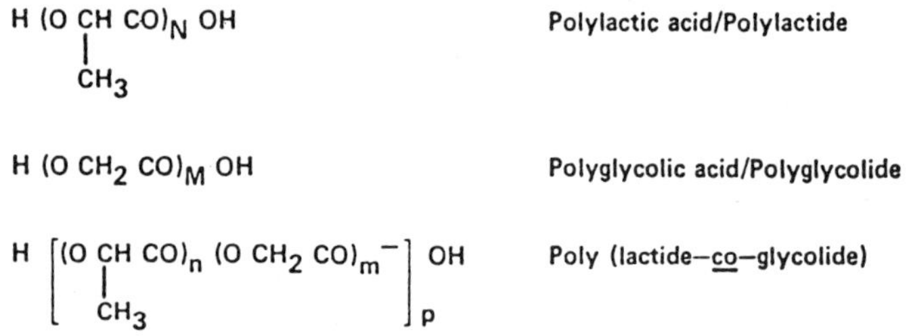

$$H\ (O\ CH\ CO)_N\ OH$$
$$\quad\ \ \ \ \ \ \ \ |$$
$$\quad\ \ \ \ \ \ \ CH_3$$

Polylactic acid/Polylactide

$$H\ (O\ CH_2\ CO)_M\ OH$$

Polyglycolic acid/Polyglycolide

$$H\ \left[(O\ CH\ CO)_n\ (O\ CH_2\ CO)_m{}^-\right]\ OH$$
$$\quad\ \ \ \ \ |$$
$$\quad\ \ \ \ CH_3 \qquad\qquad\qquad\ \ \ \ p$$

Poly (lactide–co–glycolide)

Fig 1.   Polymers and Copolymers of Lactic and Glycolic Acids

macromolecular drugs. Firstly, the mechanism most commonly used to achieve sustained release, namely controlled diffusion through a matrix or membrane, may not be appropriate for a high molecular weight polypeptide. Design of a sustained–release dosage form must take into account both the properties of the rate–controlling polymer and the drug. For diffusion of the drug through the polymer to occur it must have some limited solubility in the polymer; this is often the case with low molecular weight drugs. In contrast (Bohn, 1975) it is well established that, in the absence of specific interactions, polypeptides will either be insoluble in, or incompatible with, any polymer such as polyester, which has a totally dissimilar structure, because of entropic and enthalpic factors. Consequently, low or negligible solubility of the macromolecular drug in a polymer, such as a polyester, will prevent diffusional transport of the agent through the polymer. With regard to the properties of the drug the most important of these are its size, shape and solubility. There is an approximate log–log correlation between molecular weight (M) and diffusion coefficient (D):

$$\log D = a - b\ \log M$$

such that D decreases as the molecular weight increases. For polypeptides M is large and the diffusion coefficient becomes vanishingly small because the diffusant cannot be accommodated by the free volume of polymer arising from translational segmental movement. Consequently polymers such as polyesters, are not likely to allow partition–dependent diffusion of polypeptides to occur.

Secondly, peptides are biologically labile and can be readily degraded by tissue enzymes. They must, therefore, be effectively protected at the depot site if active drug is to released continuously. The difficulty of achieving this is emphasised by the fact that synthetic polypeptides have actually been used as biodegradable carriers for drugs such as steroids and narcotic antagonists (Mitra et al., 1979; Sidman et al., 1981).

Thirdly, excipients used to achieve sustained release of macromolecular drugs might provoke an adjuvant induced immunological response, which may be related to the nature of the excipient, the delivery rate, or profile of release. Finally, long–lasting depots might become encapsulated by fibrous tissue, thus inhibiting further release of drug. This is certainly the case for non–degradable silicone implants.

These imposing problems opposite sustained polypeptide delivery have been resolved by the design of biodegradable delivery systems based on polyesters such as poly (d,1–lactide) and poly (d,1–lactide–co–glycolide) to give formulations which allow continuous release of polypeptides over an extended period time. Although emphasis is focused on the LHRH analogue, 'Zoladex', it has been shown that the technology can also be applied to high molecular weight polypeptides.

LACTIC/GLYCOLIC ACID POLYMERS

These simple biodegradable homopolymers and copolymers were prepared at elevated temperature by the ring—opening polymerisation of dry, freshly prepared acid dimers, d,l—lactide and glycolide, by using organo—tin compounds as catalysts. Control of molecular weight was achieved by using a chain transfer agent such as d,l—lactic acid. In this way polymers of variable composition, having intrinsic viscosities in chloroform at 25°C ranging from 0.1 to >1, can be prepared. The polymers can be further characterised by size exclusion chromatography relative to polystyrene standards to define number average molecular weight (Mn), weight average molecular weight (Mw) and polydispersity (Mw/Mn), and additionally by ^{13}C n.m.r. to define the distribution of co—monomers and polymer structure.

Degradation studies on poly (d,l—lactide—co—glycolide)

Because polypeptides have high molecular weight and are water soluble their release from these polyesters by classical partition—dependent diffusion is unlikely to occur. Consequently degradation of the poly (d,l— lactide) or poly (d,l—lactide—co—glycolide) will be a critical factor in determining transport of the high molecular weight polypeptide from the dosage form. Therefore the degradation of these polymers in the absence of drug has been characterised in terms of molecular weight and its distribution, weight loss, water uptake and morphology of the hydrated and degraded polymer.

Degradation of the polymer _in vitro_ in pH 7.4 buffer results in progressive changes in molecular weight and molecular weight distribution. Under these conditions degradation is not enzyme mediated and must occur by simple hydrolytic cleavage of ester groups, and the profile of weight loss, and change in molecular weight are consistent with this. High molecular weight polymers degrade to lower molecular weights, as measured by viscosity, yet retain their water insolubility. Only after an extended time of degradation does any weight loss occur. In contrast very low molecular weight polymers can degrade with weight loss immediately. Similar results are obtained with high lactide containing polymers except that the time scale of events is more extended for these more hydrolytically stable polymers. These results are consistent with bulk hydrolysis in the _in vitro_ condition and correlates broadly with degradation of these polymers _in vivo_ suggesting that even in subcutaneous tissue enzyme mediated degradation is significantly less important than simple hydrolysis. In this event polylactides could effectively protect polypeptides at the depot site from the influence of degradative enzymes.

For these degradation experiments if the logarithm of the number average molecular weight is plotted as a function of time then for high molecular weight polymers an essentially linear relationship is seen to hold except at extended times of degradation where a discontinuity arises [Fig 2].

Other workers studying poly (d,l—lactide) have seen a similar behaviour (Pitt and Schindler, 1980) but have ignored the nature of, and reasons for, the discontinuity. In fact this arises because of water—uptake by the degrading polymer. For an amorphous polyester, water—uptake will be governed, empirically, by the intrinsic hydrophilicity of the repeat units and by end group effects. For these polyesters the end groups are alkoxylic and carboxylic and these increase as molecular weight falls. That is as degradation proceeds the essentially hydrophobic polymer becomes more hydrophilic.

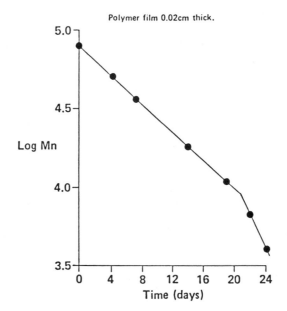

Fig 2.   In vitro Degradation of Poly (d,1—lactide—co—glycolide)
           at 37°C in pH 7.4 Buffer

Thus hydrolytic degradation is characterised by reduction in molecular
weight, enhanced water—uptake and ultimately weight loss of polymer. All
these events occur at a temperature which is below or near to the glass
transition temperature of the polyester. This in turn implies that
morphological changes are likely to occur within the polymer whilst
hydrolysis is occurring. This is confirmed by scanning electron—microscopy
of the degraded products which shows the development of porosity within the
degrading polyester.

These studies have shown that degradation of poly (d,1—lactide) and
poly (d,1— lactide—co—glycolide) is dependent on molecular weight,
polydispersity, geometry, polymer composition and polymer structure and
ultimately leads to enhanced water uptake and the generation of porosity.

Thus water soluble polypeptides may be released from these
biodegradable polyesters since enhanced water uptake and the generation of
porosity should facilitate transport of polypeptide from the dosage form.
This is likely to involve diffusion through aqueous pores generated in the
drug polymer matrix. In this event the release of polypeptide will differ
mechanistically from the processes thought to occur during release of
steroids, narcotic antagonists and antimalarials from poly (d,1—lactide) and
poly (d,1—lactide—co—glycolide) (Wise et al., 1979). Whereas these low
molecular weight drugs will diffuse, by simple partition dependent
diffusion, through intact polymer membrane in diffusion cell experiments
these same polymer membranes are totally impermeable to polypeptides.

Release studies with 'Zoladex'

Chronic administration of LH—RH analogues, such as 'Zoladex' [Fig 3]
has been shown to cause a reversible chemical castration which leads to
regression of hormone responsive animal and human mammary and prostate
tumours.

┌ Glu - His - Trp - Ser - Tyr - Gly - Leu - Arg - Pro - Gly - NH$_2$

LH-RH

┌ Glu - His - Trp - Ser - Tyr - D-Ser (Bu^t) - Leu - Arg - Pro - Azgly - NH$_2$

Zoladex ICI 118,630

Fig 3. Structures of LH—RH and 'Zoladex'

Because of low oral potency the drugs have usually been administered one or more times daily. A biodegradable formulation, based on poly (lactide—co—glycolide), either as a subdermal depot or an injectable suspension, which will deliver the drug over a period of 28 days or even longer, would be more clinically acceptable. Research was focused on 'Zoladex' (molecular weight 1269) from implants because this was thought more likely to afford a clearer understanding of the physicochemical parameters which allow transport of drug from the dosage form. In this respect 'Zoladex' is a particularly useful drug as studies both in vitro and in vivo can be undertaken. In the in vitro situation absorption of the drug into an external aqueous medium can be measured by high performance liquid chromatographic analysis of the aqueous phase to give a quantitative measure of the amount released.

Continuous release of the polypeptide in vivo can be measured qualitatively by the biological effect elicited in regularly cycling adult female rats. Normally these rats have an oestrus cycle of 4 days and the occurrence of oestrus is indicated by the presence of cornified cells in vaginal smears. In rats given subdermal implants of 'Zoladex' release of drug at an effective rate will cause a fall in circulating oestrogens, which in turn leads to a suppression of oestrus and absence of cornified smears. Rats therefore show an extended period of dioestrus.

On the basis of degradation studies, transport of drug from these depots is likely to be governed by various properties of the rate controlling polyester. These properties include polymer composition, molecular weight and distribution, level of drug incorporation, morphology of the drug/polymer mixture, degradation characteristics of the polymer and geometry. It can be shown that release of polypeptide from these biodegradable polyesters occurs by diffusion through aqueous pores generated in the dosage form. These aqueous channels, which facilitate drug release are generated by two distinct and separate mechanisms. The first involves leaching of drug from polypeptide domains at or near the surface of the delivery system and essentially is a dissolution/diffusion controlled event. However drug within the body of the implant, existing in isolated domains not continuous or contiguous to the surface cannot be released until the second mechanism becomes operative. This second mechanism involves degradation of the polyester and is associated with the generation of microporosity in, and enhanced water uptake by, the degrading polymer.

Typical parameters controlling the initial phase of release are, for example, drug loading and geometry whereas the second phase is intrinsically related to the degradation properties of the polyester. When these two phases of release do not overlap discontinuous release is observed [Fig 4 (a)].

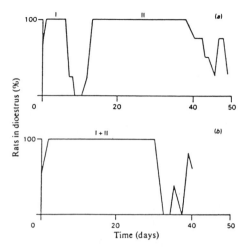

Fig 4.   Effect of Subdermal Depots Containing 300 μg of 'Zoladex'
Administered to Regularly Cycling Female Rats

(a) Depots containing 3% (w/w) 'Zoladex' in high molecular
weight polymer. (b) Depots containing 20% (w/w) 'Zoladex'
in low molecular weight polymer. I, Initial release due to
leaching from the surface; II, Degradation—induced phase.

However by controlling the properties of the polymer the initial phase
of release can be made to overlap with the second phase and depots can be
defined which give continuous release over 28 days both in vivo and in vitro
[Fig 4   ]. These depots have been used to induce a castration like effect
in rats and thereby to inhibit growth of mammary and prostate tumours (Furr
and Hutchinson, 1985).

The effect of a single subcutaneous depot containing 500 μg 'Zoladex'
on the growth of rat dimethyl benzanthracene—induced mammary tumours is
shown in Fig 5. This experiment is a model for advanced mammary cancer and
in control animals given placebo depots tumours have doubled in size in 4
weeks. In contrast tumours regress markedly in rats given the single depot.

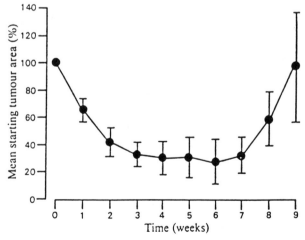

Fig 5.   Effect of a Single Subcutaneous Depot Containing 500 μg
of 'Zoladex' on the Growth of Rat Dimethylbenzanthracene—
Induced Mammary Tumours

If rats are given depots at the start of the experiment and then at weeks 4, and 8 a far more profound regression occurs [Fig 6]. By week 11 none of the tumours present at the start of the experiment are palpable. As the effect of the final depot wears off, around week 16, recovery in growth of the tumours occurs.

These depots are equally effective in animal models for prostate carcinoma. Single depots containing 1 mg 'Zoladex' given every 28 days to male rats bearing hormone—responsive Dunning R3327, transplantable prostate tumours similarly cause a marked inhibition of tumour growth. Surgical orchidectomy is a treatment for cancer of the prostate as the tumour is androgen dependent. Chemical castration using 'Zoladex' depots is shown in this animal model to cause a marked inhibition of tumour growth to values indistinguishable from those in surgically castrated animals [Fig 7].

These promising results achieved in animal studies have now been substantiated in clinical trials in patients suffering from prostatic carcinoma (Walker et al., 1984; Robinson et al., 1985).

CONCLUSION

These results indicate that by appropriate design of the carrier polymer and studies in polymer and materials science continuous sustained release of polypeptides can be achieved. Although this presentation has concentrated on 'Zoladex' it has been shown that the technology can be equally applied to other peptides with a range of molecular weights (Hutchinson, 1982; Hutchinson and Furr, 1985).

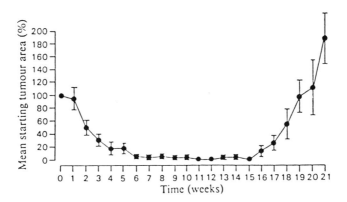

Values shown are means ± S.E.M.

Fig 6.   Effect of a Single Subcutaneous Depot Containing 500 µg of 'Zoladex' Given at Weeks 0, 4 and 8 on the Growth of Rat Dimethylbenzanthracene—Induced Mammary tumours

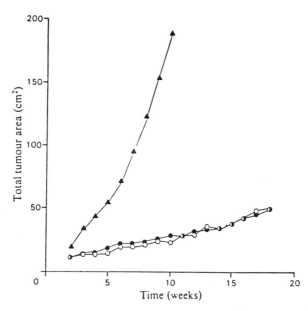

Treatment groups are placebo controls (Δ; 13 rats);
'Zoladex' (0; 12 rats) and surgically castrated
animals (0; 13 rats).

Fig 7.   Effects of a Single Subcutaneous Depot Containing 1 mg of
'Zoladex' Given Every 4 Weeks on the Growth of Hormonal—
Responsive, Transplantable, Dunning R3327, Prostate Tumours

REFERENCES

Bohn, L., 1975, Compatible polymers, in: "Polymer Handbook", 2nd Ed., J.
    Brandrup and E.H. Immergut, eds., John Wiley and Sons, New York.
Furr, B.J.A. and Hutchinson, F.G., 1985, Biodegradable sustained release
    formulations of the LH-RH analogue 'Zoladex' for the treatment of
    hormone responsive tumours. "EORTC Genitourinary Group Monograph 2,
    Part A: Therapeutic principles in metastatic prostate cancer", Alan
    R. Liss, Inc.
Hutchinson, F.G., 1982, Continuous release pharmaceutical composition.
    European Patent Application 58481.
Hutchinson, F.G. and Furr, B.J.A., 1985, Biodegradable polymers for the
    sustained release of peptides, Biochemical Society Transactions,
    13:520.
Mitra, S., Van Dress, M., Anderson, J.M., Peterson, R.V., Gregonis, D.
    and Feijen, J., 1979, Pro-drug controlled release from poly
    glutamic acid, Polymer Preparations, American Chemical Society,
    Division Polymer Chemistry, 20:32.
Pitt, C.G. and Schindler, A., 1980, The design of controlled drug deliv-
    ery systems based on biodegradable polymers, in: "Progress in con-
    traceptive delivery systems", E.S.E. Hafez and W.A.A. van Os, eds.,
    MTP Press, Lancaster.
Robinson, M.R.G., Denis, L., Mahler, C., Walker, K., Stitch, R. and
    Lunglmayr, G., 1985, An LH-RH analogue ('Zoladex') in the manage-
    ment of carcinoma of the prostate: a preliminary report comparing
    daily subcutaneous injections with monthly injections. Eur. J.
    Surg. Oncol. 11:159.

Sidman, K.R., Schwope, A.D., Steber, W.D. and Rudolph, S.E., 1981, Use of synthetic polypeptides in the preparation of biodegradable delivery systems for narcotic antagonists. <u>NIDA Research Monographs</u>, 28:214.
Walker, K.J., Turkes, A.O., Zwink, R., Beacock, C., Buck, A.C., Peeling, W.B. and Griffiths, K., 1984, Treatment of patients with advanced cancer of the prostate using a slow-release (depot) formulation of the LH-RH agonist ICI 118630. <u>J. Endocrinol.</u> 103:R1.
Wise, D.L., Fellman, T.D., Sanderson, J.E. and Wentworth, R.L., 1979, Lactic/glycolic acid polymers. <u>in</u>: "Drug carriers in biology and medicine", G. Gregoriadis, eds, Academic Press, London.

CONTROLLED DELIVERY OF NAFARELIN, AN AGONISTIC ANALOGUE OF LHRH, FROM MICROSPHERES OF POLY (D, L LACTIC-CO-GLYCOLIC) ACID

Lynda M. Sanders, Karen M. Vitale, Georgia I. Mc Rae
and Peter B. Mishky

Syntex Research
Palo Alto, CA

INTRODUCTION

The present rapid expansion of activity in development of peptide and protein drug compounds has provided a major thrust for development of novel technology for their delivery. These compounds have typically very low oral bioavailability (although this elusive goal is sufficiently attractive for it to remain an active area of exploration).

Nasal delivery has been shown, in general, to be a viable though somewhat inefficient means of administration of peptides, but is limited in being feasible only for compounds of relatively high potency. It has proven to be an effective means of delivery of the highly potent LHRH agonist nafarelin (Anik et al, 1984; Anik et al, 1986) but has not proven useful for other compounds of lower potency. Other routes, such as rectal or vaginal, may also have some utility. Nonetheless, the initial and perhaps primary dosage form for study of a novel peptide will undoubtedly remain the simple injectable solution. The dosage form of greatest ultimate practicality and utility will probably, however, be a long term controlled release parenteral system, allowing continuous controlled delivery of the compound for an extended period following a single administration.

To this end, nafarelin ([D[Nal(2)^6]LHRH) has been prepared as a controlled release injectable system (CRI) by microencapsulation in poly (d,l lactic-co-glycolic) acid (PLGA). The nature of the compound is such that this is readily feasible: it is a highly potent compound by virtue of its physiologic and metabolic profile, having a plasma $t_{1/2}$ of 5-7 times that of natural LHRH. 0.4 µg/day is sufficient to maintain suppression of estrus in the female rat (Sanders et al, 1984) and 5 µg/day has been reported to inhibit ovulation in the female rhesus monkey (Vickery and McRae, 1984). In an ongoing Phase III study, nasal administration of a dose as low as 300 µg. of nafarelin has achieved and is maintaining castrate levels of testosterone in prostatic cancer patients within 4 weeks of starting treatment (Hoffman et al, 1986). Potency of this level is mandatory to provide a controlled release delivery system of sufficiently low mass for pharmaceutical elegance and ease of administration. Nafarelin is relatively stable both chemically and physically: as a decapeptide it has no secondary or tertiary structure which would render it conformationally delicate, and it is stable to the microencapsulation process. The compound has a high thera-peutic ratio, again a necessity for this type of delivery system, and it has suitable physiochemical properties, including water solubility, to permit microencapsulation in PLGA.

The advantages of a controlled release injectable system are manifold, and include elimination of patient compliance as a variable in therapy, feasibility of treatment of pediatric or geriatric patients to whom other means of delivery would not be practicable, and greater efficiency of use of the compound. The use of a truly injectable system, which may be administered intramuscularly, has significant advantages over the alternative of a single unit monolithic subcutaneous implant, which prompted the development of microencapsulation technology for this compound.

EXPERIMENTAL

Preparation of Microspheres

Nafarelin has been microencapsulated in PLGA by a phase separation procedure. (Sanders, et al, 1984; Kent, et al, 1984) (Figure 1) An aqueous solution of nafarelin was co-emulsified with a non-aqueous solution of the PLGA, with high speed stirring. When the emulsion was well formed, a non-solvent for the polymer was pumped in, which caused the PLGA to precipitate out around the aqueous droplets, forming a suspension of semi-formed microspheres. This was then added to a larger volume of a hardening non-solvent, and the resulting microspheres collected on a filter, rinsed with an aqueous surfactant wash to impart good dry handling properties, and dried in vacuo. The process variables are determined by the physio-chemical properties of the PLGA, i.e. its composition and molecular weight profile, and by the loading level of nafarelin required, and may be adjusted to produce a good quality fairly monodisperse product in the preferred size range for optimum handling and injectability of 20-50 μm (Figure 2). Loading levels of up to 10% nafarelin have thus been achieved. The microspheres are stored under dry conditions, since PLGA is hydrolytically labile. A suspension that is readily injectable through an 18 G needle, the preferred size for intramuscular injection, may be prepared immediately before use by agitation of the microspheres with an aqueous vehicle.

The method of choice of sterilization of this system is gamma irradiation, since conventional autoclaving or dry heat sterilization will cause catastrophic degradation of the system, and other methods (such as ethylene oxide) are similarly unsuitable. Gamma irradiation decreases the molecular weight of the polymer by an appreciable amount, and it is important that this variable be accounted for in selection of the initial molecular weight of the polymer. In the rat, for example, exposure to nafarelin/PLGA microspheres to 3.3 Mrad of gamma irradiation diminished the overall duration of biological effect from 86 days to 63 days, (Sanders, et al, 1984) and even at more realistic doses (2.5 Mrad being an industry standard) the effects are proportionally reduced but not negligible.

In vitro Evaluation of Release Profile on Nafarelin

The challenges of developing an in vitro system for a controlled release product such as this are far from trivial. The ideal would provide an accelerated release with close in vivo correlation, but this is probably an unrealistic goal. One issue of practicality raised here is the need or feasibility of a routine in vitro quality control test: as the intended duration of compound release increases, the feasibility of such a test diminishes.

The in vitro release medium developed for this system comprised an ethanolic phosphate buffer of pH 7.4, in which the microspheres were agitated under mild standardized conditions. This met several significant criteria:

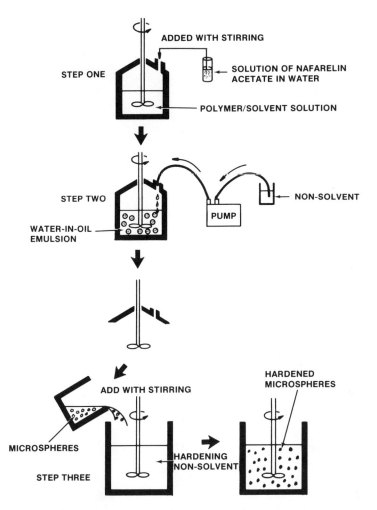

Fig. 1. Phase Separation Microencapsulation of Nafarelin
Acetate

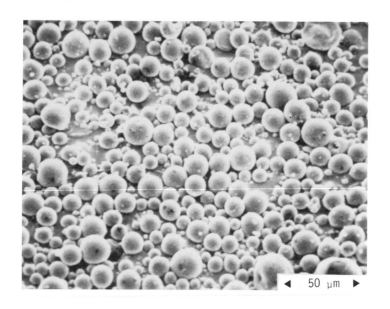

◄ 50 μm ►

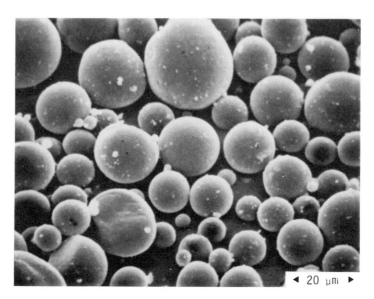

◄ 20 μm ►

Fig. 2. Microspheres of Nafarelin in PLGA

the ethanolic component .inhibited peptide degradation caused by bacterial growth, and also plasticized the polymer, reducing Tg to below 37° C. This simulated a similar phenomenon observed in vivo, in which plasticization was presumably induced by endogenous lipid components of the subcutaneous fluid. It has been observed that in a non-plasticizing buffer the degradation rate of poly (lactic) acid was two to six times less than in plasma (Mason et al, 1981), but that the addition of a plasticizer accelerated in vitro degradation. The aqueous phosphate component was at the physiological pH of 7.4, and was isotonic to simulate any osmotic effects occurring in vivo. The release rates to be quantified are low, corresponding to the high potency of the compound, and loss of material by adsorption to glass can be a significant problem in this situation. Although serum albumin and gelatin are commonly used as a competitive inhibitor of glass adsorption, it has been shown, at lease for nafarelin, that phosphate salts offer superior inhibition (Anik and Hwang, 1983) and were for this reason selected as buffering and absorption reducing agent. The composite medium provided a solubility of nafarelin of greater than 1 mg/ml, which was sufficient to maintain sink conditions.

In vivo Evaluation of Release Profile of Nafarelin

In the female rat, duration of suppression of estrus cyclicity following a single subcutaneous injection of microspheres provided information on the time for which release of nafarelin is equal to or exceeds 0.4 µg/day. In the primate, including man, plasma level determinations by radioimmunoassay provided data on release profiles of the compound, and levels of gonadotropins and estradiol, progesterone and testosterone have also been measured.

RESULTS AND DISCUSSION

Mechanism of Compound Release

It has been shown that PLGA erodes in bulk, or homogeneously, rather than superficially, or heterogeneously (Sanders, et al, 1984). A hydrophlilic compound of molecular size as large as nafarelin (1322 Daltons) has low diffusivity through intact PLGA, although one invariably observes a relatively brief phase of diffusional release, presumably from the superficial region of the microspheres. This is well illustrated by the performance in the rat of nafarelin/PLGA microspheres prepared with a 69:31 copolymer (Figure 3a). Following this primary phase, there follows a secondary phase of lower release rate, in which it may be envisaged the polymer is hydrolyzing en mass and diminishing in molecular weight. There will be insufficient gross erosion to promote release of compound during this time. When a critical molecular weight profile is reached (which will probably vary with composition of the polymer) the polymer degradation products will be sufficiently small to have significant water solubility, and erosion and consequently release of nafarelin will again be promoted, as illustrated in Figure 3a. Adjustment of the monomer ratio to a more hydrophilic 50:50 lactide: glycolide ratio resulted in the expected acceleration of point of onset of the third phase, with partial overlap of the first and third phases of efficacy (Figure 3b), and subsequent reduction of molecular weight from an intrinsic viscosity of 1.52 dl/g to 0.38 dl/g produced a further reduction in total duration of effect, and complete continuity of efficacy, (Figure 3c).

It will be appreciated that the system does not inherently provide zero order release, and the appropriate system variables require adjustment to give suitable duration and kinetics of compound release. Since release of compound is primarily erosion controlled by homogeneous degradation, size of microspheres (or surface area) would not be anticipated to be a critical system variable. This has been confirmed in the rat model (Sanders, et al, 1984).

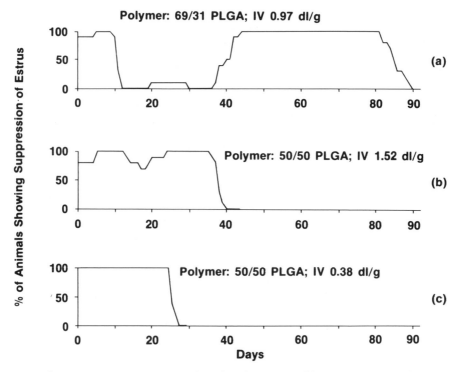

*Fig. 3.   Estrus Suppression in the Rat Following Single s/c
Injection of 300µg Nafarelin in PLGA Microspheres*

There has been a degree of controversy amongst workers in the field on
the correct description of the release mechanism described. It poses a
number of unique points: the compound is of large molecular size and is
hydrophilic, and bears little similarity to similar systems containing
steroids such as norethisterone (Beck, et al, 1983) and progesterone (Beck,
et al, 1979) in which diffusional release is predominant, either through the
intact polymer or by a 'matrix leaching' mechanism from channels created
within the polymer/compound matrix. This latter phenomenon occurs only with
relatively high loading levels of the soluble included compound, another
notable point of difference between steroid systems of high loading and the
nafarelin system of lower loading. Nonetheless, release of compound in the
primary phase is clearly diffusional, and release in the erosional tertiary
phase will be in the final analysis by diffusion of the degradation products
of the polymer, and of the nafarelin, from the disintegrating matrix (of
complex kinetics, since the matrix will present a diffusional resistance
decreasing with time). Even so, although release in the tertiary phase is
diffusional, it is not diffusion controlled, since the data clearly indicate
that polymer erosion is a rate-limiting necessary event preceding the release
of compound, and the system may therefore be accurately described as being
erosion controlled.

Physiological Properties Conferred By Continuous Release

Nafarelin has been well characterized as an agonistic LHRH analogue
(Vickery, 1986) by studies in primates including man, using
conventional means of administration such as a daily injectable solution.
It is thus established that the male cynomolgus is an unusually insensitive
specie, doses as high as 1 mg/day of nafarelin being insufficient to
suppress testosterone levels. Similarly in the female rhesus, doses of
nafarelin sufficient to prevent ovulation do not suppress circulating levels
of LH and FSH. These physiological parameters are more profoundly influenced
by continuous as opposed to intermittent delivery of nafarelin. For example,
Figure 4 illustrates plasma profiles of nafarelin in the male cynomolgus
following administration of a single i/m dose of PLGA microspheres containing
3.7 mg. nafarelin. The profile indicates the majority of compound release to
be in the latter phases of the system, with a relatively abrupt termination
of release. The levels of testosterone in 50% of the animals studied,
however, were unexpectedly dramatically suppressed after the initial agonistic stimulatory response. As here illustrated, suppression was maintained
for a period of time consistent with circulating plasma levels of nafarelin.
This was particularly surprising in light of the relative daily doses administered: 1 mg/day by daily injection failed to suppress testosterone in all
animals, whereas 3.7 mg over about 60 days, equivalent to about 60 µg/day,
when given by CRI, suppressed testosterone in 50% of the animals. There
appears to be a significant potency difference provided by the two means of
administration, to the point of providing qualitatively different pharmacological effects.

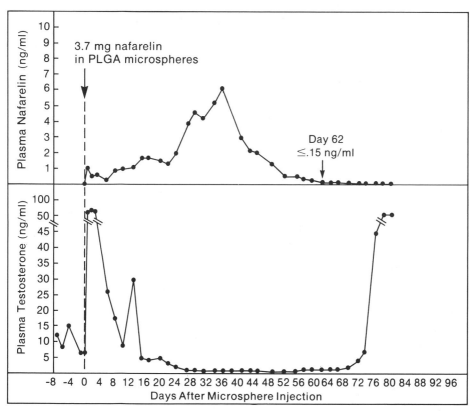

Fig. 4.   Plasma Levels of Nafarelin and Testosterone in the Male
Cynomolgus Monkey following single i/m Injection of
Nafarelin in PLGA Microspheres

A comparable phenomenon has been observed in the female rhesus (Figure 5) in which a dose of 3 mg. of nafarelin administered by CRI provided plasma levels of compound sufficient to delay ovulation (indicated by a progesterone surge) for a time consistent with circulating levels of compound. However, levels of LH and FSH are also suppressed for a similar length of time, a phenomenon again unique to the mode of delivery.

Influence of Loading Level of Compound

There are obvious clear advantages to maximizing the loading level of nafarelin in the CRI, within limits of practicality. A higher loading system would allow administration of a corresponding lower total dose of microspheres for a given compound dose, with consequent advantage in elegance of

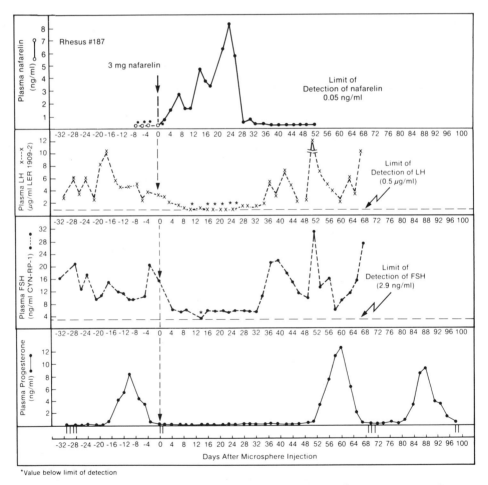

*Value below limit of detection

Fig. 5. *Plasma Levels of Nafarelin, LH, FSH and Progesterone in the Female Rhesus Monkey Following Administration of Nafarelin in PLGA Microspheres*

the system. Practical considerations such as scale up of the microencapsulation process are also of lower magnitude at a higher loading level, since a
given batch size will provide a number of therapeutic doses directly proportional to the loading level of the system. However, one would anticipate
some change in release kinetics with change in loading level. In particular,
the initial diffusional release would be expected to become more pronounced,
at partial expense of either the magnitude of the tertiary phase or the total
duration of release, or both.

Microspheres containing 2%, 4% and 8% nafarelin, prepared by
appropriate modification of the manufacturing process were administered to
male rhesus monkeys by single i/m injection of 3 mg. nafarelin. The plasma
profiles provided by these animals are illustrated in Figure 6. It may be
seen that with increase in loading level there is a clear trend to decrease
in duration of release, (Figure 7) and to increase in magnitude of the
primary diffusional phase. There is also an apparent increase in total bioavailability of compound, as indicated by area under the curve, an unexpected
phenomenon in light of the linear pharmacokinetics of nafarelin.

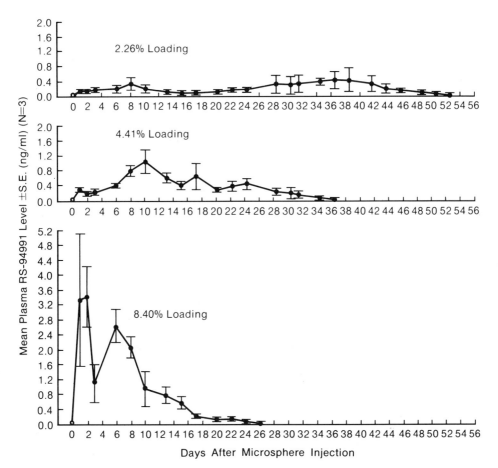

*Fig. 6. Effect of Loading Level of Nafarelin in PLGA Microspheres
on Plasma Profile of Compound in the Male Rhesus Monkey*

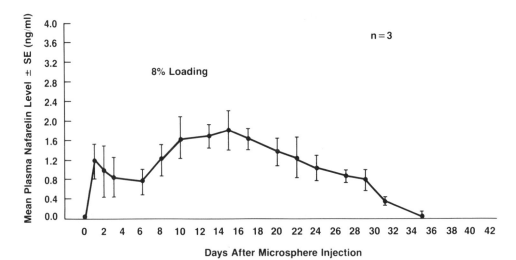

Fig. 7. Correlation of Loading Level of Nafarelin and Duration of Detectable Plasma Levels in the Male Rhesus Monkey

Similar nafarelin/PLGA microspheres containing 8% compound, when administered to male cynomolgus monkeys at a dose of 3 mg, provide significantly more linear release kinetics and a somewhat longer overall duration of release (33 days vs. 26 days in the rhesus). (Figure 8) This interspecies variation has been observed in previous studies, and poses problems in extrapolating data to the clinical situation. The reasons for the differences are not obvious: one may speculate on different endogenous lipid profiles plasticizing the PLGA to different extents, or on different degrees of fibrin deposition, a phenomenon known to occur in vivo (Sanders, et al, 1985) or upon different degrees of encapsulation. This latter effect may inhibit influx of fluids to the system or efflux of products, with con-sequent change in pH of the local environment and effect upon hydrolysis kinetics of the polymer. These considerations remain presumptive however. The system is complex and requires clinical characterization for a full understanding of its properties and potential.

In Vitro Release Profiles: Significance and In vivo Comparison

Figure 9 illustrates in vitro release of nafarelin from PLGA microspheres containing 2.3%, 4.4% and 9.2% of the compound. As seen in the in vivo situation, the release of compound in the primary diffusional phase is directly related to loading level. All those systems provide a pronounced and discrete secondary phase, during which there is minimal release of compound, in contrast to he good continuity of release seen in vivo. The point of onset and time to peak level of the tertiary erosional phase in vitro appear to increase with loading level of nafarelin, contrary to expectations. The total duration of release is about 50 d., somewhat more prolonged than that seen in vivo, and of a similar duration of each system.

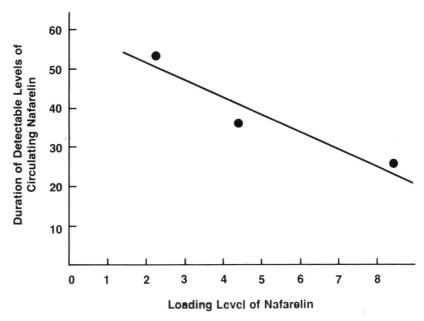

Fig. 8. Mean Plasma Levels of Nafarelin for Three Male Cynomolgus Monkeys Each Receiving a Single I/M Injection of 3 mg Nafarelin Microencapsulated in PLGA at a Level of 8%

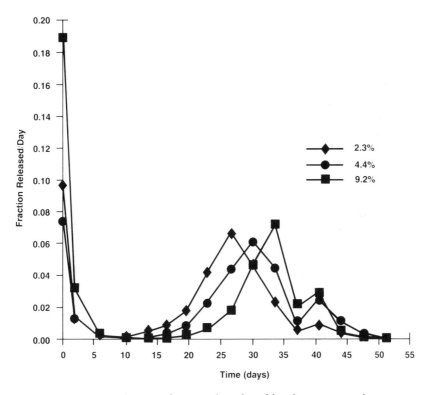

Fig. 9. In Vitro Release of Nafarelin from PLGA Microspheres: Comparison of Loading Levels

The differences in times to peak of the tertiary erosional phase for the three loading levels cannot be concluded from this study to be significant, without further data to interpolate between the critical points. Other similar studies suggest that the times to peak are indeed very close irrespective of loading level, although the relatively large differences seen in the primary phase have been observed to be very consistent between studies.

The in vitro release profiles bear comparison in some respects with the in vivo profiles, but insufficiently closely for in vitro data to be a good predictor of in vivo performance. The in vitro system is the more simple and is useful both in studying the effect of formulation parameters on compound release without compounding biological variability, and for evaluating the relative quality of different batches of the product. It does have limitations, and it will probably not prove possible to simulate the complex in vivo environment with an in vitro system. For a preparation such as this, in which there is even species variation in vivo, an in vitro system should be viewed as being no more than a model system, with utility only a sentensive as described.

Conclusions

It is clear that nafarelin microencapsulated in PLGA provides a very convenient and elegant means of continuous controlled delivery of the compound. The parameters influencing linearity of compound release have been elucidated and optimized, and significant differences in pharmacolgical properties dependant upon the mode of delivery of the compound, i.e., intermittent vs. continuous, identified. This particular phenomenon poses questions in the developmental strategy of a system such as this. It would seem to be invariably appropriate to characterize the basic biological properties of the compound prior to initiating development of a CRI, a far from trivial undertaking. This initial characterization, or even candidate drug screening, has traditionally been accomplished by use of a simple injectable solution, typically in buffered saline or a similar vehicle. The decision to carry the compound to further development, including feasibility studies on a CRI, will be based on the data thus generated. However, when prototype CRI systems are developed and tested, it may well become apparent, as with nafarelin, that the potency and/or qualitative pharmacological profile, are different when the compound is delivered by this means. It is possible that a compound very viable as a drug candidate when delivered appropriately may well not be selected from simple screening studies. Nonetheless, it is not possible to justify development of a CRI without some prior knowledge of the in vivo properties of the compound. This circular problem has no definitive resolution. It is probably an issue primarily for compounds acting on receptors that are sensitive to intermittent, or pulsed, exposure to an endogenenous compound, which is being observed with increasing frequency as the realm of peptide and protein drug compounds expands. In such cases, it would be worthwhile to be aware of the potential issue, and to initiate studies with an experimental delivery device (e.g. a continuous delivery pump) as early in the program as realistically feasible.

The development of systems such as nafarelin CRI demand skills beyond those traditionally encountered in dosage form design. They require expertise in such areas as polymer chemistry and chemical engineering as well as physical chemistry, pharmaceutics and biological sciences. The continued growth in the field, spurred by the expansion in the number of peptides and proteins requiring sophisticated drug delivery and by the successes thus far achieved, will be dependant upon the convergence of creativity and perspective from these previously loosely related areas.

REFERENCES

Anik, S.T., McRae, G.I., Nerenberg, C., Worden, A., Foreman, J., Hwang, J-Y., Kushinsky, S., Jones, R.E., and Vickery, B., 1984, Nasal Absorption of Nafarelin Acetate, the Decapeptide [D-Nal(2)^6]LHRH, in Rhesus Monkeys I, J. Pharm. Sci., 73:684.

Anik, S.T., Benjamin, E.J., Maskiewicz, R., McRae, G.I., Nerenberg, C., Hwang-Felgner, J., Schneider, J., Worden, A., and Foreman, J., 1986, Nasal Absorption of Nafarelin Acetate in Rhesus Monkeys II: Effect of Formulation Variables. Manuscript in Preparation.

Anik, S.T., and Hwang, J-Y., 1983, Adsorption of D-Nal(2)^{6}LHRH, a Decapeptide, onto Glass and Other Surfaces. Int. J. Pharm., 16:81.

Beck, L.R., Pope, V.Z., Flowers, C.E. Jr., Cowsar, D.R., Tice, T.R., Lewis, D.H., Dunn, R.L., Moore, A.B., and Gilley, R.M., 1983, Poly(DL-lactide-co-glycolide)/Norethisterone Microcapsules: An Injectable Biodegradable Contraceptive, Biol. of Rep., 28:186.

Beck, L.R., Cowsar, J.R., Lewis, D.H., Cosgrove, R.J., Riddle, C.T., Lowry, S.L., and Epperly, T., 1979. A New Long-Acting Injectable Microcapsule System for the Administration of Progesterone, Fert. Ster., 31:545.

Hoffman, P.G., Henzl, M.R., Chaplin, M.D., and Nerenberg, C.A., 1986, Phase I and II Studies: Clinical Development of Nafarelin Acetate, Adv. Contracep., In Press.

Kent, J.S., Sanders, L.M., Tice, T.R., and Lewis, D.H., 1984, Microencapsulation of the Peptide Nafarelin Acetate for Controlled Release, in "Long-Acting Contraceptive Delivery Systems", G.I. Zatuchni, A. Goldsmith, J.D. Shelton, and J.D. Sciarra, eds., Harper and Row, Philadelphia.

Mason, N.S., Miles, C.S., and Sparks, R.E., 1981, Hydrolytic Degradation of Poly DL-(lactide), Polym. Sci. Technol., 14:279.

Sanders, L.M., Kent, J.S., McRae, G.I., Vickery, B.H., Tice, T.R., and Lewis, D.H., 1984, Controlled Release of a Leuteinizing Hormone - Releasing Hormone Analogue from Poly (d,l-lactide-co-glycolide) Microspheres, J. Pharm. Sci., 73:1294.

Sanders, L.M., McRae, G.I., Vitale, K.M., and Kell, B.A., Controlled Delivery of an LHRH Analogue from Biodegradable Injectable Microspheres, 1985, J. Cont. Rel., 2:187.

Vickery, B.H., and McRae, G.I., 1984, LHRH Agonists for Control of Female Fertility: Primate Studies, in: "LHRH and its Analogs. Contraceptive and Therapeutic Applications", B.H. Vickery, J.J. Nestor Jr., E.S.E. Hafez, eds., MTP Press, Lancaster.

Vickery, B.H., 1986, Comparison of the Potential for Therapeutic Utilities with GNRH Agonists and Antagonists, Endocrine Reviews, 7:115.

THE ORAL BIOAVAILABILITY OF PEPTIDES AND RELATED DRUGS

M.J. Humphrey

Department of Drug Metabolism
Pfizer Central Research,
Sandwich, Kent, U.K. CT13 9NJ

The discovery of diverse neuro- and hormonal peptides, as well as other biologically-active peptides, has prompted investigations into their therapeutic applications and to the design of peptide drugs. However a contributing factor to the therapeutic success of a drug is the availability of an oral formulation. For peptides and proteins, oral absorption and bioavailability is generally low (as shown in Table 2) relative to that expected of non-peptide drugs (for review see Humphrey & Ringrose, 1986). The purpose of this review is to describe the various barriers to, and mechanisms of absorption of peptide drugs, as well as, to discuss the relationship between physio-chemical properties and absorption (see Table 1).

For an orally administered peptide to reach its site of action it must be resistant to chemical and enzymic degradation in the gut lumen, and then, after penetration of the mucosal membrane, avoid 'first pass' metabolism and clearance by the gut mucosa and liver. Many peptides and proteins undergo degradation by the digestive enzymes and this limits their oral activity (Weidhaup, 1981), for example tetragastrin bioavailability after intraduodenal administration is markedly increased after ligation of the common bile and pancreatic duct (Jennewein, Waldeck & Konz, 1974). One approach to overcome this problem has been to devise formulations which act as carriers and/or protect the peptides from degradation, for example the co-administration of insulin with protease inhibitors (Fujii et al., 1985). However, with an increasing knowledge of peptide design, the major approach is towards the synthesis of analogs resistant to metabolism (Veber & Freidinger, 1985; Hruby, 1985).

Table 1.   Factors Affecting Extent of Peptide Absorption

Physical	Physiological
Aqueous-pH stability profile	Regional and local pH.
Molecular size and shape	Digestive enzymes
Partition coefficient	Nature of the mucosal barrier
Electrostatic cha ge	Intestinal permeability and
Formulation	binding
	Carrier-mediated transport
	Dietary factors
	Metabolism - gut and hepatic

Table 2. Gastrointestinal Absorption of Peptides and Related Drugs

Extent of Absorption	Compound	Mol. Wt.	Reference
Very low (< 2%)	tetragastrin	483	Jennewein, Waldeck & Konz, (1974)
	pepstatinyl glycine	740	Grant, Ford & McCulloch, (1982)
	cyclo-(Pro-Phe-D Trp-Lys-Thr-Phe)	806	Bell et al., (1984)
	1-deamino-8-D-arginine vasopressin	1007	Lundin & Vilhardt, (1986)
	leuprolide	1208	Okada et al., (1982)
	empedopeptin	1250	Konishi et al., (1984)
	insulin	5700	Peters & Sibbons, (1984)
	horseradish peroxidase	40,000	Peters & Sibbons, (1984)
	bovine serum albumin	> 50,000	Warshaw et al., (1974)
Low (5%)	TRH analogs	c.a. 400	Yokohama, Yoshioka & Kitamori, (1984)
	phosphonotetrapeptides	c.a. 400	Atherton et al., (1980)
	dietary tetrapeptides	c.a. 400	Adibi & Morse, (1977)
Moderate (25-50%)	alafosfalin (phosphonodipeptide)	196	Allen et al., (1979)
	dietary di- and tri- peptides	200- 300	Silk et al., (1985)
	ampicillin	349	Jones et al., (1979)
	lysinopril	405	Ulm et al., (1982)
	cyclosporin	1203	Wood et al., (1983)
High (> 50%)	aminocephalosporins	c.a. 350	Lode et al., (1979)
	enalapril (pro-drug)	377	Ulm et al., (1982)
	talampicillin (pro-drug)	482	Jones et al., (1979)

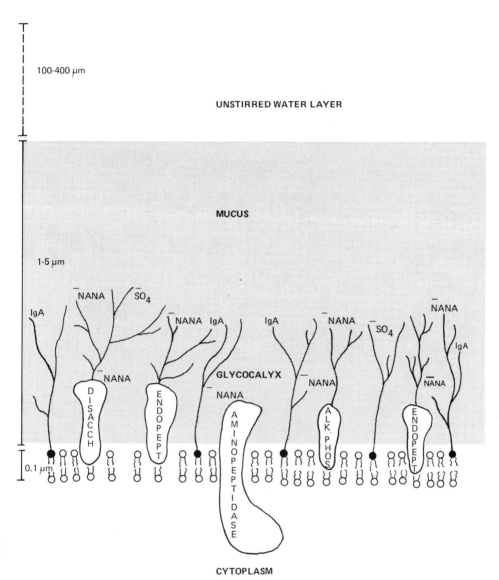

100-400 μm

UNSTIRRED WATER LAYER

MUCUS

1-5 μm

IgA $\overline{NANA}$ $\overline{SO_4}$ $\overline{NANA}$ IgA   IgA $\overline{NANA}$ $\overline{SO_4}$ $\overline{NANA}$ IgA

$\overline{NANA}$ GLYCOCALYX $\overline{NANA}$ $\overline{NANA}$

$\overline{NANA}$

DISACCH   ENDOPEPT   AMINOPEPTIDASE   ALK. PHOS.   ENDOPEPT

0.1 μm

CYTOPLASM

Figure 1.   A schematic diagram (not drawn to scale) of some of the features of the intestinal mucosal barrier. (disacch = disaccharidase; endopept. = endopeptidase; alk. phos. = alkaline phosphatase; NANA = N-acetyl neuramic acid; SO_4 = sulphated group; lgA = secreted lgA dimer).

141

The intestinal mucosa represents a complex barrier to the absorption of drugs and is depicted in Figure 1. The membrane surface of the microvillus consists of the typical trilaminar arrangement common to most biological membranes in which two molecular layers of lipid are configured with their hydrocarbon portions directed inwards while their outer hydrophilic surfaces are coated with protein. Possible modifications of this basic conformation are either when lipoproteins form the central region or where there are globular protein units embedded in the bimolecular lipid leaflet. The outer membranes of adjacent cells are fused at the basal membrane forming 'tight junctions' which form an effective barrier between intestinal lumen and the intercelluar spaces. However some spaces in the membrane are formed when cells are extruded into the intestinal lumen and may represent a major site for the absorption of drugs (salicylate and cephalexin, Yamashita et al., 1984:) via paracellular diffusion (Csaky, 1984).

An integral and dynamic part of the apical membrane is the glycocalyx, which is a uniform layer of filamentous glycoprotein (Egberts et al., 1984). The carbohydrate chains are covalently linked to the polypeptide chains in the core and contain the following monosaccharides : acetylglucosamine, acetylgalactosamine, galactose, fucose, mannose, glucose and sialic acid. This glycoprotein layer has a negative charge at physiological pH largely due to the presence of the sialic acids which always occupy a terminal position in the carbohydrate chain. Sulphation of sugars also contributes to the acidity of the glycoproteins and therefore to the negative charge of the glycocalyx.

The glycocalyx is up to 0.5um in thickness, but is less prominent over goblet cells and M-cells (Peyer's patches). Superimposed on this surface coat is the mucus layer which is an order of magnitude thicker. Some interaction of peptide molecules with the protein and mucopolysaccharides of the coat would seem inevitable, whilst the strong electronegative charge carried by the acidic microclimate is maintained within an unstirred water layer (UWL), which is much thicker (approximately 400um) than the mucus layer, and is discrete from the rest of the gut contents (Thomson & Dietschy, 1984). The movement of peptides through this unstirred layer will involve simple diffusion and can be rate-limiting to the absorption of hydrophobic molecules. For polar molecules the mucus and glycocalyx surface coat, may represent a diffusional barrier because of its viscosity and electronegative charge, (Smithson et al., 1981; Esposito et al., 1983), although there is some evidence to dispute this view (Westergaard & Dietschy, 1974).

The absorption of intact dietary peptides and peptide drugs has been reported to occur to varying extents (Gardner, 1984; Silk et al., 1985; Humphrey and Ringrose, 1986). Some of the putative routes and mechanisms of passage of peptides and proteins across the mucosal barrier are:-

1) **PARACELLULAR ROUTE** : movement between the tight junctions between cells and/or across the spaces formed when cells are extruded into the intestinal lumen.

2) **TRANSCELLULAR ROUTE** : passage through the membrane by direct permeation of the lipid layer or by channels (aqueous pores or otherwise) or pinocytosis. The latter two routes probably involving carrier-mediated transport.

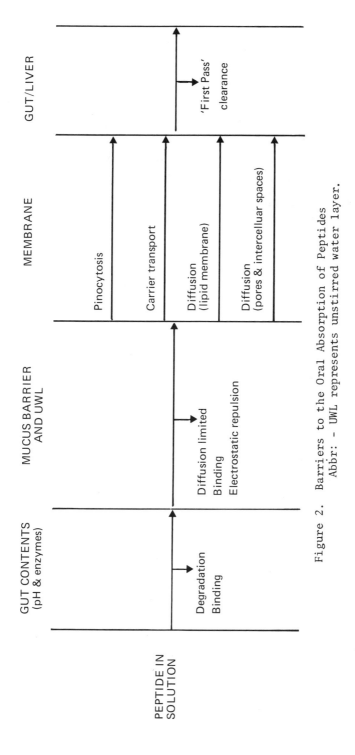

Figure 2. Barriers to the Oral Absorption of Peptides
Abbr: - UWL represents unstirred water layer.

For small peptides it is probable that the extent of absorption will involve a contribution from a number of mechanisms (see Fig. 2) all working in parallel. For instance, cephalexin absorption is believed to involve both the trans- and para-cellular routes while the direct passage of the drug through the membrane includes an involvement from a saturable transport process (Yamashita et al., 1984).

The mode of absorption of protein digestion products has been extensively reviewed and in the main is thought to involve hydrolysis of oligopeptides at the surface of the microvilli to yield amino acids, di- and tri-peptides which then undergo carrier-mediated transport. As there are some 8000 possible dietary tripeptides it has not been possible to study the absorption mechanism of each in turn. However, some guidelines for carrier-mediated transport have been reported (Matthews, 1975 and 1983). The transport processes for di- and tri-peptides are stereochemically specific; peptides of the unnatural D configuation are poorly taken up and are slowly hydrolysed. For effective recognition of the L-amino acid peptides an alpha peptide bond is preferred while substitution of either the N- or C- terminus decreases affinity for transport. Little evidence for the intact absorption of tetrapeptides has been reported, (Adibi & Morse, 1977, Burston, Taylor & Matthews, 1979, Kerchner & Geary, 1983).

Table 3   Oral Bioavailability of TRH and Analogs

COMPOUND & DOSE (mg/kg)	ABSOLUTE BIOAVAILABILITY (% dose)	
	RAT	DOG
TRH (1)		
pGlu-His-Pro-NH$_2$		
2	–	12.6
10	–	9.8
20	1.5	5.6
100	0.4	3.5
250	0.2	–
DN-1417 (2)		
carboxy-butyrolactone-His-Pro-NH$_2$		
2	–	12.0
20	1.8	15.7
100	2.0	9.3
500	3.8	–
(3)		
pGlu-L-2-pyridylalanine-Pro-NH$_2$		
40	4.0	21.1
(3)		
pGlu-D-2-pyridylalanine-Pro-NH$_2$		
40	4.2	23.6

(1) Data from Yokohama et al., (1984).
(2) Data from Yokohama, Yoshioka & Kitamori, (1984).
(3) Unpublished data, Pfizer Central Research.

Interestingly, a number of peptide drugs have been shown to be absorbed by a similar process to that reported for dietary di- and tri- peptides and include β-lactam antibiotics (Kimura et al., 1983; Nakashima et al., 1984), alafosfalin (Allen et al., 1979) and thyrotrophin-releasing hormone (TRH) (Yokohama et al., 1984). The importance of this mechanism to the absorption of TRH is illustrated by apparent saturation with increasing dose in both rat and dog (see Table 3). It is also noticeable that there is an apparent species difference in the extent of absorption; in dog absorption appears to be an order of magnitude greater than in rat. A similar species difference in the absorption of TRH analogs has also been observed (see Table 3), although the fact that the analogs containing an unnatural amino acid (D or L pyridylalanine) also show the difference suggest that it may result for some reason other than a carrier-mediated process.

It is well established that the absorption of most drugs takes place by passive diffusion though the lipid membrane and that the rate of passage is correlated to the partition coefficient of the molecule (for review see Houston and Wood, 1980). A similar situation has been observed for the peptide-like β-lactam antibiotics where a log P value between 1.9 and 3.3 was associated with good absorption (Yoshimura & Kakeya, 1983). There is, however, a notable exception with the phenylglycine analog, ampicillin, which is a polar molecule, present in zwitterionic form, showing good absorption. The favourable effects of a neutral or electropositive charge on absorption are discussed later.

The range of sizes and shapes of peptide molecules is diverse and the relevance of these properties to absorption should be discussed. The diffusion coefficient (D) and also the permeability coefficient (P) for a barrier of known thickness, decreases as the molecular weight of the solute (M) increases according to the following equation:

(1) DM^{β} = constant

The value of β is not constant and depends on the molecular weight of the diffusing compound and on the nature of the membrane or medium (Stein, 1967; Stein & Lieb, 1974). For diffusion in water β has a value of 0.5. However, for diffusion through pores, extrusion zones, lipid membranes or more viscous matrices like the mucosal barrier, molecular weight will become an increasingly important determinant of absorption i.e. β will be greater than 0.5. For a somatostatin hexapeptide analog, insulin and horseradish peroxidase with molecular weights of 806, 6000 and 40,000 respectively, absorption (0.35, 0.05 and <0.02% dose respectively) decreased in an approximately proportionate manner with increasing molecular weight (Peters & Sibbons, 1984), that is β appears to have a value of unity.

The lipid nature of the intestinal membrane must also be taken into account for more lipophilic peptides for which diffusion through the membrane is an important route. Assuming rapid equilibrium between the aqueous phase of the UWL with the lipid membrane, equation (1) can be written as follows:

(2) $\dfrac{PM^{\beta}}{q}$ = constant

where P is the permeability coefficient and q is the partition coefficient (Capraro, 1984). Thus high lipophilicity which many peptides lack, is an important determinant of permeability. Binding interactions with the mucosal layer are also important as the rate of absorption (n) is dependent on the concentration gradient according to the following equation:

$$(3) \quad n = AP (Co - Ci)$$

where A is the surface area and Co and Ci represent the concentrations of the molecule in the aqueous–membrane interface and in the cell interior respectively. Any binding to the external mucus barrier will effectively reduce Co and therefore will limit the concentration gradient and rate of absorption.

Another physico–chemical property which needs to be considered is the electrostatic charge of the molecule. It is well accepted that peptide–like molecules like the α–carboxy β–lactam antibiotics, such as carbenicillin, or the N–carboxyalkyl dipeptide inhibitors of angiotensin converting enzyme (ACE), which have two carboxylate anions at physiological pH, are poorly absorbed. For these compounds mono–esterification results in markedly improved absorption (Clayton et al., 1975; Wyvratt & Parchett, 1985). Such chemical modification will improve lipophilicity and thus absorption, but other factors like reducing the degree of electrostatic repulsion by the electronegatively charged mucosal barrier may be involved.

Some insight into the role of overall charge and conformation of the molecule on absorption of peptides can be obtained by analysis of the ACE inhibitors. Enalaprilat has poor oral activity in rat, dog and man (Tocco et al., 1982; Ulm et al., 1982), while the molecule (see Fig. 3) has a basic –NH– group and two carboxyl groups and an octanol:aqueous buffer (pH 6.5) partition coefficient of <0.01.

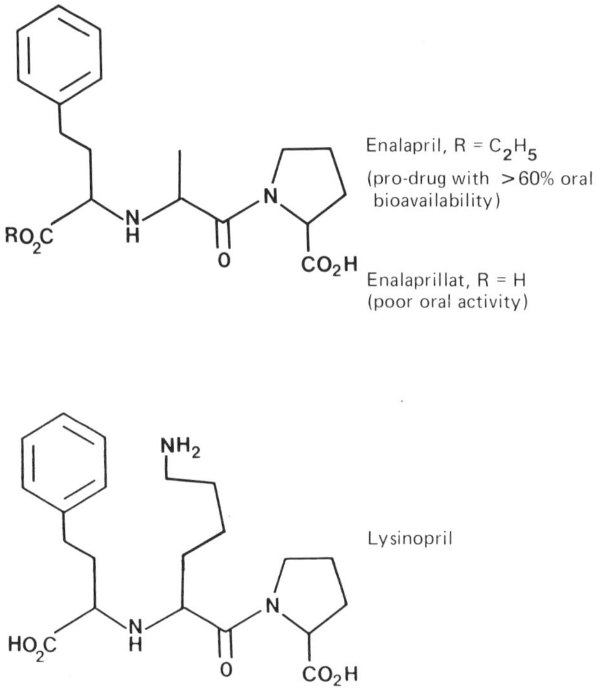

Enalapril, R = C_2H_5
(pro-drug with >60% oral bioavailability)

Enalaprillat, R = H
(poor oral activity)

Lysinopril

Figure 3.   Angiotensin Converting Enzyme Inhibitors with Good Oral Bioavailability

The mono-ethyl ester of enalaprilat (enalapril) has excellent oral activity and it is believed that the dominant effects of esterification is to lower the basicity of the -NH- group (enalapril, pKa 5.5; enalaprilat, pKa 7.6) and to remove the charge of one carboxyl, both of which should reduce overall charge and assist membrane transport (Wyvratt & Patchett, 1985). Indeed the partition coefficient (value 0.22 in octanol:aqueous buffer, pH 6.5) and absorption of enalapril is pH-dependent with maximum intestinal absorption being demonstrated in situ in the pH4-5 range (Gardner, 1985). Overall, the enalapril molecule can be considered to have a neutral charge and greater lipophilicity than the parent diacid (enalaprilat). Similarly, the lysylproline analog of the diacid (see Fig. 3 for lysinopril and enalaprilat) which is electrostatically neutral, also exhibits good absorption (Ulm et al., 1982), despite a lack of lipophilicity (partition coeffient, 0.02).

The observation in our laboratories that some structural analogs of enalapril and lysinopril, are not well absorbed, either as diacids or mono ethyl esters, is indicative that conformation of the molecule, or some other structural feature as yet not understood, is important for the absorption of these peptides.

Overall few peptide drugs seem to have the optimum lipophilicity, size/shape or electrostatic charge for good oral absorption by passive diffusion. Only di- and tri-peptides seem to have a general potential to exhibit good absorption and this sometimes involves a carrier-mediated transport process. One exception to this is cyclosporin, a cyclic undecapetide which has been shown to be up to 50% absorbed. Cyclosporin is a neutral peptide which is extremely lipophilic having an octanol:water partition coefficient of about 1000. Although lipophilicity may be an important factor in cyclosporin absorption, the compound surprisingly does not cross the lipid membrane of the blood brain barrier (Pardridge, 1985). The poor aqueous solubility of cyclosporin necessitates that a solution formulation is used for optimum absorption; the clinical drug formulation consists of olive oil : peglicol 5 oleate : ethanol (40:42:18 v/v).

Since there has only been limited success to date in designing peptide drugs with good oral absorption and activity, the possibility of using adjuvants to modify the mucosal barrier needs to be considered. It has been reported that polar drugs, and thus perhaps peptides, are more rapidly absorbed with increasing water flux (Ochsenfahrt & Winne, 1974; Kitazawa et al., 1976). Increased hydration of the membrane or transport through water channels have been postulated as the mechanisms involved. However, the use of agents which promote water absorption, for example various alcohols which increase theophylline absorption (Harrigan & Levy, 1975), do not seem to have been evaluated as adjuvants for peptide absorption. Methoxysalicylate is one adjuvant which has been reported to greatly enhance the absorption of a variety of peptides (Peters & Sibbons, 1984: Nishihata, Takahagi & Higuchi, 1983). Although this compound causes mucosal damage, it is thought that it has some other effect which promotes absorption. However, the suitability of methoxysalicylate as an adjuvant is diminished by the large doses (up to 300mg/kg) required.

Improvement in cefmetazole oral bioavailability from 6% to 65% has been reported (Sekine et al, 1985) when it is co-administered with a medium chain glyceride base (CGB). Interestingly best results were obtained when the cefmetazole formulation was enteric coated to ensure high local concentrations of drug and adjuvant in the upper small intestine. How widely CGB is applicable as an adjuvant to the absorption of peptides is not known, but it is interesting to note that it is a constituent, in the commercial formulation of cyclosporin (vide supra.).

In summary, there are some examples of drugs and dietary di-and tri-peptides which have been shown to be well absorbed from the gut. These compounds may pass through the mucosal barrier by one or more routes and possess structural features which either aid passive diffusion or are required by some carrier-mediated transport system. For larger peptides, absorption is extremely poor, although there are exceptions as exemplified by cyclosporin. Clearly we need to understand the mechanisms by which small and large peptides are absorbed and to evaluate the use of adjuvants as modifiers of the mucosal barrier. By these means, we may be able to fully exploit the therapeutical potential of peptides administered by the oral route.

Acknowledgements

I would like to thank Drs. Rance and Wicks for their data on TRH analogs and ACE inhibitors respectively, and to my colleagues in the Drug Metabolism Department for many useful discussion on the absorption of peptide drugs. The efforts of Mrs. C. Deeley in typing this manuscript are also much appreciated.

References

Adibi, S. A., and Morse, E. L., 1977, The number of glycine residues which limit intact absorption of glycine oligopeptides in human jejunum, J. Clin. Invest., 60 : 1008.

Allen, J. G., Havas, L., Leicht, E., Lenox-Smith, J., and Nisbet L. J., 1979, Phosphonopeptides as antibacterial agents : metabolism and pharmacokinetics of alafosfalin in animals and humans, Antimicrob. Agents, Chemo., 16 : 306.

Atherton, F. A., Hall, M. J., Hasall, C. H., Holmes, S. W., Lambert, R. W., Lloyd, W. J., and Ringrose, P. S., 1980, Phosphonopeptide antibacterial agents related to alafosfalin : design, synthesis and structure-activity relationships, Antimicrob. Agents. Chemo., 18 : 897.

Bell, J., Peters, G. E., McMartin, C., Thomas, N. W., and Wilson, C. G., 1984, Estimation of gut absorption of peptides by biliary sampling, J. Pharm. Pharmacol., 36 : 88P.

Burston, D., Taylor, E., and Matthews, D. M., 1979, Intestinal handling of two tetrapeptides by rodent small intestine in vitro, Biochem. Biophy. Acta., 553 : 175.

Capraro, V., 1984, Permeability and related phenomenon : basic concepts, in : "Pharmacology of Intestinal Permeation I", T.Z. Csaky ed., Springer-Verlag, Berlin.

Clayton, J. P., Cole, M., Elson, S. W., Hardy, K. D., Mizen, L. W., and Sutherland, R., 1975, Preparation, hydrolysis and oral absorption of alpha-carboxy esters of carbenicillin, J. Med. Chem., 18 : 172.

Csaky, T. Z., (1984), Intestinal Permeation and Permeability : an overview, in : "Pharmacology of Intestinal Permeation I", T. Z. Csaky ed., Springer-Verlag, Berlin.

Egberts, H. J., Koninkx, J. F., Dijk, J. and Mouwen, J. M., 1984, Biological and pathobiological aspects of the glycocalx of the small intestinal epithelium - a review, Vet. Quat., 6 : 186.

Esposito, G., Faelli, A., Tosco, M., Orsenigo, M., De Gasperi, R., and Pacces, N., 1983, Influence of the enteric surface coat on the unidirectional flux of acetamide across the wall of the rat small imtestine, Experimentia., 39 : 149.

Fujii, S., Yokayama, T., Ikegaya, K., Sato, F., and Yokoo, N., 1985, Promoting effect of the new chymotrypsin inhibitor FK-448 on the intestinal absorption of insulin in rats and dogs, J. Pharm. Pharmacol., 37 : 545.

Gardner, C. R., 1985, Gastrointestinal barrier to oral drug delivery, in : "Directed Drug Delivery", R. Borchardt, A. J. Repta and V. J. Stella, eds. Humana Press, New Jersey.

Gardner, M.L., 1984, Intestinal assimilation of intact peptides and proteins from the diet - a neglected field, Biol. Rev., 59:289.

Grant, D. A., Ford, T. F., and McCulloch, R. J., 1982, Distribution of pepstatin and statine following oral and intravenous administration in rats. Tissue localisation by whole body autoradiography, Biochem. Pharmacol., 31 : 2302.

Harrigan, D. J., and Levy, G., 1975, Concentration dependence of ethanol effect on intestinal absorption of theophylline in rats, J. Pharm. Sci., 64 : 897.

Houston, J. B., and Wood, S. G., 1980, Gastronintestinal absorption of drugs, in : "Progress in Drug Metabolism", J.W. Bridges and L. F. Chasseaud, eds., John Wiley and Sons, New York.

Hruby, V. J., 1985, Design of peptide hormone and neurotransmitter analogs, Trends in Pharm. Sci., June : 259.

Humphrey, M. J. and Ringrose, P. S., 1986, Peptides and related drugs: a review of their absorption metabolism and excretion, Drug Met. Rev., accepted for publication.

Jennewein, H. M., Waldeck, F., and Konz, W. 1974, The absorption of tetragastrin from different sites in rats and dogs, Arzneim. Forsch., 24 : 1225.

Jones, K. H., Langley, P.F., and Lees, L. J. 1978, Bioavailability and metabolism of talampicillin, Chemotherapy., 24 : 217.

Kerchner, G.A., and Geary, L.E., 1983, Studies on the transport of enkephalin-like oligopeptides in rat intestinal mucosa, J. Pharmacol. Exp. Ther., 226 : 33.

Kimura, T., Yamamoto, T., Mizuno, M., Suga, Y., Kitade, S., and Sezaki, H. 1983, Characterisation of aminocephalosporin transport across rat small intestine, J. Pharm. Dyn., 6 : 246.

Kitazawa, S., Ishizu, M., and Arakawa, E., 1976, Effect of perfusate constituents on transmucosal fluid, movement and drug absorption in rat small intestine, Chem. Pharm. Bull., 24 : 3169.

Konishi, M., Sugawara, K., Hanada, M., Tomita, K., and Tomatsu, K., 1984, Empedopeptin (BMY-28117), a new depsipeptide antibiotic. I. Production, Isolation and Properties. II. Structure Determination, J. Antibiot., 37 : 949.

Lundin, S., and Vilhardt, H., 1986, Absorption of intragastrically administered DDAVP on conscious dogs, Life Sci., 38 : 703.

Matthews, D.M., 1975, Intestinal absorption of peptides, Physiol. Rev., 55 : 537.

Matthews, D.M., 1983, Intestinal absorption of peptides, Biochem. Soc. Trans., 11 : 808.

Nakashima, E., Tsuji, A., Kagatani, S., and Yamana, T. 1984, Intestinal absorption mechanism of amino-β-lactam antibiotics. III. Kinetics of carrier-mediated transport across the rat small intestine in situ, J. Pharm. Dyn., 7 : 452.

Nishihata, T., Takahagi, H., and Higuchi, T., 1983, Enhanced small intestinal absorption of cefmetazole and cefoxitin in rats in the presence of non-surfactant adjuvants, J. Pharm. Pharmacol., 35 : 124.

Ochsenfarht, H., and Winne, D., 1974, Contribution of solvent drag to intestinal-absorption of basic drugs amidopyrine and antipyrine from jejunum of rat, Arch. Pharmacol., 281 : 175.

Okada, H., Yamazaki, I., Ogawa, Y., Hirai, S., Yashiki, T., and Mima, H., 1982, Vaginal absorption of a potent luteinizing hormone-releasing hormone analog (leuprolide) in rats, I : Absorption by various routes and absorption enhancement, J. Pharm. Sci., 71 : 1367.

Pardridge, W. M., Strategy for drug delivery through the blood-brain barrier, in : "Directed Drug Delivery", R. Borchardt., A. J. Repta., and V. J. Stella, eds. Humana Press, New Jersey, (1985).

Peters, G. E., and Sibbons, P.D., 1984, Macromolecule absorption in a vascularly perfused rat gut preparation in vivo, Second Eur. Congress. Biopharm. and Pharmacokin., 2 : 424.

Sekine, M., Terashima, H., Sasahara, K., Nishimura, K., Okada, R., and Awazu, S., 1985, Improvement of bioavailability of poorly absorbed drugs. II. Effect of medium chain glyceride base on the intestinal absorption of cefmetazole sodium in rats and dogs, J. Pharmacobio-Dyn., 8 : 286.

Silk, D. B., Grimble, G. K., and Rees, R.G., 1985, Protein digestion and amino acid and peptide absorption, Proc. Nutrit. Soc., 44 : 63.

Smithson, K. W., Millar, D., Jacobs, L. and Gray, G. 1981, Intestinal Diffusion Barrier : Unstirred water layer or membrane surface mucous coat, Science, 214 : 1241.

Stein, W. D., 1967, "The Movement of molecules across cell membranes", Academic Press, New York.

Stein, W., and Lieb, W., 1974, How molecules pass through membranes, New Scientist, January 10 : 77.

Thomson, A. B. R. and Dietschy, J. M., 1984, The role of the unstirred water layer in intestinal permeation, in : "Pharmacology of Intestinal permeation II", T.Z. Csaky, ed., Springer-Verlag, Berlin.

Tocco, D. J., de Luna, A., Duncan, A. E., Vassil, T. C., and Ulm, E. H., 1982, The physiological disposition and metabolism of enalapril maleate in laboratory animals, Drug Met. Disp., 10 : 15.

Ulm, E. H., Hichens, M., Gomez, H.J., Till, A. E., Hand, E., Vassil, T.C., Biollaz, J., Brunner, H. R., and Schelling J. L., 1982, Enalapril maleate and a lysine analogue (MK-521) : disposition in man, Br. J. Clin. Pharmacol., 14 : 357.

Veber, D. F. and Freidinger, R. M., 1985, The design of metabolically-stable peptide analogs, Trends Neuro. Sci., Sept. : 392.

Warshaw, A. L., Walker, W. A., and Isselbacher, K. J., 1974, Protein uptake by the intestine : evidence for absorption of intact macromolecules, Gastroenterol., 66 : 987.

Westergaard, H., and Dietschy, J.M., 1974, Delineation of the dimensions and permeability characteristics of the two major diffusion barriers to passive mucosal uptake in the rabbit intestine, J. Clin. Invest., 54 : 718.

Wiedhaup, K., The stability of small peptides in the gastrointestinal tract, in : "Topics in Pharmaceutical Sciences", D. Bremmer, and P. Spiser, eds., Elservier, North Holland Biomedical Press, (1981).

Wood, A. J., Maurer, G., Niederberger, W., and Beveridge, T., 1983, Cyclosporine : pharmacokinetics, metabolism and drug interactions, Transplant. Proc., 15 : 2409.

Wyvratt, M. J., and Patchett, A., 1985, Recent developments in the design of angiotensin-converting enzyme inhibitors, Med. Res. Rev., 5 : 483.

Yamashita, S., Yamazaki, Y., Mizuno, M., Masada, M., Nadai, T., Kimura, T. and Sezaki, H., 1984, Further investigations on the transport mechanisms of cephalexin and ampicillin across rat jejunum, J. Pharm. Dyn., 7 : 227.

Yokohama, S., Yoshioka, T., and Kitamori, N., 1984, Absorption of
    γ-butyrolactone-γ-carbonyl-L-histidyl-L-prolinamide citrate
    (DN-1417), an analog of thyrotrophin-releasing hormone, in rats
    and dogs, J. Pharm. Dyn., 7 : 527.
Yokohama, S., Yoshioka, T., Yamashita, K., and Kitamori, N., 1984,
    Intestinal absorption mechanisms of thyrotrophin releasing
    hormone, J. Pharm. Dyn., 7 : 445.
Yoshimura, Y., and Kakeya, N., 1983, Structure - gastrointestinal
    absorption relationship of penicillins, Int. J. Pharm.,
    17 : 47.

ORAL DELIVERY OF PEPTIDE DRUGS

Karl-Erik Falk and Jan-Erik Löfroth

Physical Pharmacy
AB Hässle
S-431 83 Mölndal
Sweden

INTRODUCTION

Peptides of various sizes and compositions will become an important class of drugs in the future. Recent advances in molecular biology and pharmacology have shown that peptides can be developed as highly effective therapeutic agents in a number of different areas. As with many other drugs, however, the therapeutic efficacy is often diminished by their inability to reach the site of action in adequate amounts, and the choice of administration route is therefore important.

The oral route presents a severe obstacle for peptide drugs due to the enzymatic and cellular barriers of the intestinal tract. However, the oral dosage form of a drug is for several reasons the most popular way of administration. One reason is patient compliance, which merits special attention in long time therapy with potent drugs. Since peptides and peptidelike substances most likely in the future will belong to the more important class of drugs in such therapy, an oral controlled release delivery form of these drugs would be of utmost need and importance. Also, the intestinal tract is intended for absorption, in contrast to, e.g., the nasal cavity. Using other routes than the oral for administration for a long time might therefore induce unpredictable side effects.

The understanding of the mechanisms of peptide hydrolysis and absorption in the gastrointestinal tract is, in our opinion, a prerequisite for rational work towards a commercially available oral dosage form of peptides. Also, basic research is equally needed for the understanding of the importance of components in the formulation and their roles in absorption enhancement and protection against degradation.

The present contribution is based upon some studies of the literature on peptide hydrolysis and absorption. In no way is it intended to be an exhaustive review, but merely one enlightening some problems which have been identified and presenting some ideas which so far have emerged.

153

HYDROLYSIS AND ABSORPTION OF PEPTIDES IN THE GI-TRACT

By definition, peptides are molecules composed by amino acids linked by peptide bonds. Thus, although metabolic products are in principle predictable to a fairly high degree of confidence, which is an advantage, peptides are sensitive to the hydrolytic activities of the peptidases found in the stomach and the lumen, brush border, and cells of the intestine. These enzymes cover a wide spectrum of substrate specificity but unfortunately no comprehensive, systematic classifications of gastrointestinal peptidases seem to have been presented, except for a few reviews. Neither have mechanistic aspects been adressed of more considerable proportions concerning the absorption of larger peptides.

The "Enzyme Handbook", edited by T.E.Barman (1969,1974), however, is one example, where peptidases are classified according to their specificity and which also provides physicochemical and kinetic data. This handbook is useful once the peptidases of interest have been identified. However, when trying to describe the scenario of peptides in the gastrointestinal tract, two strategies may in principle be taken: either research is carried out from the point of view of the peptide or the peptidases. The first approach tries to identify and characterize the peptidases which show activity against a particular peptide, while in the second case the strategy is to identify peptidases and their specificity in general. Since around 400 dipeptides and about 8000 tripeptides theoretically may be composed, the first approach seems to be more attractive experimentally when studying peptides composed by more than two amino acids. Nevertheless, intelligent approaches have been taken to handle the problems associated with classifying of peptidases in general. Stratford and Lee (1986) identified and compared aminopeptidases from various mucosa homogenates by utilizing combinations of special amino acid derivates, inhibitors and activators. It was found that the absolute activity,defined as moles of substrate hydrolyzed per second, per weight protein did not appreciably differ between homogenates of different origin. Since, e.g., nasal formulations of peptides are known to work in vivo the results indicate that good possibilities exist to develop oral dosage forms of such drugs. Similar studies of an activity concept based on amount of peptidase per total area would be highly interesting and valuable for such work. These problems have been identified and are further discussed elsewhere in this volume (Lee, in press).

A similar report on di- and tripeptidases, although in investigations by biopsy methods, was also recently presented by Tobey et al.(1986), who has earlier reported on methods to assay these enzymes (Tobey et al., 1985). The main interest concerned the enzymes of the brush border and the purposes of the studies were

i) to detect all human brush border di-and tripeptidases,

ii) to find discriminating substrates for the development of assay methods, and

iii) to classify the enzymes biochemically.

In addition to four intrinsic brush border dipeptidases, at least three other peptidases also hydrolyzing tripeptides were found. Although enzymes like, e.g. oligopeptidases, were not assayed in these studies, other reports have indicated that such peptidases may preferentially be associated with the brush border and not the cytosol preparations that were used (Kim et al, 1974).

Reports on the distribution of peptidases along the gastrointestinal tract have been presented. Triadou et al.(1983) reported that the ileum showed higher brush border activity than the jejunum of the assayed enzymes, neutral and acid aminopeptidase and dipeptidyl peptidase. A similar distribution of activity was reported by Silk et al.(1976), who found that the dipeptides were more efficiently hydrolyzed by the brush border enzymes in preparations from the rat ileum than from the jejunum. On the other hand, the investigation showed that the jejunal activity was dominated by enzymes in the cytoplasm of the mucosal cells. Further studies, e.g. based on cytochemical methods as suggested and shown by Gossrau (1985) are important in the investigations of enzymes in different parts of the gastrointestinal tract.

The second approach outlined above for the study of hydrolysis of peptides was to look for peptidases which hydro-lyze a given peptide. This may be the method of choice when studying a particular peptide as a drug. As judged by the literature such studies seem to be closely associated with the question of absorption. However, only in a few cases has the mechanism of transport of peptides other than di- and tripep-tides been discussed. Gardner has, as part of a larger article, reviewed the investigations carried out on absorption of biologically active peptides (Gardner, 1984). It was reported that in some cases a protective group at the amino terminus may explain the fact that significant absorption of the peptide occured. This was the case for, e.g., LHRH (luteinizing hormone releasing hormone) and TRH (thyrotropin releasing hormone). A comparison of different routes of admin-istration was presented by Okada et al. (1982) in their studies of a LHRH-analog. Although absorption enhancers like polybasic carboxylic acids and surfactants were used, only the vaginal route gave sufficient bioavailability, the nasal and intestinal absorptions being unacceptable. Saffran et al. (1979,1982) discussed the oral administration of insulin, vasopressin, and desmopressin, and showed that studies of absorption of intact molecules could be carried out by using different approaches, e.g., co-administration of protease inhibitors. However, absorption of other oligopeptides has also been studied, e.g. by Smithson and Gray (1977). It was concluded that the uptake of the studied tetrapeptide was a two step process; hydrolysis was followed by transport of hydrolytic products. The hydrolysis could be attributed to a brush border amino peptidase.

Thus, oligopeptides may in certain cases be absorbed as such, while mostly the uptake seems to be governed by a first step involving hydrolysis. The vast literature in nutrition sciences shows that this is the case. Several reviews have been presented, where both the questions of protein digestion and absorption have been addressed. One of the latest compre-hensive reviews has been given by Gardner (1984) who discussed both protein and peptide hydrolysis as well as mechanisms of transport. Silk et al. (1985) summarized the present knowledge in these questions, while Silk (1981) discussed mainly transport phenomena, which also were discussed by Matthews and Adibi (1976). A more detailed review of both intestinal mucosal peptidases and di- and tripeptide transport was presented by Adibi and Kim (1981) (see e.g.table 2 of that paper).

The main conclusions from these studies about protein digestion, peptide hydrolysis and absorption of small peptides can be summarized as follows:

i)   oligopeptides (products from the luminal digestion processes in the stomach and the duodenum) undergo hydrolysis mainly by the action of brush border aminopeptidases;

ii)   the products (di- and tripeptides) undergo further hydrolysis by cytoplasmic or brush border intestinal enzymes;

iii) specialized carrier-mediated and active transport systems may exist;

iv)   when a peptide is absorbed, bulky peptides and peptides with bulky residues are less easily absorbed than non-bulky ones.

Also, these studies underline the necessity to investigate and utilize derivates of oligopeptides which are not hydrolized, in order to clarify the roles of diffusion and active transport mechanisms in absorption.

CONCLUDING REMARKS

In the development of an oral dosage form of a peptide drug three aspects must be particularly addressed:

i)   the peptide must be protected from the hydrolytic enzymes in the gastrointestinal tract;

ii)   the physical absorption, i.e. the transport, of the peptide must in many cases be improved;

iii) a controlled release form is in many cases desirable.

In this contribution we have given a short review reflecting some studies of the first of these aspects. It seems that many researchers are now working in this area and we can therefore expect that the necessary basic knowledge of peptide degradation will increase. When it then comes to designing a formulation that protects the peptide drug from degradation in the intestinal lumen, we feel that there exist a number of possible pharmaceutical tools. It is for the passage through the cellular barrier that we need new and innovative approaches to be able to keep the peptide intact.

The second aspect, decreased or hindered absorption, is a feature present also for many other substances and seems not to be exclusive for peptides. In this field it is strikingly apparent that basic research on transport and absorption processes is needed, before any rational approach to enhancing and controlling the rate of absorption can be taken. Much information can be found from the absorption mechanisms of, e.g., natural food stuff, but basic research concerning transport mechanisms on a molecular and cellular level is needed.

Thirdly, peptides can have very short lifetimes in the circulation and it is therefore important to design a formulation that delivers the drug not only intact and with a high bioavailability but also one providing a long duration. It is today difficult to see all aspects which may need our attention but it seems at present to be a problem of less magnitude than the others associated with transport improvement and protection. Post absorption phenomena like liver metabolism and biliary excretion are sometimes important in reducing the effect of a peptide drug (K.J.Hoffman and C.G.Regårdh, personal communication), and must therefore be considered in the pharmaceutical work. This point has been clearly amplified by Stratford and Lee (1986) in their recent article: "The implication of these possibilities is that oral peptide delivery would be feasable provided peptide release is confined to the vicinity of the mucosal surface in a region of the small intestine that favours peptide uptake into the lymphatic circulation".

The aim to present a commercially available delivery system for peptide drugs seems at a first sight to set up an insuperable obstacle. However, a careful investigation of knowledge presented by scientists within, e.g., biochemistry, pharmacology, pharmacy, and physical chemistry, supported by basic research should constitute a solid basis for future successful work.

REFERENCES

Adibi, S.A., and Kim, Y.S., 1981, Peptide absorption and hydrolysis, in: "Physiology of the Gastrointestinal Tract," L.R.Johnson, ed., Raven Press, New York.
Barman, T.E., 1969,1974, "Enzyme Handbook, vol. I, II, and Supplement I," Springer Verlag, Berlin, Heidelberg.
Gardner, M.L.G., 1984, Intestinal assimilation of intact peptides and proteins from the diet - a neglected field?, Biol. Rev., 59:289.
Gossrau, R., 1985, Cytochemistry of membrane proteases, Histochem. J., 17:737.
Hoffmann, K.-J., and Regårdh, C.-G., personal communications, AB Hässle.
Kim, Y.S., Kim, Y.W., and Sleisenger, M.H., 1974, Studies on the properties of peptide hydrolases in the brush-border and soluble fractions of small intestinal mucosa of rat and man, Biochim. Biophys. Acta, 370:283.

Lee, V.H.L., (in press), Enzymatic barrier to peptide and
    protein absorption and use of penetration enhancers to
    modify absorption, in: "Advanced Drug Delivery Systems
    for Peptides and Proteins," S.S. Davis, L. Illum, and E.
    Tomlinson, eds., NATO ARW, Copenhagen, Plenum Press, New
    York.
Matthews, D.M., and Adibi, S.A., 1976, Peptide absorption,
    Gastroenterology, 71:151.
Okadfa, H., Yamazaki, I., Ogawa, Y., Hirai, S., Yashiki, T.,
    and Mima, H., 1982, Vaginal absorption of a potent
    luteinizing hormone-releasing hormone analog (Leuprolide)
    in rats I: absorption by various routes and absorption
    enhancement, J. Pharm. Sci., 71:1367.
Saffran, M., Franco-Saenz, R., Kong, A., Papahadjopoulus, D.,
    and Szoka, F., 1979, A model for the study of the oral
    administration of peptide hormones, Can. J. Biochem.,
    57:548.
Saffran, M., 1982, Oral administration of peptides,
    Endochrim. Experim., 16:327.
Silk, D.B.A., Nicholson, J.A., and Kim, Y.S., 1976, Hydrolysis
    of peptides within lumen of small intestine, Am. J.
    Physiol., 231:1322.
Silk, D.B.A., 1981, Peptide transport, Clin. Sci., 60:607.
Silk, D.B.A., Grimble, G.K., and Rees, R.G., 1985, Protein
    digestion and amino acid and peptide absorption, Proc.
    Nutr. Soc., 44:63.
Smithson, K.W., and Gray, G.M., 1977, Intestinal assimilation
    of a tetrapeptide in the rat: Obligate function of brush
    border aminopeptidase, J. Clin. Invest., 60:665.
Stratford, R.E., Jr, and Lee, V.H.L., 1986, Aminopeptidase
    activity in homogenates of various absorptive mucosae in
    the albino rabbit; implications in peptide delivery, Int.
    J. Pharm., 39:73.
Tobey, N.A., Heizer, W., Yeh, R., Huang, T.-I., and Hoffner,
    C., 1985, Human intestinal brush border peptidases,
    Gastroenterlogy, 88:913.
Tobey, N.A., Lyn-Cook, L.E., Uhlsen, M.H., and Heizer, W.D.,
    1986, Intestinal brush-border peptidases: Activities in
    normal and abnormal peroral intestinal biopsy specimens,
    J. Lab. Clin. Med., March:221.
Triadou, N., Bataille, J., and Schmitz, J., 1983, Longitudinal
    study of the human intestinal brush border membrane
    proteins, Gastroenterology, 85:1326.

DRUG DELIVERY OF PEPTIDES:

THE BUCCAL ROUTE

Hans P. Merkle[*], Reinhold Anders[*,+], Jürgen Sandow[+],
and Werner Schurr[#]

[*]Pharmazeutisches Institut der Universität, Pharmazeu-
tische Technologie, D-5300 Bonn 1, [+]Hoechst AG, D-6230
Frankfurt aM 80, and [#]Abteilung Innere Medizin VI
Universitätspoliklinik, D-6900 Heidelberg

INTRODUCTION

Peptides and proteins are currently emerging as a major class of future drugs. So far the research in this field is mainly focused on basic research covering isolation, synthesis, analysis, and biological and clinical effects. However, increasing attention is now also given to considerations regarding suitable dosage forms and routes of absorption. It is widely accepted that the most common dosage forms and routes, i.e. solid dosage forms for peroral application and sterile preparations for parenteral application, will not provide a realistic basis for a widespread use of these drugs in the future. This is because (i) most oligopeptides and proteins are not readily absorbed in the gastrointestinal tract, e.g. due to the presence of proteolytic enzymes and the low permeability of the gut membranes to such often hydrophilic compounds. And also (ii) parenteral application, certainly, is of limited suitability to long term treatments and frequent use of drugs.

Recently, however, alternative mucous membranes were evaluated for peptide absorption. The nasal (Chien, 1985), the rectal (Yoshioka et al., 1982), and the vaginal (Nishi et al., 1975; Okada et al., 1982; Okada et al., 1983) membrane were discussed as efficient absorption sites. Even the ocular cornea and the skin are under consideration. The scope of this report, however, is restricted to the buccal mucosa. The sublingual or the gingival mucosa may be similar to the buccal membrane, but only the buccal route will be further elaborated in this paper.

As demonstrated by a number of reports, recently reviewed by Su (1986), the nasal route is currently the route of choice for peptides. However, the nasal site does have distinct limitations. Upon long term treatments there might be a pathologic change of the nasal mucosa (Su, 1986), or, as a side effect, the preservative added to the preparation might interfere with the ciliary activity (Van de Donk et al., 1982) of the membrane. Moreover, there

is a debate on the consequences of vast individual variations in mucous secretion and turnover on the extent and rate of absorption; and finally, proteases and peptidases present in the mucus or associated with the nasal
membrane may act as an enzymatic barrier to peptide absorption as found with
other mucosal sites (Stratford and Lee, 1985). It may thus be concluded that
in spite of many promising aspects the nasal route may have its shortcomings
and not be the ultimate answer to every peptide absorption problem.

Information on the buccal absorption of peptides is rather scarce, except for a body of knowledge on the buccal absorption of oxytocin (e.g.
Wespi and Rehsteiner, 1966; Bergsjoe and Jenssen, 1969) as early as in the
nineteen-sixties. Generally, however, the oral mucosa is an established
absorption organ, as demonstrated for a variety of possible drugs. Recently
more peptides were investigated and it was shown that the buccal mucosa
might provide a promising absorption site for small peptides (Anders, 1984;
Anders et al., 1984; Merkle et al., 1985). In comparison to other non-parenteral absorption sites the buccal mucosa shows a number of distinct advantages. Buccal peptide absorption may not be as efficient as the nasal
alternative, but the buccal mucosa is definitely less sensitive than the
nasal one. According to its natural function the buccal mucosa is routinely
exposed to a multitude of different foreign compounds which is likely to
make it less prone to irreversible irritation or damage. Because of the
excellent accessibility of the oral mucosa appropriate dosage forms may be
easily attached and removed at any time, if necessary. It is not a sex-
specific absorption site like the vaginal membrane and patients may comply
better to buccal than to nasal, rectal or vaginal formulations.

DOSAGE FORM CONSIDERATIONS

The most common way to deliver a peptide to the oral mucosa would be to
use aqueous solutions or conventional buccal or sublingual tablets. The risk
to exclude a major part of the drug from absorption by (i) accidental swallowing of the solution or even the tablet, or (ii) by the salivary wash-out
of the tablet appears to be quite high. Therefore, alternative dosage forms
have been designed to retain the dosage form in the oral cavity and in intimate contact with the mucosa, either buccally, sublingually or on the
gingiva. Among the different concepts approached is the use of self-adhesive
dosage forms for close attachment to the mucosa. The adhesion mechanism
operating is the intercalation of the polymer chains of both the polymer
used as dosage form excipient and the glycoproteins of the mucosal membrane,
leading to non-specific and/or specific interactions of the two polymeric
species (Ch'ng et al., 1985; Park and Robinson, 1986; Peppas et al., 1986).

A collection of four different self-adhesive set-ups is given in Fig.
1. It shows that different approaches may be used ranging from simple self-
adhesive disks to laminated systems (Davis et al., 1982; Ishida et al.,
1982; Offenl. DE 2908847 (1980); Offenl. DE 3237945 A 1 (1983); Anders,
1984). The adhesive polymer may work as the drug carrier itself (Case a and
d), on the other hand it may act as an adhesive link between a drug loaded
layer and the mucosa (Case c). Also a drug containing disk may be fixed to
the mucosa by using a self-adhesive shield (Case b).

An important difference may be seen with respect to the directions open
for drug release. Case a and c allow for a bi-directional release of the
drug, i.e. the drug is not only delivered to the mucosa but also to the oral
cavity, or the saliva, respectively. This may lead, however, as we have
seen, to a substantial loss of the drug due to involuntary swallowing of saliva. On the other hand the total surface of the oral cavity is now available for absorption. Drug loss to the saliva may be decreased by using a
self-adhesive protective shield (Case b) or a non-permeable backing layer

(Case d); however, the main absorption site now remaining is the rather limited mucosal area covered by the dosage form itself. Further spreading of
the drug across the oral buccal mucosa may increase the effective area for
peptide absorption. This may happen either by squeezing-out effects of individual jaw movements or may be due to a slow floating motion of the device
across the mucosal surface. The size of such systems is variable, but the
maximum size suitable for buccal administration will be around 10 to 15 cm^2
at the most.

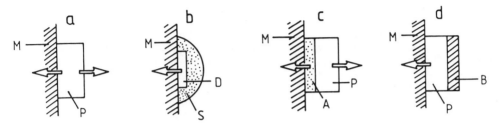

Fig. 1. Schematic view of four different types of self-adhesive patches
         for buccal peptide delivery. Case a: bi-directional release from
         adhesive patch by dissolution or diffusion. Case b: uni-direc-
         tional release from patch embedded in adhesive shield. Case c:
         bi-directional release from laminated patch. Case d: uni-direc-
         tional release from laminated patch. M, mucosa; P, polymer with
         peptide; D, drug depot; S, adhesive shield; A, adhesive layer;
         B, impermeable backing layer

All systems may be additionally loaded with any additive needed. A
major advantage of those systems carrying a non-permeable protective shield
or layer is that the effect of these additives can be restricted to the very
site of application. A local microenvironment may thus be created between
the dosage form and the mucosa which may be able to establish more favorable
absorption conditions than the natural mucosal site, e.g. by adjustment of a
specific pH, or by providing an absorption enhancer, if available. Any irritation or damage exerted to the mucosa by the drug or any of the dosage form
excipients is, therefore, restricted to a rather limited area and not to the
complete oral mucosa as it would be the case without the protective shield
or layer. Subsequent recoverage of reversibly damaged sites appears to be
possible, even during long term treatments, since the application site may
be varied across the total surface available and damaged areas will be
small. Anyway, all additives released to the oral cavity have to be rather
critically evaluated since the oral mucosa is the site of a complex bacterial microflora whose composition and viability is essential for its health
and appearance.

With regard to the choice of polymers for buccal self-adhesive devices
there exists a body of knowledge from other mucosal sites (Park and Robinson, 1986; Peppas and Buri, 1986). It appears that a variety of polymers can
be used, including all kinds of water-soluble and insoluble hydrocolloid
polymers from both the ionic and non-ionic type. Drug release from soluble
polymers is accompanied by the gradual erosion-type dissolution of the polymer. Polymer dissolution and drug diffusion may, therefore, determine the
overall release mechanism. In addition, non-soluble hydrogels may be used as

well. The most common polymer applied is the anionic polyacrylate-type of hydrogel (Ch'ng et al., 1985). Drug release from such hydrogels should follow fickian or non-fickian diffusion kinetics (Lee, 1986). Most of the polymers suggested are commonly used in drug formulation. But there is yet no detailed knowledge of how these polymers will affect the oral mucosa upon long term treatments.

Depending on the pharmacodynamics of the peptides various buccal dosage forms of different release rates may be designed. In some cases fast release of the peptide may be required; for other peptides a sustained release may be desirable. To achieve sustained release a number of standard strategies are at hand, e.g. matrix diffusion control, membrane controlled transport of the peptide, or polymer erosion control. In many cases, however, instantaneous release of the peptide may be desired, which requires rapidly eroding or highly permeably carriers. The maximum application time span for self-adhesive mucosal dosage forms appears to be in the order of several days (Nagai, 1986). But special delivery devices with mechanical attachment to the teeth may be designed to release for weeks or months. In most cases, however, the maximum buccal residence time should not exceed several hours. This is due to the fact that buccal devices may possibly interfere with drinking, eating and even talking. Buccal patches for treatments of several hours have to be perfectly formulated in order to motivate patients to comply with. A smooth surface and good flexibility are prerequisites to prevent mechanical irritation or local discomfort.

It should, finally, be noted that most of these dosage form considerations are provided on a mainly theoretical or even speculative basis. Only few practical results are at hand that support one or the other idea, and much more work has to be done to make self-adhesive polymeric disks or laminated patches an established dosage form for buccal peptide delivery.

MATERIALS AND METHODS

All materials and methods used in the subsequent study were described elsewhere in detail (Anders, 1984).

Peptides. Protirelin (TRH, thyroliberin), buserelin and calcitonin were used as model peptides.

Self-adhesive patches. For buccal delivery of peptides two-ply laminates were studied, consisting of a backing layer which was impermeable to the drug and a hydrocolloid layer containing the peptide. Hydroxyethylcellulose was used as the main hydrocolloid polymer. The two-ply laminates were made by a casting procedure applying suitable polymer/peptide solutions. For human experiments ellipsoid type patches were used with an area of up to 12 cm^2. For rats circular patches were prepared with an area of up to 0.4 cm^2. Preliminary experiments in humans were also carried out using a polytef-disk with a central circular depression to receive a filter paper disk which was soaked with a concentrated aqueous peptide preparation.

Additives. Citric acid and Na-5-methoxysalicylate were used as potential absorption enhancers.

In vivo release and absorption studies in humans. In humans both in vivo peptide release studies and peptide absorption studies were performed. In vivo release was followed in healthy human subjects using protirelin loaded self-adhesive patches or patches loaded with Na-salicylate as a marker. The patches were removed after certain time periods and the peptide or marker remaining in the patch was analyzed. Data obtained after different time periods were collected and used to establish in vivo drug release profiles.

In vivo absorption was studied using the preliminary polytef-disk method and/or self-adhesive patches. Absorption of protirelin was evaluated by monitoring pituitary thyrotropin (TSH) and prolactin (PRL) plasma levels as the pharmacodynamic response. With calcitonin only a preliminary study was run in human subjects, using the polytef-disk approach.

Absorption studies in rats. Additional in vivo studies mainly with protirelin and also with buserelin were performed in anaethetized rats. Self-adhesive patches of ca. 5 - 6 mm diameter were attached to the buccal mucosa of the rats. Continous sampling of blood, separation of serum for analysis by centrifugation, and recirculation of blood cells into the animals allowed for a continous monitoring of thyrotropin after administration of protirelin patches; upon buserelin patches both plasma buserelin and lutropin were analyzed.

Peptide analysis. Peptide analysis in plasma was performed by using commercial or otherwise provided radioimmunoassay methods (RIA) of thyrotropin (TSH), prolactin (PRL), buserelin, lutropin (LH) and calcitonin. If possible protirelin (TRH) and buserelin were also analyzed by HPLC.

RESULTS AND DISCUSSION

Human Absorption Studies

Preliminary studies. Preliminary studies in humans using the polytef-disk approach demonstrated that protirelin (MW=362) was readily absorbed via the buccal mucosa, as shown by significant increases of pituitary thyrotropin and prolactin, whereas calcitonin (MW=3500) could not be found to pass the buccal mucosa at all. This is most obviously due to the large difference of the molecular weights of both peptides which is likely to result in vastly different permeabilities of the buccal mucosa. Exact knowledge about the viability of this hypothesis needs further studies. The fact that oxytocin (MW=1007), having a molecular weight between the two other peptides, can efficiently pass the oral mucosa (Wespi and Rehsteiner, 1966), supports this hypothesis, but not the negative result on buccal buserelin (MW=1239; Sandow and Petri, 1985). This indicates that predictions on mucosal permeabilities cannot be based on a single parameter only.

Protirelin, being a tripeptide, can also be absorbed, to some extent, in the gastrointestinal tract. So it might have been possible that the absorption observed could have occurred partly or even totally due to GI absorption rather than buccal absorption. To exclude these doubts, additional experiments were run with the same set-up, but with the subjects' saliva being constantly withdrawn by aspiration. The same thyrotropin and prolactin stimulation pattern as before resulted from these experiments demonstrating that buccal absorption was indeed the major route.

Protirelin absorption from self-adhesive patches. Experiments on the basis of self-adhesive buccal patches showed the same pharmacodynamic response as the preliminary studies run with the polytef-disk approach. The result is shown in Fig. 2. Between 48 and 72% of the peptide were recovered in the patches and, therefore, not available for absorption within the 30 min contact time. In order to increase the rate of release of the peptide from the patch the polymer fraction of the patch was decreased by two thirds. At the same time the protirelin dose was also reduced from 20 mg per dose to 10 mg. Both high and low viscosity grade HEC was used as the polymer. The study was run with female and male healthy subjects. The result of

163

the test is demonstrated in Fig. 3. As expected females showed higher thyro-tropin and prolactin levels than males. The fraction of peptide remaining in the patch after 30 min mucosal contact was in the range of 0 - 15% for the low viscosity grade polymer and 0 - 50% in case of the high viscosity grade polymer. In spite of the obviously higher release rate of the low viscosity polymer patch the thyrotropin and prolactin stimulation was not statisti-cally different between the polymers used. But in the case of prolactin found in female subjects and for the high viscosity HEC only there was a clear correlation between the pharmacodynamic response and the amount of peptide released after 30 min, as indicated by a statistically significant Spearman rank order correlation coefficient (P = 0.05). This is one of several occasions in this work where a correlation of the peptide release pattern and the pharmacodynamic response upon application was detected.

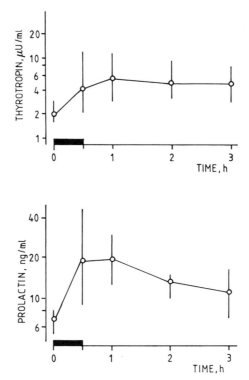

Fig. 2.   Plasma thyrotropin and prolactin concentrations upon buccal
          application of self-adhesive protirelin patches. Dose: 20 mg
          protirelin in high viscosity HEC-patch; bars indicate time of
          mucosal contact; data from N = 4 human subjects

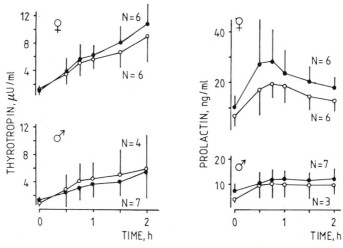

Fig. 3.   Plasma thyrotropin and prolactin concentrations upon buccal
application of self-adhesive protirelin patches. Dose: 10 mg
protirelin in high viscosity (closed circles) and low viscosity
(open circles) HEC patches; data from female and male human
subjects

Comparing buccal protirelin absorption with other routes. In a comparative study buccal protirelin was evaluated in comparison to iv, nasal
and peroral administration (Schurr et al., 1985). With respect to the protirelin dose required to achieve significant thyrotropin and prolactin incremental increases, the nasal application was about 10 times more efficient
than the buccal route. The effective buccal dose, however, was only about
one quarter of the peroral dose. No side effects of the treatment were
noticed with the buccal patches, whereas minor effects were caused by the
nasal application, and the side effects of the iv injection included nausea,
flushing and urinary urgency for a majority of the subjects investigated.
This is another demonstration of the much more moderate pituitary stimulation kinetics of buccal protirelin, as compared to the iv and nasal route.
It remains an open question whether this aspect might be a relevant factor
for drug formulation of other peptides as well.

Rat Absorption Studies

Animal models are prerequisites for the investigation of peptide absorption phenomena. Here we report on a rat technique for buccal peptide
absorption which will be the basic tool for forthcoming studies in this
laboratory. The purpose of this technique is twofold: (i) to optimize
possible formulation effects with self-adhesive buccal peptide patches, and
(ii) to evaluate potential absorption enhancers for oral mucosal transport
of peptides. Further progress in buccal peptide delivery in humans will
definitely be related to such base-line studies. Moreover, rat studies will

help to find peptides of sufficient buccal permeability and to evaluate possible absorption enhancers.

Studying absorption in rats is a common instrument in the investigation of the nasal absorption of peptides and has been thoroughly reviewed previously (Chien and Chang, 1985; Hussain et al., 1985; Su and Campanale, 1985; Sandow and Petri, 1985). Other potential animal models are the dog (Ishida et al., 1981) or sheep (Davis, 1985). The suitability of the rat as a model to study buccal peptide absorption has quite recently been assessed by the authors (Anders, 1984; Merkle et al., 1986). The peptides so far investigated were protirelin and buserelin. The buccal patches administered to the rats were similar to the two-ply laminate type tested in human studies, except for their size, which was 5 - 7 mm in diameter. The patches could be easily attached to the mucosa of the buccal pouch of the anaesthetized rat. Upon continuous blood sampling the absorption process was followed by monitoring peptide plasma levels or its pharmacodynamic response.

Protirelin absorption. Two techniques were used, i.e. without and with triiodothyronine pretreatment of the rats previous to the absorption experiment. By means of a negative feed back thriiodothyronine pretreatment leads to a strong reduction of endogenous protirelin and thyrotropin. The result without such pretreatment is shown in Fig. 4. There is a clear indication that protirelin is readily absorbed via the buccal mucosa, since plasma thyrotropin levels are greatly increased above the normal physiologic level. More experiments were run with triiodothyronine pretreated animals. This set-up was regarded to represent the more reliable and robust test method as compared to the method without pretreatment. Erratic thyrotropin level fluctuations in the test animals under stress and/or anaesthesia may thus be excluded. Again, there was excellent experimental proof that protirelin is

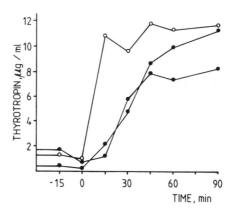

Fig. 4.   Thyrotropin stimulation in rats upon buccal application of self-adhesive buccal protirelin patches. Dose: 931 µg protirelin in high viscosity HEC patch; open circles: 5.5 mm diameter patch; closed circles: 6.7 mm diameter patch

buccaly absorbed. It is interesting to note that there was a statistically
significant rank order correlation (Spearman, P = 0.05) between the individual amounts of drug released to the mucosa of the rats during the experiment and the corresponding pharmocodynamic responses in terms of the maximum
thyrotropin plasma levels observed (Table 1). Thus, the dosage form used
needs to be further optimized by trying to attain faster and more reproducible release rates of the peptide in order to achieve high pharmacodynamic

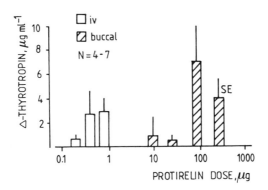

Fig. 5.   Dose effects of pharmacodynamics of iv and buccal protirelin in
          rats

response at low peptide doses. No information is so far available to explain
the vast variation in drug release between different animals. In humans we
were able to show that the release of peptides from such patches is far more
reproducible (Anders, 1984). The design of appropriate formulations and experimental assessments by in vitro dissolution studies should help to find a
more suitable and reproducible release behavior.

Table 1. Spearman rank order correlation[a] of protirelin released from
patch and maximum pituitary thyrotropin in rats

| Protirelin, released | | Maximum thyrotropin | | Patch diameter |
%	/ Rank	µg/ml	/ Rank	mm
97.2	1	7.44	1	5.5
74.9	2	5.79	2	5.5
69.7	3	3.50	5	5.5
34.1	4	4.65	4	6.7
32.9	5	5.57	3	6.7
3.2	6	2.03	6	6.7

[a]Spearman rank order correlation coefficient r_s = 0.771 (P = 0.05)

Dose effects upon buccal protirelin and other routes. A comparison of
the pharmacodynamic effects upon buccal protirelin and iv protirelin in rats
is given in Fig. 5. The graph shows that the buccal dose required to achieve
an equivalent pharmacodynamic response is about 200 times higher than that
for iv injection of the peptide. It must, however, be kept in mind that this
relation does not allow calculation of the fraction of the peptide absorbed.
The efficiency of peptide absorption with respect to its pharmacodynamic
response is not only a matter of the total dose absorbed but is also influenced by the rate of appearance of the peptide at the target organ. This
depends on the rate of absorption, and it is also affected by the hydrody-
namics of the transport in the bloodstream and the simultaneous metabolism
in the blood. The latter is highly significant with peptides of extremely
short biological half-lifes like protirelin.

An iv bolus injection of protirelin is followed by a sharp incremental
rise of the drug's concentration at the target site, i.e. the pituitary
gland, resulting in a pronounced pharmacodynamic response. In case of the
buccal route, however, the mucosal membrane transport and distribution im-
pedes the incremental rise of protirelin at the target, and, therefore, buccal doses have to be much higher than iv doses in order to achieve the same
pharmacodynamic response. It would have been an erroneous conclusion to regard the data in Fig. 5 as a means to derive first estimations of the total
fraction of protirelin buccaly absorbed. But it is safe to conclude that the
pharmacodynamic efficiency of buccal protirelin was around two hundred times
less than that of iv protirelin.

Another interesting relation can be observed by comparing the iv and
buccal data in Fig. 5 with the results of Sandow and Petri (1985) on nasal
protirelin absorption. Using the same animal model a 2 µg nasal dose gave a
peak thryrotropin concentration of ca. 4 µg/ml. Based on the pharmacodynamic
effects observed, the nasal dose, therefore, had to be about five times
higher than the iv dose, wheras the buccal dose required was 40 times the
nasal one. This result is in close agreement with the results found in human
subjects (Schurr et al., 1985) and does indeed strengthen our confidence in
the rat model for future studies.

It is additionally interesting to note that the maximum thyrotropin responses found upon buccal protirelin, although requiring higher doses, were
about twice as high as those found upon iv or nasal protirelin. It appears
that this may be the result of a more sustained type pituitary stimulation
in the course of buccal absorption, as compared to the iv and nasal application. At this time no further evidence can be given to support this hypothesis. For a complete understanding more should be known about buccal pep-

tide absorption kinetics and its effects on pituitary pharmacodynamics in man and in rats. This may have interesting therapeutic implications in the future.

Effects of additives. In order to improve the permeability of the buccal membrane and the efficacy of buccal peptide administration it appears to be indispensible to find highly effective, biocompatible and non-toxic absorption enhancers. No such additives have yet been tested for buccal absorption improvement. As a first step two potential absorption enhancers were investigated, i.e. citric acid and Na-5-methoxysalicylate. These compounds were previously reported to increase the vaginal absorption of Leuprolid (Okada et al., 1982), and the rectal absorption of Insulin (Nishihata et al., 1981), respectively. The opening of mucosal pores, loaded with calcium ions, is the most probable mechanism for these additives. Both compounds were studied using patches of both high and low viscosity HEC as the polymeric carrier .

In the case of citric acid a ca. 100% increase of the means of maximum thyrotropin concentrations was found with both polymers. Na-5-methoxysalicylate gave a similar increase of the means of maximum thyrotropin, but with tho low viscosity polymer only, and not with the high viscosity type. None of these effects, however, was ohown to be statistically significant (t-test of means of maximum concentrations). This appears to be due to the low number of animals available in the study and the rather high statistical variation of the pharmacodynamic response between animals. In addition, the protirelin dose used for this study, i.e. 84 µg, was a dose which turned out to show an already maximum pharmacodynamic response (see Fig. 5). Further effects by addition of absorption enhancers, therefore, are not likely to be detected. Future studies with more animals and a more sensitive experimental design, i.e. testing at lower peptide doses, will clarify these points and help to further evaluate possible enhancers. Still, it has to pointed out that the thyrotropin concentrations found upon addition of both additives to the polymeric patches are the highest ever found in the whole study. In conclusion, more studies in the field of possible absorption promoting additives appear to be worthwhile; but the preliminary results so far obtained do not yet allow a full understanding of all the effects encountered.

Buserelin absorption. In addition to the absorption studies with protirelin, preliminary rat absorption studies were also run with buserelin, i.e. an LHRH agonist. The same experimental design as with protirelin was used. The outcome of an absorption study with adhesive patches loaded with 0.7 mg of the peptide is given in Fig. 6. This result shows that there is only a minute absorption of buserelin as indicated by the low plasma buserelin recovered and the resulting lutropin levels from pituitary stimulation. So in this form buccal buserelin patches are not suitable for efficient buserelin delivery to the systemic circulation.

It is, however, interesting to note that there was a rather constant lutropin stimulation pattern with three animals, whereas one animal failed to respond. Detailed inspection of the percentage of buserelin released during the experiment, and the amount renally excreted and the maximum lutropin concentration achieved, respectively, for the four rats investigated showed that there is a significant rank order correlation (Spearman, P = 0.05) between these variables (Table 2). This implies a direct relationship of the amount and/or rate of peptide released from the polymeric patch and the resulting pharmacokinetics and pharmacodynamics.

Obviously, the release of the peptide from the polymeric patches should be improved. A similar finding was observed with protirelin. The patches should be designed in such a way that the peptide is released fully and reproducibly after application of the patch onto the buccal mucosa. It remains

169

to be clarified what the effect of an optimized patch onto buccal peptide
efficiency and efficacy would be. But further optimization of such patches
is currently being sought in this laboratory.

Table 2. Rank order correlations of buserelin amount released from patch
          and renally excreted buserelin, and maximum pituitary lutropin,
          respectively, in rats

Buserelin, released			Buserelin[a], renally excreted			Maximum lutropin[b]		
%	/	Rank	ng	/	Rank	ng/ml	/	Rank
49.2		1	12.79		1	1160.5		1
47.4		2	3.09		3	1001.3		2
27.1		3	3.87		2	862.1		3
13.0		4	0.83		4	99.8		4

[a]Spearman correlation coefficient r_s = 0.800 (P = 0.05)

[b]Spearman correlation coefficient r_s = 1.000 (P < 0.05)

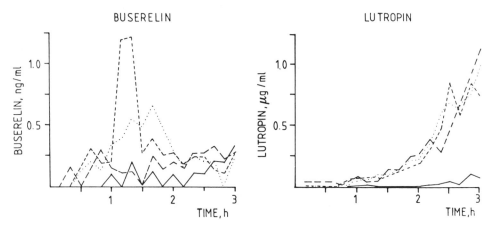

Fig. 6. Plasma buserelin and lutropin levels following buccal buserelin
         in rats

Human Release Studies

Formulation aspects. There are two principal options for polymers to
formulate self-adhesive polymeric patches as defined by Fig. 1 (Case d),
i.e. insoluble hydrogels and water-soluble hydrocolloids. So far experimental results from these authors are only available for patches based on
the use of water-soluble hydrocolloids. A full experimental description of
the work done is given by Anders and Merkle (1986). Below only a few out-
lines of the results are given. All of the results are based on in vivo release studies in human subjects. Variables were the type of polymers used,
the viscosity grade of the polymers, and the amount of polymer per unit

square of the patch. Absolutely no local irritations or other damage to the oral mucosa whatsoever were so far observed with these patches.

The polymers used were hydroxyethylcellulose (HEC; Natrosol 250L and Natrosol 250G, from Hercules), and polyvinylpyrrolidon (PVP; Kollidon 30 and Kollidon 90, from BASF), i.e. both polymers were tested for two viscosity grade levels each. The release was studied by means of sub-therapeutic doses of protirelin or by Na-salicylate as a marker.

Types of in vivo release profiles. The types of release that were observed with the buccal patches studied are shown in Fig. 7. All experiments were run with the same subject. As demonstrated by the graphs the release of the marker can be controlled over a wide range. Expectedly, an increase of the viscosity grade sustains the release of the marker from the patch. If the amount of polymer per unit square is increased the release of the marker is slowed down. It is interesting to note that with low amounts of polymer per unit square the amount of marker remaining in the patch appears to decrease exponentially, whereas higher amounts approach an almost linear release profile, e.g. with PVP 90. Studies currently performed in this laboratory at even higher polymer amounts, show that the release profiles are indeed essentially linear. We also found that the rate of polymer erosion is the rate-determining step of the release process of the drug.

The efficiency of the two polymers studied, regarding the sustainment of the release, is highly different. The high viscosity HEC only needs about one third of the amount of the high viscosity PVP patch to obtain the same degree of sustainment.

Within-subject variability of release. Moreover, the data in Fig. 7 supply some information regarding the within-subject variability of drug release from this type of buccal patch. Since the release profiles resulted from totally independent runs in one subject, each run being represented by a single data point and with three runs for each time period, the range of variation seen in Fig. 7 represents the within-subject variability of these patches. So, buccal release from such polymeric laminates appears to be rather reproducible, which is in contrast to the previous rat studies.

Between-subject variability of release. Data regarding the variation between subjects is given in Figs. 8 and 9. Fig. 8 shows the fraction of protirelin, as a model peptide, remaining in the patch after staying in contact to the buccal mucosa for 30 min in 4 up to 11 subjects. Three different patch formulations were evaluated. Depending on the amount of polymer employed and the viscosity grade of the polymer, slow, medium or fast release of the drug can be obtained. Obviously, this result shows that the release rates of self-adhesive patches can be individually tailored to meet the specific requirements of a certain peptide or therapy. The variations found between subjects were substantial, but within a tolerable range.

More information on the between-subject variations of drug release is given in Fig. 9. Here the release of a marker was studied in five subjects following complete release profiles. Each data point of the graph represents an independent run. Again, there is a substantial amount of variability in the data. It is more pronounced than the within-subject variability, but stays in a normally tolerable range. The variations may be explained by individual habits in saliva flow or jaw movements of the subjects, resulting in different dissolution rates of the hydrocolloid polymer. Further studies on the optimum site for application are currently under way. It appears that the area facing the 6th or 7th molar of the upper jaw are to be preferred.

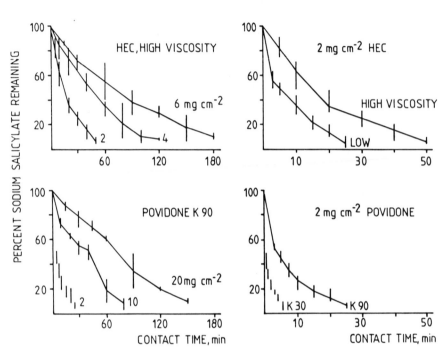

Fig. 7. Effect of polymers, viscosity grades and amounts of polymer per unit
square on the buccal release of a marker (Na-salicylate) from self-
adhesive polymeric patches. Three independent experiments were run
on each of the contact times. Bars indicate total range of values
obtained.

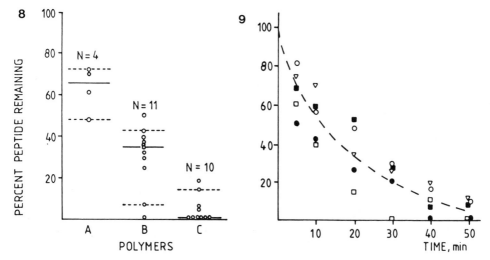

Fig. 8. (Left graph) Percent protirelin remaining in buccal patch after 30 min of buccal contact in human subjects; protirelin content of patch: 1–2 mg/cm^2; HEC polymer content: (A) 6.2 mg/cm^2 high viscosity, (B) 2.2 mg/cm^2 high viscosity, (C) 2.1 mg/cm^2 low viscosity; solid line: median; broken lines: 5% confidence limits

Fig. 9. (Right graph) Release profile of marker (Na–salicylate) from buccal patch in five subjects; symbols indicating subjects; marker content of patch: 1 mg/cm^2; 2.1 mg/cm^2 high viscosity HEC.

REFERENCES

Anders, R., Merkle, H.P., Schurr, W., Ziegler, R., 1983, Buccal Absorption of protirelin: an effective way to stimulate thyrotropin and prolactin, J. Pharm. Sci., 72:1481.
Anders, R., 1984, Ph.D. Thesis: Selbsthaftende Polymerfilme zur bukkalen Applikation von Peptiden, Universität Bonn, Bonn.
Anders, R., and Merkle. H.P., 1986, Arzneiformung selbsthaftender Polymerfilme zur bukkalen Applikation, manuscript in preparation.
Bergjoe, P., and Jenssen, H., 1969, Nasal and buccal oxytocin for the introduction of labour: a clinical trial, J. Obstet. Gynaec. Brit. Cwlth., 76:131.
Chien, Y.W., ed., 1985, Transnasal Systemic Medications, Elsevier, Amsterdam.
Chien, Y.W., and Chang, S.F., 1985, Historic development of transnasal systemic medications, in: "Transnasal systemic medications", Y.W. Chien, ed., Elsevier, Amsterdam, 1.

Ch'ng, H.S., Park, H., Kelly, P., and Robinson, J.R., 1985, Bioadhesive polymers as platforms for oral controlled drug delivery II: synthesis and evaluation of some swelling, water-insoluble bioadhesive polymers, J. Pharm. Sci., 74:399.

Davis, S.S., Daly, P.B., Kennerley, J.W., Frier, M., Hardy, J.G., and Wilson, C.G., 1982, Design and evaluation of sustained release formulations for oral and buccal administration, in: "Controlled release nitroglycerin in buccal and oral form", W.-D. Bussmann, R.-D. Dries, and W. Wagner, eds., Advances in Pharmacotherapy, Vol. 1, Karger, Basel, 17.

Davis, S.S., 1985, personal communication.

Ishida, M., Machida, Y., Nambu, N., and Nagai, T., 1981, New mucosal dosage form of insulin, Chem. Pharm. Bull., 29:810.

Ishida, M., Nambu, N., Nagai, T., 1982, Mucosal dosage form of lidocain for toothache using hydroxypropyl cellulose and carbopol, Chem. Pharm. Bull., 30:980.

Hussain, A.A., Bawarshi-Nassar, R., Huang, C.H., 1985, Physicochemical considerations in intranasal drug administration, in: "Transnasal systemic medications", Y.W. Chien, ed., Elsevier, Amsterdam, 121.

Lee, P., 1986, Kinetics of drug release from hydrogel matrices, in: "Advances in drug delivery systems", J.M. Anderson and S.W. Kim, eds., Elsevier, Amsterdam, 277.

Merkle, H.P., Anders, R., Sandow, J., Schurr, W., 1985, Self-adhesive patches for buccal delivery of peptides, Proceed. Intern. Symp. Control. Rel. Bioact. Mater., 12:85.

Merkle, H.P., Anders, R., and Sandow, J., 1986, Abstract: Buccal Absorption of peptides in rats, Proceed. 32th annual congress of APV, Mainz, 57.

Nagai, T., 1986, Adhesive topical drug delivery systems, in: "Advances in drug delivery systems", J.M. Anderson, S.W. Kim, eds., Elsevier, Amsterdam, 121.

Nishi, N., Arimura, A., Coy, D.H., Vilches-Martinez, J.A., Schally, A.V., 1975, The effect of oral and vaginal administration of synthetic LHRH and (D-Ala(6)-DesGly(10)-NH$_2$)-LHRH ethylamid on serum LH-levels on ovariectomized, steroid blocked rats, Proc. Soc. Exp. Biol. Med., 148:1009.

Nishihata, T., Rytting, J.H., Higuchi, T., Caldwell, L., 1981, Enhanced rectal absorption of insulin and heparin in rats in the presence of non-surfactant adjuvants, J. Pharm. Sci., 33:334.

Okada, H., Yamazaki, I., Ogawa, Y., Hirai, S., Yashiki, T., Mima, H., 1982, Vaginal absorption of a potent luteinizing hormone-releasing analogue (Leuprolide) in rats I: absorption by various routes and absorption enhancement, J. Pharm. Sci., 71:1367.

Okada, H., Yamazaki, I., Yashiki, T., Mima, H., 1983, Vaginal absorption of a potent luteinizing hormone-releasing analogue (Leuprolide) in rats II: mechanism of absorption enhancement, J. Pharm. Sci., 72:75.

Park, H., and Robinson, J.R., 1986, Physico-chemical properties of water insoluble polymers important to mucin/epithelial adhesion, in: "Advances in drug delivery systems", J.M. Anderson, and S.W. Kim, eds., Elsevier, Amsterdam, 47.

Peppas, N.A., and Buri, P.A., 1986, Surface, interfacial and molecular aspects of polymer bioadhesion on soft tissues, in: "Advances in drug delivery systems", J.M. Anderson, and S.W. Kim, eds., Elsevier, Amsterdam, 257.

Sandow, J., and Petri, W., 1985, Intranasal administration of peptides biological activity and therapeutic efficacy, in: "Transnasal Systemic Medications", Y.W. Chien, ed., Elsevier, Amsterdam, 183.

Schurr, W., Knoll, B., Ziegler, R., Anders, R., and Merkle, H.P., 1985, Comparative study of intravenous, nasal, oral and buccal TRH administration among healthy subjects, J. Endocrin. Invest., 8:41.

Stratford, R.E., and Lee, V.H.L., 1985, Aminopeptidase activity in albino
    rabbit extraocular tissues relative to the small intestine, J. Pharm.
    Sci., 74:731
Su, K.S.E., 1986, Intranasal delivery of peptides and proteins, Pharm.
    Int., 7:8.
Su, K.S.E., and Campanale, K.M., 1985, Nasal drug delivery systems re-
    quirements, development and evaluations, in: "Transnasal Systemic
    medications", Y.W. Chien, ed., Elsevier, Amsterdam, 139.
Van de Donk, H.J.M., Van den Heuvel, A.G.M., Zuidema, J., and Merkus, F.W.
    H.M., 1982, The effects of nasal drops and their additives on human,
    nasal mucociliary clearance, Rhinology, 20:127.
Wespi, H.J., and Rehsteiner, H.P., 1966, Erfahrungen mit Syntocinon- und
    ODA-Buccaltabletten, Gynaecologia, 162:414.
Yoshioka, S., Caldwell, L., and Higuchi, T., 1982, Enhanced rectal bio-
    availability of polypeptides using sodium 5-methoxysalicylate as
    an absorption promotor, J. Pharm. Sci., 71:593.

ENHANCED ABSORPTION AND LYMPHATIC TRANSPORT

OF MACROMOLECULES VIA THE RECTAL ROUTE

Shozo Muranishi, Kanji Takada, Hiroshi Yoshikawa,
and Masahiro Murakami
Kyoto Pharmaceutical University
Misasagi, Yamashina
Kyoto, Japan

INTRODUCTION

The rectal route has long been known as a specific absorption means for the delivery of lipophilic small molecules. In general rectal delivery exhibits several advantages as summarized in Table 1.

Orally administered polypeptide drugs are degraded or metabolized by acid and/or enzymes in the stomach and small intestine, or are absorbed poorly, and thus have lowered bioavailability. By contrast, bioconversion of polypeptides hardly occurs in the lower digestive tract due to low enzymatic activity and neutral pH. However, the normal adult lower intestine is an impermeable barrier to the uptake of macromolecules (Dalmark, 1968; Warshaw et al., 1977; Taniguchi et al., 1980), and for effective drug therapy, the form of the drug must be modified to improve absorption, and to make delivery safe and efficient.

CHARACTERISTICS OF ENHANCED ABSORPTION BY PROMOTERS

Various investigations are being made presently towards enhancing the rectal absorption of poorly absorbable drugs, (for example see Nishihata et al. (1981)). Our first report in 1977 showed that the absorption of heparin through the large intestine was greater than that through the small intestine if aided by an adjuvant; a lipid-bile salt mixed micellar system (Muranishi et al., 1977).

At the beginning of the study we intended to apply the potential adjuvant effect to oral medication, but our results strongly suggested

Table 1. Advantages of Rectal Administration

---

1. Safe and convenient administration, painless
2. Possible way to reduce drug degradation in gastrointestinal tract
3. By passing of the liver to avoid "first pass" elimination of high clearance drugs
4. Convenience to administer a large dose

---

that rectal administration was more suitable for inducing the absorption of macromolecules. Although we have used an aqueous solution or colloidal suspension of the promoters in animal experiments, a dosage formulation for rectal administration can be designed for therapeutic use as shown in Fig. 1.

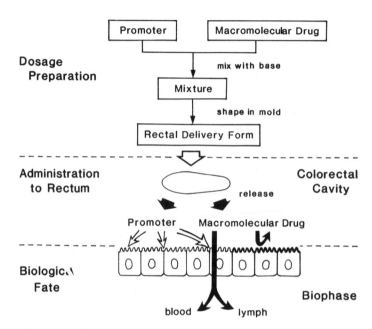

Fig. 1. Strategy for getting potential absorption of macromolecules

When the designed suppository is administered to the rectal cavity, the macromolecular drug and promoter are released to be in close contact with the rectal and colonic mucous membranes. The promoters, such as monoolein, oleic acid, linoleic acid, capric acid, salicylic acid or their salts can act on the epithelial cells to allow permeation of the macromolecules. The molecules can then pass through the cells and enter both the blood and lymph capillaries.

Most promoters are lipophilic compounds which have a small hydrophilic moiety such as a carboxyl group. Some seem to have a surfactant action on the biomembrane (the mucous surface) and thereby modify the epithelium. However, it is evident by many experimental results that the absorption enhancing effect by these safe adjuvants is essentially different from the action of surfactants. Microscopic observations have failed to show severe damage such as disruption and loss of the surface of the mucosal cell membrane, on exposure to the promoters. As shown in

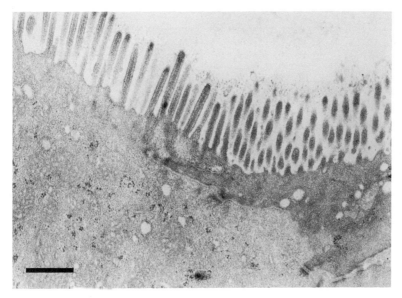

Fig. 2. Electron micrograph of rat colonic epithelium after
exposure of the colonic mucosa to 0.5% linoleic
acid - 0.8% HCO 60 (non-ionic surfactant) mixed
micellar solution for 5 min. (Magnification   x
15,000. Scale bar, 500 nm.)

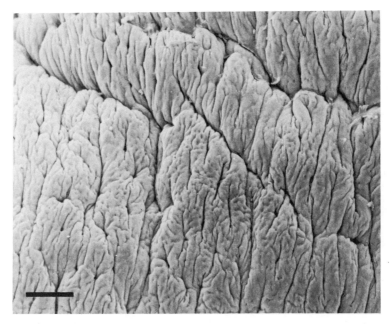

Fig. 3. Scanning electron micrograph of colonic surface of
rat after exposure of the colonic mucosa to 0.5%
linoleic acid -0.8% HCO 60 mixed micellar solution
for 2 h. (Magnification x 160. Scale bar, 100 µm.)

Table 2. Examples of large Molecules adsorbed
from the Colorectum

	Molecular weight
Bleomycin	~ 1500
Insulin	~ 6000
Heparin	~ 6000
Interferon α, β	25000 ~ 35000
Dextrans	20000 - 70000
Dextran sulfate	~ 500000

Figs. 2 and 3, electron microscopy also revealed that the colonic mucosal cells were completely intact after administration of linoleic acid - HCO 60 mixed micellar solution (MM).

Surfactants such as sodium lauryl sulfate or BL-9EX when used to treat the intestine, cause the breakdown of the mucous layer covering the epithelium and a long-lasting increase in absorption. Such membrane damage may be directly relevant to the enhancing effect of surfactants on drug absorption (Attwood and Florence, 1983). Regeneration of epithelial cells of the intestine usually takes 6-10 hrs. On the other hand, the promoters mentioned above are characterized by a transient effect on the biomembrane.

When 10 mM oleic acid - HCO in a pH 7.4 phosphate buffer MM was perfused into the large intestine, the increase of permeation of a solute began about 10-15 min after the start of perfusion. Furthermore when the promoter solution was washed out with saline, the enhanced permeability gradually disappeared, and returned to the value for an impermeable membrane about 15-20 min after washing (Muranishi et al., 1980). This transient and reversible nature of the promoter effect is the most important and distinct difference from that of simple surfactant action.

The strength of the enhancing effect for the polar lipid - surfactant MM system differs greatly with the site in the digestive tract. In short, the mucosal sensitivity to the promoter along the gastrointestinal tract is in the following order: rectum > colon > small intestine > stomach. The highest sensitivity seen for the colorectal area was surprising, but is very attractive for the rectal delivery of macromolecules (Muranishi, 1985).

BLOOD - LYMPH UPTAKE OF MACROMOLECULES: MOLECULAR WEIGHT CONSIDERATIONS

Among therapeutic drugs, there are many water-soluble, poorly absorbable high molecular weight compounds such as the polypeptides. The compounds tested for absorption have been large with a molecular weight of from 1500 to 500000 as shown in Table 2.

The first example of a large molecule is bleomycin, an anticancer agent and cationic glycopeptide of MW 1500. In the presence of 40 mM lipid - bile salt MM, bleomycin levels in blood and lymph increased rapidly and reached a maximum at about 30-45 min, at which time the concentrations were over 10 fold of those for the experiment without adjuvant (Fig. 4, Yoshikawa et al., 1981). It is considered likely that the small peptide may be transported into both fluids at equal concentrations after passing through the mucosal cells.

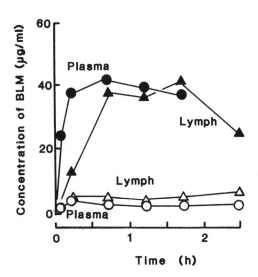

Fig. 4. Concentrations of bleomycin in plasma and thoracic duct lymph after administration with 40 mM monoolein - taurocholate MM into the large intestine. Open symbol; no adjuvant, closed symbol; plus promoter

FITC-labelled dextrans (FD) of various molecular weights above 10000 were chosen as water soluble macromolecules in order to evaluate the blood-lymph selection mechanism for higher molecular weight compounds. As shown in Fig. 5, the maximum plasma levels decreased with an increase in molecular weight, whereas the maximum lymph levels remained high irrespective of molecular weight. Therefore, the lymph/plasma ratio was elevated by an increase in molecular size. The absorption rate and amount seemed to be lowered with an increase in the molecular weight, since the lymph levels showed a slower rise with the larger molecules.

The lymph levels of FD with MW higher than about 20000 were significantly higher than their plasma levels. From these results we can conclude that the marked increase in lymph/plasma ratios of FD, with increase in their molecular weight, is responsible for the difficulty in delivering FD into the blood circulation (Muranishi, 1984). The result of this blood-lymph selectivity is likely to be non-active and a simple molecular sieving mechanism.

Fig. 6 shows the movement of molecules in the biophase after rectal administration. If neither phagocytosis nor binding to tissue and biomacromolecules occurs locally, small molecules can transfer directly into both the blood and lymph capillaries. Large molecules and particles that can pass through the epithelium do not readily enter the blood vessels but instead easily pass into the lymphatic channels through clefts in the lymphatic endothelium. A polypeptide smaller than MW 10000 may be transferred into both fluids at about the same concentrations, while a protein over approximately MW 20000, like albumin, may enter principally into the lymphatic fluid. It will enter the jugular/subclavian vein through the thoracic duct near the heart, thereby avoiding the liver.

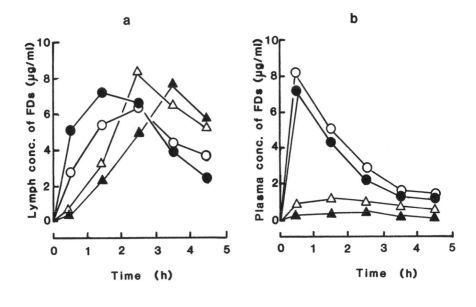

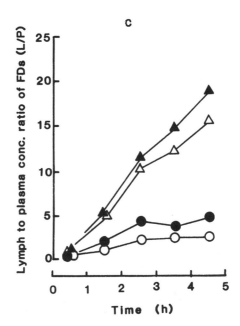

Fig. 5. Lymph and plasma concentrations of FDs after administration with lipid – surfactant mixed micelles into the large intestine. (a) Lymph concentration, (b) Plasma concentration, (c) Lymph/Plasma concentration ratio. ● FD10, o FD20, Δ FD40, ▲ FD70.

Fluorescent microscope observations of a colon containing FD 70 (Fig. 7) clearly demonstrate that the dextran can pass through the colonic epithelium in the presence of a promoter. Thus, we will consider the transfer routes of uptake of macromolecules by the mucosal epithelium in order to clarify the trans-epithelium mechanisms.

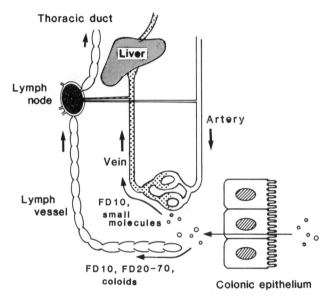

Fig. 6.   Schematic view of the passage of a molecule or particle from an intraluminal administration site into blood and lymph.

Fig. 8 depicts the events presumed to occur within the epithelium for the uptake and transport of a macromolecule. There could be at least two routes: the transcellular and the paracellular, in the enhanced state of absorption obtained with MM. To elucidate this transport process, we have used three kinds of colorectal material: everted loop, isolated epithelial cells, and brush border vesicles.

The experiment using the perfused everted loop involved permeation through two routes. In contrast, the uptake into isolated epithelial cells involves only transmembrane movement and includes brush border membrane transport as well as basolaterial membrane transport. The uptake into brush border membrane vesicles, prepared by the method Kessler et al., involves only permeation of the mucosal surface membrane of the cells (Kessler et al., 1978).

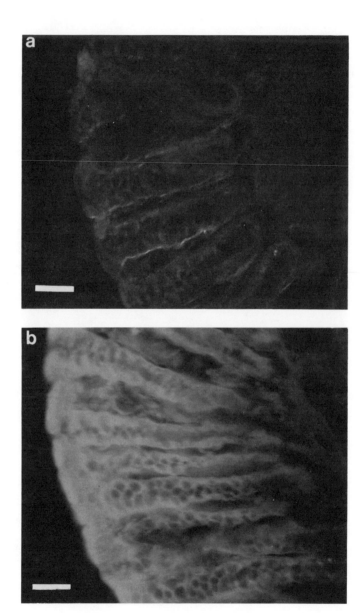

Fig. 7. Fluorescence microphotographs of rat colon after
         exposure to (a) 60 μg/ml FD 70 aqueous solution for 5
         min, and (b) the same concentration of FD 70 with
         0.5% linoleic acid - HCO 60 MM for 5 min. (Scale bar,
         20 μm.)

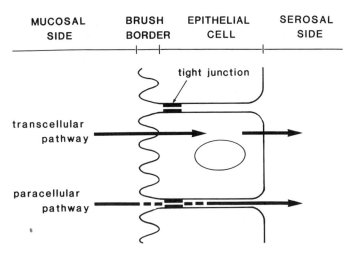

Fig. 8.   Diagrammatic representation of permeation across
          intestinal barriers

Table 3.   Permeated Amounts of FDs from Mucosal Side through
           the Everted Wall of Rat Large Intestine after 2 h

	FD10	FD20	FD40	FD70
None (ng)	1234	1295	361	162
MM (ng)	7679	5140	1054	390

Table 4.   Uptakes of FDs into the Isolated Epithelial Cells
           of Rat Large Intestine after 30 min

	FD10	FD20	FD40	FD70
None (μg/mg protein)	5.57	2.63	1.78	1.34
MM (μg mg/protein)	11.58	4.04	3.99	1.34

Table 3 shows the permeated amounts of FD into serosal fluid 2 hrs after administration into the everted loop. The permeated amounts decreased inversely with the increasing molecular weight either with or without MM. However, the enhancement effect was stronger for the smaller dextrans than for the larger ones. In the study of isolated cells, the uptake of smaller FDs was also promoted by MM, but the largest molecule (FD 70) did not show an apparent promotion (Table 4).

The ratios of FD permeated or taken up with MM, to that without MM, were calculated and compared (Fig. 9). The uptake into isolated cells was less than that for the everted loop. There were some differences in the two systems for any given FD; the biggest being for FD 10 and a slight difference was found even for FD 70. In the study of brush border membrane vesicles, the uptake of FDs smaller than MW 40000 was promoted as shown in Table 5. These results suggested that the brush border membrane of epithelial cells could become permeable to the macromolecules in the presence of MM. Based on the above permeation study, the participation of paracellular as well as transcellular transport can be considered important in the enhancing effect of MM on the colorectal absorption of macromolecules.

ENHANCED UPTAKE OF COLLOIDS

The sizes of various FDs and colloidal particles are summarized in Table 6. Compared with the colloidal materials, FD 10 would correspond to colloidal gold G-5, and FD 70 would be smaller than colloidal gold G-20. We have used dialysed commercial ink colloids and colloidal golds to study enhanced absorption of colloids in the colorectum.

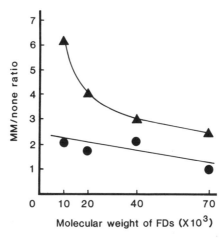

Fig. 9. Comparison of enhancing effect by MM between isolated cells and everted loop.
o, isolated cells, Δ, everted loop

Table 5. Uptakes of FDs into Brush Border Membrane Vesicles of Rat Large Intestine

	FD10	FD20	FD40	FD70
None (µg/mg protein)	16.02	16.59	2.37	2.21
MM (µg/mg protein)	60.41	46.35	5.61	2.50

Table 6. Sizes of Test Colloids and Macromolecules (diameter, nm)

Colloid		Macromolecule**	
Platinum ink	2.4-10*	FD10	4.6
Colloidal gold G-5	5	FD20	6.4
G-20	20	FD40	8.8
G-40	40	FD70	11.6
Rotring ink	100-800*		

* Determined by ultrafiltration.
**Calculated from Stokes radius.

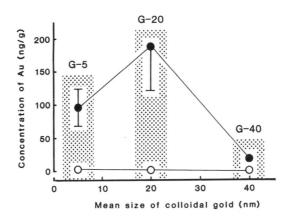

Fig. 10. Effect of MM on the large intestinal absorption of colloidal golds at 2 hrs after dosing.
o, Regional lymph nodes, o, Plasma

After administration of platinum ink a black stain was visualized in the iliac lymph nodes and thoracic duct lymph, while coloring did not appear after the administration of Rotring ink. Furthermore, at 2 hrs after administration of colloidal golds of different sizes, measurable concentrations of gold could be determined in the lymph nodes and plasma. As shown in Fig. 10, much higher concentrations of gold were detected in the regional lymph nodes as compared to the plasma. However, high levels in the lymph nodes were not observed for colloidal gold G-40, indicating that a limitation for absorbable size may be around 40 nm.

When the absorption sites were examined in more detail, higher concentrations in lymph nodes were observed following administration to the area of rectum as compared to the colon. Apparently, small nondegradable and insoluble colloidal particles can be traversed across the mucosal barrier into lymphatic fluid and retained in the regional lymph nodes. These findings on colloidal particles support those on the the movement of macromolecules.

CONCLUSION

Rectal dosage design using promoters provides the possibility of enhancing the absorption of macromolecules. Such systems could be useful for delivery of polypeptides such as insulin and interferon (Yoshikawa et al., 1985). The water soluble molecules of a size larger than approximately MW 20000 had lymphotropic properties. The size limitation size in promoted absorption may be as large as 40 nm diameter. Bacteria and rickettsia should be too large to permeate the colorectal barrier and consequently, the rectal delivery might be a highly safe method of administering macromolecules.

REFERENCES

Attwood, D. and Florence, A.T., 1983, Interaction of surfactants with membranes and membrane components, in: "Surfactant Systems," Chapman and Hall, London.

Dalmark, M., 1968, Plasma radioactivity after rectal instillation of radioiodine-labeled human albumin in normal subjects and in patients with ulcerative colitis, Scand. J. Gastroent., 3:490

Kessler, M., Acuto, O., Storelli, C., Murer, H., Muller, M., and Semenza, G., 1978, A modified procedure for the rapid preparation of efficiently transporting vesicles from small intestinal brush border membranes, Biochim. Biophys. Acta, 506:136.

Nishihata, T., Rytting, J.H., and Higuchi, T., 1981, Enhanced rectal absorption of insulin and heparin in the presence of non-surfactant adjuvants, J. Pharm. Pharmacol., 33:334.

Muranishi, S., Tokunaga, Y., Taniguchi, K., and Sezaki, H., 1977, Potential absorption of heparin from the small intestine and the large intestine in the presence of monoolein mixed micelles, Chem. Pharm. Bull., 25:1159.

Muranishi, S., 1984, Characteristics of drug absorption via rectal route, Meth. and Find. Exptl. Clin. Pharmacol., 6:763.

Muranishi, S., 1985, Modification of intestinal absorption of drugs by lipoidal adjuvants, Pharm. Res., 3:108.

Muranishi, N., Kinugawa, M., Nakajima, Y., Muranishi, S., and Sezaki, H., 1980, Mechanism for inducement of the intestinal absorption of poorly absorbed drugs by mixed micelles I. Effects of various lipid - bile salt mixed micelles on the intestinal absorption of streptomycin in rat, Int. J. Pharm., 4:271.

Taniguchi, K., Muranishi, S., and Sezaki, H., 1980, Enhanced intestinal permeability to macromolecules II. Improvement of the large intestinal absorption of heparin by lipid - surfactant mixed micelles in rat, Int. J. Pharm., 4:219.

Warshaw, A.L., Bellini, C.A., and Warker, W.A., 1977, The intestinal mucosal barrier to intact antigenic protein:difference between colon and small intestine, Am. J. Surg., 133:55.

Yoshikawa, H., Muranishi, S., Kato, C., and Sezaki, H., 1981, Bifunctional delivery system for selective transfer of bleomycin into lymphatics via enteral route, Int. J. Pharm., 8:291.

Yoshikawa, H., Satoh, Y., Naruse, N., Takada, K., Muranishi, S., 1985, Comparison of disappearance from blood and lymphatic delivery of human fibroblast interferon in rat by different administration routes, J. Pharmacobio-Dyn., 8:206.

BIOPHARMACEUTICAL ASPECTS ON THE INTRANASAL ADMINISTRATION OF PEPTIDES

A. S. Harris

Ferring AB
P O Box 30561
S-200 62 MALMÖ, Sweden

INTRODUCTION

The intranasal route for administering peptides is probably one of the most neglected methods of delivery to the systemic circulation. Yet because of its high surface area available for absorption, its highly vasculized bed of mucosa and the fact that the nasal cavity appears to have very little metabolizing capacity all indicate that absorption across the nasal membranes is a reasonable proposition. The increasing importance which has been attached to peptides as new therapeutic agents is a consequence of the isolation and structural characterisation of various peptides, including the discovery of hypothalamic releasing hormones and pituitary hormones. The advantages of the naturally occuring peptide hormones as drug candidates have mainly been attributed to their potent pharmacological activity and their good biological tolerance. However, the disadvantages have been their broad pharmacological activity (which is often masked by a singular potent effect) and their relative short biological halflife (Table 1). However, with the introduction of peptide

Table 1. Characterisation of naturally occurring peptide hormones as candidates for administration by the nasal route.

PEPTIDE HORMONES AS DRUG CANDIDATES

- Broad pharmacological activity
- Short half-life
- Good biological tolerance
- Often prescribed for chronic and life-long diseases
- Often used in substitutionen therapy
- Poor stability in G.I. fluids
- Undergo extensive first-pass elimination
- Parenteral administration is most common route

analogues the spectrum of their biological activities have been markedly changed and improved in terms of more potent, more specific effects with longer biological halflives.

WHICH PEPTIDES HAVE BEEN ADMINISTERED BY THE NASAL ROUTE?

The earliest examples of nasal administration of peptides were the use of pituitary hormones such as oxytocin, vasopressin and its analogues. More recently, the range of compounds which have been found to cross the nasal mucosa has been extended to include polypeptides such as insulin (Morimoto et al., 1985), luteinizing hormone releasing hormone (LHRH) (Anik et al., 1984), secretin (Ohwaki et al., 1985), and growth releasing factors (GRF) (Evans et al., 1983). However, among all these previously named compounds only the pituitary hormones and LHRH are presently licensed by international regulatory authorities for therapeutic use by the intranasal route (Table 2).

WHAT IS THE THE CLINICAL EXPERIENCE?

The pituitary hormones, oxytocin, vasopressin and its analogues have been administered by the nasal route for many years. Oxytocin is the drug of choice for the induction of labour once the pregnancy is at term; it is used to assist an ongoing abortion, or to increase milk flow to the infant (Hoover, 1971). Vasopressin or antidiuretic hormone (ADH), is a polypeptide with 9 amino acid residues. Vasopressin promotes water retention but also increases excretion of sodium and chloride. When there is a defect in the hypothalamic secretion of ADH, diabetes insipidus develops. Polyuria and polydipsia are the major symptoms. Longterm treatment of diabetes insipidus has been either the intramuscular injection of pitressin tannate or the nasal insufflation of crude posterior pituitary powder (Fraser and Scott, 1963). Lysopressin, the synthetic analogue of vasopressin has been administered by nasal spray. This preparation is effective in patients with diabetes insipidus and its use was first described in 1963 (Barltrop, 1963). Desmopressin (DDAVP or

Table 2. A list of peptides which are in <u>routine</u> clinical use for various therapeutic indications and are given by the nasal route.

PEPTIDE	THERAPEUTIC INDICATION
Oxytocin (PARTOCON®) (SYTOCINON®)	• stimulate lactation • induction of labour
Vasopressin/Lypressin (POSTACTON®)	• diabetes insipidus
Desmopressin/DDAVP (MINIRIN®)	• diabetes insipidus • primary nocturnal enuresis • release Factor VIII
Gonadotropin-releasing hormone, LHRH-agonist (BUSERELIN®)	• prostate carcinoma • testis retention • endometriosis

l-deamino-8-D-arginine vasopressin) is a synthetic analogue of vasopressin. Vavra et al (1968) reported that in rats, dogs and humans, desmopressin has a greater antidiuretic potency than either the natural hormone or any other known synthetic analogue and that it also produces a prolonged antidiuresis. The pressor activities normally associated with vasopressin were simultaneously reduced to very low values. Furthermore, in comparison with vasopressin it has a better biological tolerance and longer halflife and greater duration of therapeutic effect (Fig 1). On the basis of a slow metabolic clearance, good absorption through the nasal mucosa and lack of side effects, desmopressin is the drug of choice for the treatment of vasopressin sensitive diabetes insipidus (Edwards et al., 1973) (Figure 1).

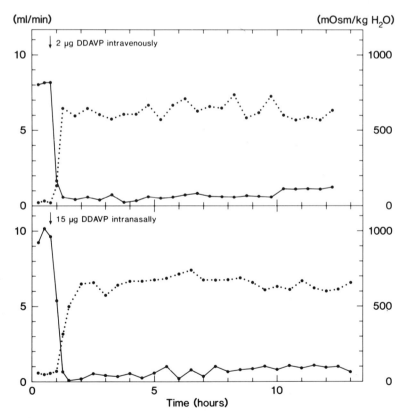

Fig. 1.   The clinical effect of DDAVP given intravenously and intranasally on urine volume (•——•) and urine osmolality (•----•) in six patients with diabetes insipidus.

WHAT IS THE BIOAVAILABILITY AFTER NASAL ADMINISTRATION?

Present evidence seems to suggest that nasal administration of peptides has a bioavailability trend between 1 - 20% depending on molecular weight and physiochemical properties of the peptide. The fact that some absorption of GRF, a peptide with 44 amino acids has been described is very encouraging (Table 3).

Next to the parenteral route, administration by the nasal route may be the most efficient means of achieving systemic effect. For LHRH and its agonists, for example, although the nasal route may require a 100 fold multiple of the parenteral dose, administration by the rectal and vaginal route are 4 - 6 times less effective. Furthermore, oral bioavailability of LHRH is extremely low, requiring a 30 - 100 higher dose than by the nasal route (Sandow and Petri, 1985) (Table 4).

Table 3. Bioavailability of peptides following nasal administration: Effect of molecular weight.

RELATIONSHIP BETWEEN
NASAL BIOAVAILABILITY AND MOLECULAR WEIGHT

Peptides	Absorption (%)	No of amino acids
Thyrotropin-releasing hormone (TRH)	20	3
Vasopressin analogs	6-12	9
LHRH, agonists and antagonists	1-10	9-10
ACTH analogs	12	17-18
Growth hormone-releasing factor (GRF)	1-2	40-44

Table 4. Relationship between route of administration and relative efficacy of LHRH in the induction of ovulation in rats

EFFECT OF LHRH IN THE INDUCTION OF OVULATION

Route of administration	Relative effective dose Ovulation
S.c./I.v.	1
Nasal	100
Rectal	400
Vaginal	600
Oral	3 000

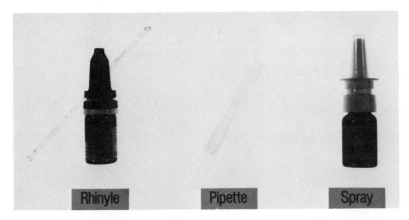

Fig. 2. Three types of delivery systems currently used for nasal administration

WHICH DELIVERY FORMS ARE AVAILABLE?

The standard method of administration has been in the form of sprays or drops being delivered using rhinyle catheters, single dose pipettes, and metered dose spray pumps (Figure 2). The rhinyle catheter was the first system to be introduced and has the advantage that the catheter is graduated for different doses as required by the patient. The advantage of the disposal pipette is that it is suitable for single dose administration and therefore does not require a preservative to be added which is one of the most singular causes of nasal irritation and allergic rhinitis in patients on long term nasal therapy. The spray pump is simple to use and allows multiple dosing of any given dose.

WHICH FACTORS AFFECT SYSTEMIC ABSORPTION?

There are many factors which affect the systemic uptake of nasally administered peptides. These factors can be grouped into either a function of the peptide itself, of the nasal mucosa or influenced by the choice of delivery system and formulation (Table 5).

It has been postulated that the site of absorption and rate of clearance of the drug influence the absorption and therefore its therapeutic effect. A study by Hardy et al (1985) compared the deposition and clearance of solutions administered by spray (100 μl) and by one (30 μl) or three nasal drops (90 μl). The nasal spray was found to deposit anteriorly in the nasal atrium in contrast to the drops which dispersed throughout the length of the nasal cavity. In consequence the spray was found to clear more slowly than the drops since most of the sprays deposited on non-cilated regions.

Although these previous studies have investigated in some detail the method and technique of nasal administration, no work has been done on the relationship between deposition and in vivo absorption on the one hand and the effect of nasal delivery systems on resulting biological response on the other hand. Using the peptide desmopressin as a model, a study was designed to compare various methods of intranasal delivery by measuring

Table 5. Physiochemical, physiological and
pharmaceutical factors which influence
systemic absorption of peptides given
by the nasal route.

Which factors affect systemic absorption?

PEPTIDE EFFECT

- Molecular size
- Hydrophilic/lipophilic characteristics
- Local enzymatic degradation in the nasal cavity

NASAL EFFECT

- Rhinitis
- Local pathological changes in the nasal cavity
- Colds

DELIVERY EFFECT

- Formulation
- Choice of delivery system
- Deposition and clearance

deposition and clearance using gamma and scintigraphy, by measuring systemic absorption using a specific radioimmunoassay and, by determining the effect on circulating levels of Factor VIII, its consequent biological response.

EXPERIMENTAL

Nasal formulations

Desmopressin solutions containing ^{99m}Tc-labelled human serum albumin were administered intranasally as sprays using two types of metered dose spray pumps or as drops using a rhinyle catheter or a pipette. The rhinyle delivery device was a calibrated plastic catheter designed to give a dose of 200 µl or 300 µg of a solution of 1.5 mg/ml desmopressin. The single dose pipette contained 200 µl or 300 µg desmopressin. Two nasal sprays were tested: one gave a volume of 100 µl or 150 µg of 1.5 mg/ml desmopressin, the other gave a volume of 50 µl or 150 µg of 3.0 mg/ml desmopressin per actuation. Radiolabelling of each device was done by addition of 1 mg human serum albumin radiolabelled with 100 – 200 MBq ^{99m}Tc. Each dose contained 2 – 4 MBq ^{99m}Tc.

Deposition Studies

The nasal solutions were administered to six healthy volunteers, all male of 30 years or more. None of the subjects had nasal problems and all were free from colds. Separated by an interval of at least three days, each subject received all four methods of delivery which were allocated in a blind, randomised sequence using coded, sealed envelopes. In this way, a total of 24 administrations were made. The study was approved by the hospital ethical committee and radioisotope committee, and each subject gave written informed consent prior to entry into the study.

All nasal solutions were administered with the subjects sitting in an upright position and into the same nostril on each occcasion. A standard dose of 300 µg desmopressin was self-administered in every case. The rhinyle was administered by first filling 0.2 ml solution into the tube.

One end of the rhinyle was then put into the mouth, the other end was introduced 5 - 10 mm into the nostril and delivery was accomplished by blowing. The pipette was administered by the following procedure: the subject's head was tilted back and individual drops were dispensed into the nostril during normal breathing. The head was turned to the right and left and then back to the original position before the subject assumed a normal sitting position. The two nasal sprays were designed to give accurate doses of 50 µl and 100 µl respectively. Prior to administration, each spray device was primed by activating the pump five times. The applicator tip was introduced 5 - 10 mm into the nostril and two doses of 100 µl or 50 µl were dispensed during normal inhalation, with the contralateral nostril open.

Throughout the study, and at each monitoring period, the subjects continued to breath normally but did not blow their noses or sneeze. Food and drink were withdrawn for the first hour, thereafter ad libertum.

At the instance of dosing, each subject was seated adjacent the gamma camera head. Immediately after dosing, the tracer was monitored repeatedly by the gamma camera and a lateral view of the head recorded for 10 min. Additional images were recorded at 15 min intervals for the first hour and then at hourly or two-hourly intervals up to 8 hours.

The data were recorded by computer (PDP (11/34), Gamma II V3.1) for subsequent analysis. Each image was displayed on a monitor and regions of interest were demarcated. The count rate at each monitoring period was corrected for radioactive decay. Each count rate in each region of interest was expressed as a percentage of the initial count rate taken immediately after dosing.

Blood Collection and Plasma Collection

Blood samples were collected by vein puncture (21-gauge needles) at times 0, 15, 30, 45 and 60 min and 2, 4 and 8 hours after administration. Blood was collected in a 3.8% trisodium citrate solution at a ratio of 9 to 1. Platelet poor plasma was obtained after centrifugation at 2000 x g for 10 min at 4°C and stored frozen at -50°C until tested.

Assay methods

Plasma DDAVP was assayed using a sensitive and specific radioimmunoassay (RIA). Antiserum to DDAVP was developed as described by Sofroniew et al (1978). Since DDAVP lacks the N-terminal amino group it was necessary to use 8-D-AVP, and this analogue was then coupled to thyroglobulin (Lundin et al., 1985). Monoiodinated DDAVP was produced by the chloramin T method (Greenwood et al., 1963). Briefly, 5 µmoles of DDAVP (0.25 mg/ml in 0.05 M sodium phosphate buffer, pH 7.5) were added to 1mCi of Na^{125}I (IMS 30, Amersham) and incubated for 60 s. The monoiodinated tracer was immediately isolated by reversed phase HPLC (27% acetonitrile in 0.1% trifluoroacetic acid) to a specific activity of at least 1600 mCi/µmol. The RIA contained 100 µl of standard (5.0 pg/ml to 640 pg/ml) or sample diluted five times with assay buffer, 100 µl of tracer (approximately 500 cpm) and 200 µl of antiserum (1/100 000). 100 µl of normal human serum diluted five times was added to the standard and 100 µl assay buffer was added to the sample tubes. Incubation were carried out for 48 h at 4°C followed by separation of bound and free radioactivity by addition of 1 ml plasma-coated charcoal. The assay diluent was 0.05 M sodium phosphate buffer, pH 7.5, containing 0.01% sodium acid and 0.1% human serum albumin. F VIII coagulant activity (F VIII:C) was measured by chromogenic substrate assay (Coatest®, KabiVitrum, Stockholm, Sweden)

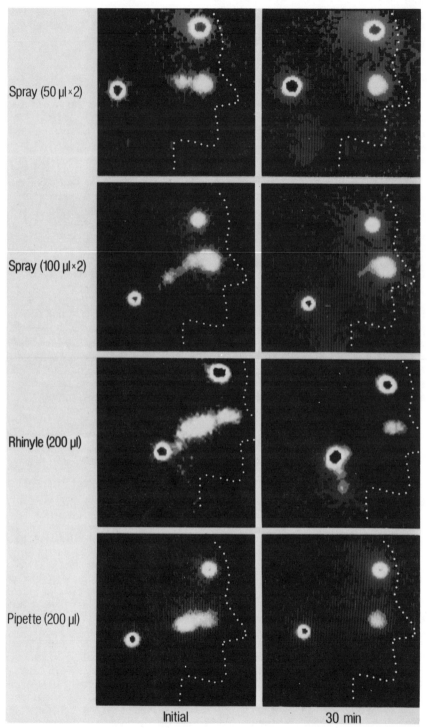

Fig. 3. Gamma scintigraphy images of sites of deposition and patterns of clearance following administration of sprays by two nasal pumps and drops by rhinyle and pipette. Each pair of images is of the same subject, but the four pairs are of different subjects.

according to Rosen et al (1984). F VIII/von Willebrand factor (F vWF) was measured by immunoradiometric assay (IRMA) according to Ruggeri et al (1976). To eliminate the large systematic differences observed between subjects, the samples obtained before administration were given an arbitrary potency of 100% for F VIII:C and F vWF.

Statistical methods

Friedman's two-way analysis of variance by ranks and Wilcoxon matched-pairs, signed rank test were used where appropriate. In addition t max, C max and ½ t were calculated for plasma profiles of desmopressin after each method of administration. AUC were determined for plasma desmopressin verses time course. Linear regression was calculated using the least squares method.

RESULTS AND DISCUSSION

Deposition studies

Analysis of the data revealed a distinct difference in the pattern of deposition and clearance between the nasal sprays and nasal drops. On the one hand, the pipette and rhinyle appeared to deposit solution towards the rear of the nasal cavity at the site of the nasopharynx while, on the other hand, the nasal sprays tended to deposit anteriorly in the nasal cavity (Fig 3). As the images were taken continually for the first ten minutes, it was possible to visualize the dynamic clearance of each solution from its site of deposition. It was apparent that the major bulk of the pipette and rhinyle drops was cleared very rapidly whilst the nasal sprays tended to break-up into small portions from its site of deposition and were cleared at a slower rate as cilary movement transported these small portions back along to the nasopharynx.

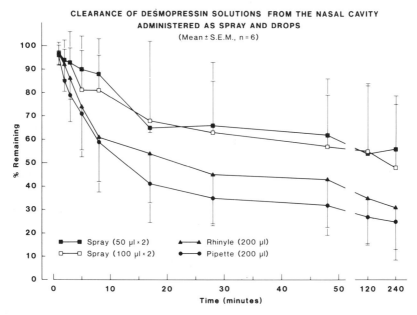

Fig. 4. Nasal clearance of the ^{99m}Tc radiolabelled tracer from the nasal cavity after administration of 100 µl spray, 200 µl spray, rhinyle and pipette each to six subjects (Mean ± SEM).

These qualitative findings were complimented by qualitative data on the relative rate of clearance of each solution. The curves revealed a biphasic pattern of clearance, a fast initial clearance followed by a slower, more prolonged second phase (Fig 4). It was the initial, fast phase that clearly distinguished the nasal drops of the pipette and rhinyle from the spray drops. This showed a 50% clearance by 14 and 20 minutes for the pipette and rhinyle respectively in contrast to 120 and 240 minutes for the 200 μl and 100 μl sprays respectively. These results are in agreement with the findings of Aoki and Crawley (1976) who showed that drops were cleared faster than sprays. However, in contrast, our data shows the rate of clearance to be much faster for all solutions but specifically so for the nasal drops. Indeed, many subjects commented subjectively on a sensation of swallowing the drops when given by pipette and rhinyle as they were rapidly cleared in large portions into the throat. These differences may be due to the method of delivery as our subjects were sitting upright in contrast to the supine position described by Aoki and Crawley (1976). It is our experience, however, that most patients prefer to take their nasal medicine in a sitting position as it is more convenient especially for patients who need medication on a life-long basis.

Plasma profile

The plasma profile of desmopressin after each method of administration is shown in figure 5. The results show a clear distinction in plasma levels between the nasal sprays and nasal drops. Peak plasma levels were significantly greater after nasal sprays than after nasal drops (p < 0.001). The pharmacokinetic data show a significantly greater AUC after nasal spray administration than after nasal drops (p < 0.001) indicating a two to three fold greater bioavailability. No significant difference in plasma levels or AUC between the nasal sprays were recorded although it was interesting to observe a greater response after the 100 μl

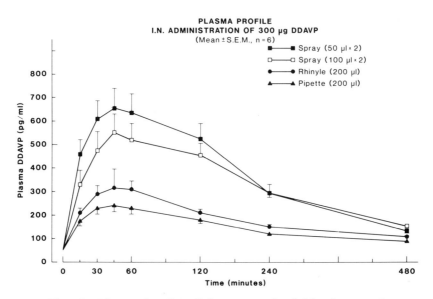

Fig. 5. Plasma levels of desmopressin following nasal administration of 300 μg desmopressin in 100 μl spray, 200 μl spray and 200 μl drops by rhinyle and pipette each to six subjects (Mean ± SEM).

dose than with the 200 µl dose indicating that dose concentration may be important. Plasma half-life ranged between 2.8 and 3.6 hours and did not differ significantly between methods. Time to peak plasma levels was approximately 50 minutes for all solutions. It is apparent therefore that the drug may be continued to be absorbed for at least this period, which indicates the importance of retaining sufficient drug in the nasal cavity for this period of time.

Biological Response

The effects of the different methods of administration on circulating levels of F VIII:C and F vWF are shown in figs 6 and 7 respectively. Figure 6 shows the response in F VIII:C activity and, again, highlights the difference between the nasal sprays and drops. Peak response was 388 ± 170% and 269 ± 27% for the 100 µl and 200 µl nasal sprays respectively. In contrast, the nasal drops of the rhinyle and pipette resulted in maximum activity of 209 ± 118% and 201 ± 100% respectively. This difference in maximum biological response between the nasal sprays and drops was highly significant (p < 0.001). Figure 7 shows a similar effect on F vWF activity although the magnitude of response to all nasal administrations was less pronounced. This phenomena is well known and has been described after intravenous administration of desmopressin (Mannucci et al., 1981). The difference in peak activity between the nasal sprays and drops was again highly significant (p < 0.001). On plotting the individual maximum plasma levels against corresponding maximum rises in F VIII:C activity, a linear correlation was found (r = 0.859, p < 0.001) indicating that the biological response to desmopressin is indeed a function of its nasal absorption.

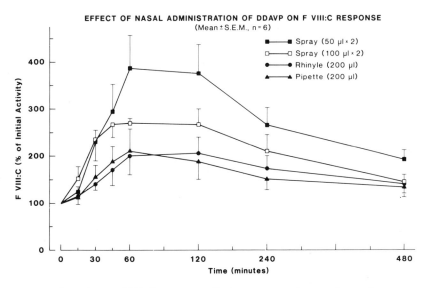

EFFECT OF NASAL ADMINISTRATION OF DDAVP ON F VIII:C RESPONSE
(Mean ± S.E.M., n = 6)

- Spray (50 µl × 2)
- Spray (100 µl × 2)
- Rhinyle (200 µl)
- Pipette (200 µl)

Fig. 6. F VIII:C expressed as a percentage rise of pre-administration levels following nasal administration of 300 µg desmopressin by 100 µl·spray, 200 µl spray, rhinyle and pipette each to six subjects (Mean ± SEM).

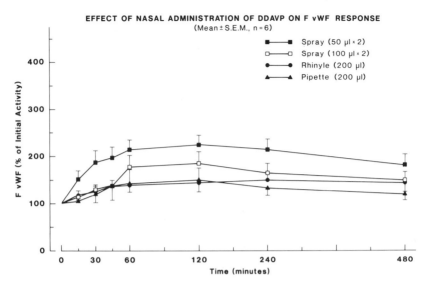

EFFECT OF NASAL ADMINISTRATION OF DDAVP ON F vWF RESPONSE
(Mean ± S.E.M., n = 6)

Spray (50 µl × 2)
Spray (100 µl × 2)
Rhinyle (200 µl)
Pipette (200 µl)

Fig. 7. F vWF expressed as a percentage rise of pre-administration levels following nasal administration of 300 µg desmopressin by spray and drops each to six subjects (Mean ± SEM).

What is also evident is that the deposition and clearance data after nasal delivery by spray and drops can, for the first time, be interpreted in terms of their effect on drug absorption and biological response. These data suggest that a strong relationship exists between the rate of clearance and its absorption. Our findings indicate that the sprays, which were cleared at a slower rate than the drops, were better absorbed and therefore produced a more pronounced biological effect.

The increase in relative bioavailability seen after spray administration of desmopressin can be of considerable advantage to its therapeutic use. Desmopressin, the synthetic analogue of the naturally occuring antidiuretic hormone, vasopressin, has for many years been the drug of choice in the treatment of diabetes insipidus (Richardson and Robinson, 1985). Traditionally, it has been delivered by the intranasal route using the rhinyle method and was one of the first examples of a peptide which could be given by the nasal route as a means of delivery to the systemic circulation. Recently, because of its ability to raise circulating levels of F VIII/F vWF, it has an increasing place in the treatment of bleeding disorders such as haemophilia A and von Willebrand's disease (Mannucci et al., 1977). It is in these indications that a greater magnitude of response has its most beneficial effect as the levels of F VIII/vWF are strongly correlated with the bleeding tendency in these diseases. Previously, however, desmopressin has been administered by the parenteral route (Kobrinsky et al., 1984) as earlier studies on the intranasal route gave unpredictable results with many poor responses. We have now established that the biological response is a function of nasal deposition, clearance and absorption and that absorption can be improved dramatically using sprays. Indeed, the levels attained here approach those described after intravenous administration of the recommended dose of 0.4 µg/kg bodyweight (Nilsson et al., 1982).

The nasal sprays used in this study were of a better quality than those described elsewhere (Hardy et al., 1985). For example, when testing 10 samples of each spray pump an average of five activations were necessary to prime the pumps after which a series of accurate doses of 49 ± 3 µl and 101 ± 3 µl were achieved.

CONCLUSIONS

There are, of course, many factors which may affect absorption and biological response to peptides administered nasally. Unfortunately, many factors are outside our control, i.e., the state of the nasal function and accompanying pathologies such as allergic and chronic rhinitis. Indeed, it has been shown that even trivial conditions such as the common cold can alter clearance rates and thereby affect efficacy (Bond et al., 1984). For this reason it is important to elucidate those factors which we can control, i.e., the method and technique of administration. In conclusion, this study shows that an intranasal spray device can deposit well controlled doses into the nostril and allow for delivery to the required site in the desired volume and concentration. Sprays are cleared at a slower rate than large drops from either intranasal pipettes or rhinyle catheters thereby producing a clear enhancement in absorption and bioavailability.

REFERENCES

Anik, S., McRae, G., Nerenberg, C., Worden, A., Foreman, J., JiinYu, H., Kushinsky, S., Jones, R. and Vickery, B., 1984, Nasal absorption of nasarelin acetate, the decapeptide [D-Nal(2)[6]] LHRH, in resus monkeys. I.,
J. Pharm. Sci., 73:684
Aoki, F.Y. and Crawley, J.C.W., 1976, Distribution and removal of human serum albumin – technetium 99m instilled intranasally,
Br. J. Clin. Pharmacol., 3:869
Barltrop, D., 1963, Diabetes insipidus treated with synthetic lysine vasopressin,
Lancet, i:276
Bond, S.W., Hardy, J.G. and Wilson C.G., 1984, Deposition and clearance of nasal sprays,
Proceedings of the Second European Congress of Biopharmaceutics and Pharmacokinetics, Salamanca, Spain, 93
Edwards, C.R.W., Kitau, M.J., Chard, T. and Besser G.M., 1973, Vasopressin analogue DDAVP in diabetes insipidus: Clinical and laboratory studies,
Br. Med. J., 3:375
Evans, W.S., Borges, L.C., Kaiser, D.L., Vance, M.L., Sellers, R.P., Macleod R.M., Vale W., Rivier, J. and Thorner, M.O., 1983, Intranasal administration of human pancreatic tumor GH-release in normal men,
J. Clin. Endocr. Metab., 57:1081.
Fraser, R. and Scott, D.J., 1963, Nasal spray of synthetic vasopressin for the treatment of diabetes insipidus,
Lancet, i:1159
Greenwood, F.C., Hunter, W.M. and Glover, J.S., 1963, The preparation of ^{131}I-labelled human growth hormone of high specific radioactivity,
Biochem. J., 89:114
Hardy, J.G., Lee, S.W.S. and Wilson, C.G., 1985, Intranasal drug delivery by spray and drops,
J. Pharm. Pharmacol., 37:294

Hoover, R.T., 1971, Intranasal oxytocin in eighteen hundred patients: A study on its safety as used in a community hospital, Am. J. Obstet. Gynec., 110:778

Kobrinsky, N.L., Israels, E.D., Gerrard J.M., Cheang, M.S., Watson, C.M., Bishop, A.J. and Schroeder, M.L., 1984, Shortening of bleeding time by 1-deamino-8-D-arginine vasopressin in various bleeding disorders Lancet, i:1145

Lundin, S., Melin, P. and Vilhardt H., 1985, Plasma concentrations of 1-deamino-8-D-arginine vasopressin after intragastric administration in the rat, Acta Endocrinol., 108:179

Mannucci, P.M., Canciani, M.T., Rota, L. and Donovan, B.S., 1981, Response of factor VIII/von Willebrand factor to DDAVP in healthy subjects and patients with haemophilia A and von Willebrand's disease, Br. J. Haematol., 47:283

Mannucci, P.M., Ruggeri, Z.M., Pareti, F.I. and Capitanio, A., 1977, 1-deamino-8-D-arginine vasopressin: a new pharmacological approach to the management of haemophilia and von Willebrand's disease, Lancet, i:869

Morimoto, K., Morisaka, K. and Kamada, A., 1985, Enhancement of nasal absorption of insulin and calciotonin using polyacrylic acid gel, J. Pharm. Pharmacol., 37:134

Nilsson, I.M., Vilhardt, H., Holmberg, L., Åstedt, B., 1982, Association between factor VIII related antigen and plasminogen activator, Acta Med. Scand., 211:105

Ohwaki, T., Ando, H., Watanabe, S. and Miyake, Y., 1985, Effects of Dose, pH, and Osmolarity on Nasal Absorption of Secretin in Rats, J. Pharm. Sci., 74:550

Richardson, D.W. and Robinson A.G., 1985, Desmopressin, Ann. Int. Med., 103:228

Rosén, S., Owaldsson, U., Blombäck, M., Larrieu, M., Nilsson I.M. and Vinazzer H., 1984, Evaluation of a chromogenic method for determining F VIII:C in hemophiliacs, von Willebrand patients and F VIII concentrate, Scand. J. Haematol., Suppl 40, 33:93

Ruggeri, Z.M., Mannucci, P.M., Jeffcoate, S.L. and Ingram, G.I.C., 1976, Immunoradiometric assay of factor VIII related antigen, with observations in 32 patients with von Willebrand's disease, Br. J. Haematol., 33:221

Sandow, J. and Petri W., 1985, Intranasal administration of peptides biological activity and therapeutic efficacy, in: "Transnasal Systemic Medications," Y.W. Chien, ed., Elsevier Science Publishers B.V., Amsterdam

Sofroniew, M.W., Madler, M., Müller, O.H. and Scriba, P.C., 1978, A method for the consistent production of high quality antisera to small peptide hormones, Fresenius Z. Anal. Chem., 290:163

Vavra, I., Machova, A., Holecek, V., Cort, J.H., Zaoral, M. and Sorm, F., 1968, Effect of a synthetic analogue of vasopressin in animals and in patients with diabetes insipidus Lancet, i:948

MICROSPHERES AS A POTENTIAL CONTROLLED RELEASE NASAL DRUG DELIVERY SYSTEM

Lisbeth Illum

Depart. of Pharmaceutics
Royal Danish School of Pharmacy
2 Universitetsparken
DK-2100 Copenhagen, Denmark

INTRODUCTION

The epithelial cells of the nasal mucosa are for the main part of the nasal cavity covered with numerous microvilli thereby increasing considerably the surface available for drug absorption. Furthermore, the subepithelial layer is highly vascularized with large and fenestrated capillaries specially designed for rapid passage of fluid through the vascular wall (Mygind, 1978). Unlike absorption from the gastrointestinal tract the venous blood draining from the nose passes directly into the systemic circulation and not into the portal circulation and thence to the liver. Thus, the nose is well suited for the absorption of drugs, especially those that are extensively metabolized in the gastrointestinal fluids and the gut wall or are subjected to an extensive first pass hepatic metabolism. The various regulatory peptides and proteins are good examples.

The bioavailability of a wide range of drugs administered via the nasal route including peptides and proteins, has been studied in the recent years. For some drugs, such as propranolol (Hussain et al, 1979, 1980a,b), progesterone (Hussain et al, 1979; David et al, 1981) and enkephalins (Su et al, 1985) this route of administration was found to be comparable to the intravenous route in terms of absorption efficiency. However, generally for most peptides and proteins evaluated (such as insulin, analogues of luteinizing hormone releasing hormone and growth hormone releasing factor) the absorption efficiency is much lower intranasally than for the intravenous route (Moses et al, 1983; Saltzman et al, 1985; Berquist et al, 1979; Evans et al, 1983).

In order to increase the bioavailability by the nasal route these "difficult" drugs have been administered in combination with penetration enhancers such as surfactants (e.g. polyoxyethylene-9-lauryl ether) and bile salts (e.g. sodium glycocholate). The absorption promoting effect of these enhancers has been shown to be due to their ability to increase membrane fluidity by extracting proteins from the nasal membrane and for bile salt also to the ability of these enhancers to inhibit enzyme activity (e.g. aminopeptidases, proteases) in the membrane (Hirai et al, 1981). However, while it has been shown that penetration enhancers can increase the absorption of drugs quite dramatically in many cases, there is still debate about the long term toxicological consequences.

An alternative strategy for increasing the bioavailability of intranasally administered drugs is that of prolonging the contact of the drug with the absorptive surface by means of an appropriate delivery system.

The mucocilliary functions of the nasal mucosa will clear applied material at the average rate of 5 mm/min from the turbinates into the nasophrynx. In contrast, clearance from the non- or sparcely ciliated anterior region of the nasal cavity is slower and results from the mucous layer being dragged into the ciliated region (Proctor et al, 1973). Thus, when nasal sprays, drops or powders are applied to the nasal cavity this mucocilliary function will normally clear the applied material from the nose rapidly. Studies on the clearance rate of technetium labelled human serum albumin applied as nasal sprays or drops showed the time for 50% clearance to be in the order of 20-30 min depending on the form of application and droplet size (Aoki and Crawley, 1976, Hardy et al, 1985).

Thus, it can be argued that this rapid mucucilliary clearance mechanism leaving little time for contact between the drug and the mucosa can be considered as an important factor when low absorption values are obtained for various peptides and proteins. The degradation of administered macromolecules by enzymes could be an additional consideration. As a consequence we have investigated methods whereby the clearance of administered drug could be delayed by using microspheres as a delivery system.

Bioadhesive microsphere delivery system

In order to increase the total absorption of drugs through the nasal mucosa and thereby the bioavailability we have explored the possibility of developing a delivery system for the nose that would ensure an increased time of contact between the delivery system and the mucosa by a process of bioadhesion with the possibility of additionally releasing the drug from the system in a sustained and controlled manner. It is also possible that such a system would protect the drug from enzymatic degradation in the nasal cavity.

The mechanism of adhesion of bioadhesive polymers to soft tissues has been discussed by Peppas and Buri (1985) and Park and Robinson (1984) and involves both chemical and physical binding. The mechanisms involve development of weak or strong interactions (van der Waals interaction, hydrogen bonding and ionic bonding) between certain types of chemical groups on the polymer (e.g. hydroxyl or carboxyl groups) and the glycoprotein network of the mucous layer.

In order for strong adhesive bonds to develop the establishment of intimate molecular contact between the polymer and glycoprotein chains is essential (Peppas and Buri, 1985). Thus, an important requirement for bioadhesive polymers is their ability to swell by absorbing water (from the mucous layer in the nasal cavity) thereby forming a gel like structure in which environment the interpenetration of polymer and glycoprotein chains can take place and the bondings can form rapidly. These important physical factors for a bioadhesive delivery system to include microspheres are outlined in Fig. 1.

NASAL DRUG DELIVERY SYSTEM

- PARTICLE DIAMETER
- SWELLING
- VISCOSITY
- ADHESIVENESS

Fig. 1. Important parameters
for a nasal drug
delivery system.

Table 1. Properties of bioadhesive delivery systems for the nose

Microsphere System	Swelled Size (µm)	Degree of Swelling	Bioadhesive Properties	Binding
Albumin	40-60	ca. 40%	good	hydrogen bonding
Starch-Spherex®	48	0.6-8.4 ml/g	good	hydrogen bonding
DEAE-Sephadex®	40-60	swells readily	good	ionic bonding

We have chosen microspheres made from materials that are known to swell in contact with an aqueous medium and form a gel-like layer and, due to the adherence to the nasal mucosa, should be cleared slowly while renewing the surface of contact. The bioadhesive properties and the physical characteristic of the microsphere delivery systems are given in Table 1.

The applicability of these proposals for a nasal delivery system has been investigated in vivo measuring the rate of clearance of the different microsphere systems and two controls in human volunteers by means of gamma scintigraphy.

Human studies

Experimental

The microsphere systems selected for human studies were: (i) albumin microspheres, (ii) starch microspheres, (iii) DEAE-dextran microspheres. As standard references two registered drug-formulations were used, one as a powder, the other as a solution: (iv) nasal powder, (v) nasal spray.

Albumin microspheres were produced by a method previously described by (Illum et al, 1986). The particle size range of the swollen microspheres in the selected crude batches was 32.5-51.6 µm as measured by a Coulter Counter.

Starch microspheres (Spherex®) were obtained from Pharmacia AB (Uppsala, Sweden). The swollen microspheres had a volume-mean-diameter of 48 µm, the dry volume-mean-diameter was approximately 20 µm.

DEAE-dextran microspheres (DEAE-Sephadex®) from Pharmacia AB (Uppsala, Sweden) were fractionated and a size range of 40-60 µm was obtained. The nasal powder and the nasal nebulogenum were obtained commercially.

The microsphere systems were labelled with technetium 99m by the standard stannous chloride method (Hardy et al, 1985). The labelling efficiency was found to be not less than 97%. The stability of the labelling was measured by suspending the microspheres in normal saline and determining the activity in the supernatant. Less than 3% of the activity was released after 60 min.

The microspheres were freeze-dried overnight and appeared afterwards as free flowing powders that were filled into capsules with 10 mg in each capsule. The labelling of the spheres had been performed so that the activity of 10 mg microspheres was approximately 50 µCi, which was the dose applied to the volunteers in each test.

The spray and powder formulations were labelled by adding a solution of DTPA-Tc-99m (diethylenetriamine penta acetic acid) or freeze-dried DTPA-Tc-99m, respectively. The latter was filled into capsules as above. It has been shown by Dudley et al (1980) that DTPA in solution is absorbed readily from the nasal mucosa.   Thus, this label can be used as a good model for an absorbable drug.

Gamma Scintigraphy

Each preparation was given to a group of 6 healthy human volunteers (20-30 years of age) in turn leaving at least two days between the studies.

The three microsphere systems and the nasal powder were applied to the nose of the volunteer using the nasal insufflator. The total content of one capsule (10 mg - 50 μCi) was applied evenly to the mucosal surface of the right half of the nose. Puffs were given during inhalation to the upper and the lower part of the nasal cavity in turn until the capsule was empty. This required 5-6 puffs. The nasal spray was applied with the normal pump-spray with one puff (0.13 ml) given during inhalation to the right half of the nose.

The deposition and subsequent clearance of all the different preparations were monitored immediately after application by gamma scintigraphy. Later views of the head were recorded dynamically for 15 minutes (each image of 60 sec. duration) and later images were taken at appropriate time intervals up till 180 min. each of which was recorded for three minutes. The nostril containing the tracer was nearest the collimator, and a Perspex rod attached to the collimator was used to ensure accurate repositioning. The images were recorded for subsequent quantification.

Regions of interest were drawn around the site of application and the total activity in this area followed with time and corrected for decay (Fig. 2).

Upon administration to the nose the microsphere formulations and the powder formulation were mainly deposited in the anterior part of the nasal cavity with little of the dose reaching the turbinates initially. In contrast, the solution was dispersed from the atrium to the nasopharynx after application by spray.

The activity-time profiles given in Fig. 3 show that both the solution and powder formulations were cleared quite rapidly with a half time of clearance from the site of deposition of the order of 15 min, whereas the microsphere systems had much longer clearance times. After 3 hours 50% of the initial activity combined with the albumin and starch microspheres and 60% combined with the DEAE-Sephadex® were still at the site of application. The half time of clearance from the initial deposition site for DEAE-Sephadex® microspheres were calculated to be about 4 hours.

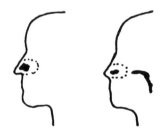

Fig. 2. Spreading of applied
material in the nose
as measured by gamma
scintigraphy. (i) ini-
tial scintigraph (ii)
later scintigraph

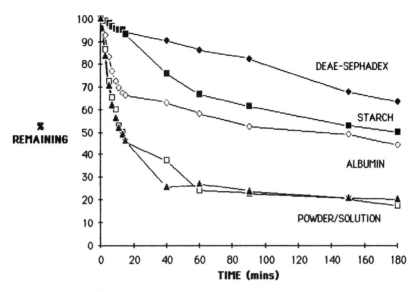

Fig. 3. The clearance of different microsphere systems and of two control systems from the nose.

Discussion

As reported by others (Hardy et al, 1985) the clearance of the solution and powder formulation occurred quite rapidly whereas our microspheres formulations were cleared much more slowly. The reasons for this difference between the microsphere formulations and the controls can be attributed to the fact that the microspheres undergo a process of imbibing water and swelling thereby forming a mucoadhesive system that is cleared slowly. The observed variations between the different microsphere systems can be related to their chemical properties and swelling characteristics. These factors will be explored in detail in future in vitro studies.

Proposed in vivo studies to be performed in human subjects will explore whether the microsphere system will provide an enhancement of the bioavailability of selected drugs to include peptides and proteins. Modifications to the physical properties of the microspheres (e.g. crosslinking) should allow these systems to demonstrate controlled release behaviour. Studies will also be conducted to evaluate the ability of microsphere systems to protect sensitive compounds against enzymatic degradation. It is also appreciated that such microsphere systems could be used to deliver not only pharmacological active substances but also absorption modifiers. It is interesting to note that Nagai et al (1984) have increased the absorption of insulin after nasal application in dogs using a gelling formulation containing materials such as hydroxypropyl cellulose and neutralized polyacrylic acid (Carbopol 934). The use of a nasal gel to enhance the absorption of insulin and calcitonin in the rat has been described by Morimoto et al (1984). Once again polyacrylic acid was the material of choice.

We believe that our microsphere systems should provide similar or even better effects. Their physical properties should also allow for better administration and deposition behaviour since it is possible to prepare such systems in a variety of sizes.

REFERENCES

Aoki, F.Y. and Crawley, J.C.W., 1976, Distribution and removal of human serum albumin - technetium 99m instilled intranasally, Br. J. Clin. Pharmac., 3:869.

Berquist, C., Nillins, S.J. and Wide, L., 1979, Intranasal gonadotropin-releasing hormone agonist as a contraceptive agent, Lancet, 2:215.

David, G.F.X., Puri, C.P. and Anaud Kumar, T.C:, 1981, Bioavailability of progesterone enhanced by intranasal spraying, Experientia 37:533.

Dudley, R.E., Muggenburg, B.A., Cuddihy, R.G. and McClellan, R.O., 1980, Nasal absorption of DTPA in rats, Health Phys. 38:763.

Evans, W.S., Borges, J.L.C., Kaiser, D.L., Vance, M.L., Seller, R.P., Macleod, R.M., Vale, W., Rivier, J. and Thorner, M.O. 1983, Intranasal administration of human pancreatic tumor GH-releasing factor-40 stimulates GH release in normal men. J. Clin. Endocrinol. Metab., 57:1081.

Hardy, J.G., Lee, S.W. and Wilson, C.G., 1985, Intranasal drug delivery by sprays and drops, J. Pharm. Pharmacol. 37:294.

Hirai, S., Yashiki, T. and Mima, H., 1981, Mechanisms for the enhancement of the nasal absorption of insulin by surfactants, Int. J. Pharm., 9:173.

Hussain, A., Foster, T., Hirai, S., Kashihara, T., Batenhorst, R. and Jones, M., 1980a, Nasal absorption of propranolol in humans, J. Pharm. Sci., 69:1240.

Hussain, A., Hirai, S. and Bawarski, R., 1979, Nasal absorption of propranolol in rats, J. Pharm. Sci., 68:1196.

Hussain, A., Hirai, S. and Bawarski, R., 1980b, Nasal absorption of propranolol from different dosage forms by rats and dogs, J. Pharm. Sci., 69:1411.

Illum, L., Jørgensen, H., Bisgaard, H., Krogsgaard, O. and Rossing, N., Bioadhesive microspheres as a potential nasal drug delivery system (to be published).

Morimoto, K., Morisaka, K. and Kamada, A., 1985, Enhancement of nasal absorption of insulin and calcitonin using polyacrylic acid gel, J. Pharm. Pharmacol. 37:134.

Moses, A.C., Gordon, G.S., Carey, M.C. and Flier, J.S., 1983, Insulin administered intranasally as an insulin-bile salt aerosol: effectiveness and reproducibility in normal and diabetic subjects. Diabetes, 32:1040.

Mygind, N., 1978, "Nasal Allergy", Blackwell Scientific Publications, Oxford

Nagai, T., Nishimoto, Y., Nambu, N., Suzuki, Y. and Sekine, K., 1984, Powder dosage form of insulin for nasal administration, J. Control. Rel. 1:15.

Salzman, R., Manson, J.E., Griffing, G.T., Kimmerle, R., Ruderman, N., McCall, A., Stoltz, E.I., Mullin, C., Small, D., Armstrong, J. and Melby, J.C:, 1985, Intranasal aerosolized insulin, N. Eng. J. Med., 312:1078.

Su, K.S.E., Campanale, K.M., Mendelsohn, L.G., Kerchner, G.A. and Gries, C.L., 1985, Nasal delivery of polypeptides, I: nasal absorption of enkephalins, J. Pharm. Sci., 74:394.

NAZLIN[R] - TRANSNASAL SYSTEMIC DELIVERY OF INSULIN

John P. Longenecker

California Biotechnology, Inc.
2450 Bayshore Parkway
Mountain View, CA   94043

INTRODUCTION

I recently had a discussion with a scientist from a major "Eastern
Establishment" pharmaceutical company in the U.S. The topic of our discussion was the success of this young upstart biotechnology industry.
Although we were in agreement that biotechnology allows for a more
rational approach to design of therapeutic agents, he argued that, "you
cannot make it in the pharmaceutical industry simply on injectable
hormones". Whether or not the economic argument is valid, it is clear
that widespread, patient-controlled use of therapeutic proteins and peptides demands an alternative to parenteral administration. The most
likely route of administration for this relatively new and rapidly expand-
ing class of therapeutic agents is via the nasal cavity. The highly
vascularized mucosal surfaces of the nasal passages, the ease of administration, potential advantages of no first pass metabolism and the rapid
kinetics of absorption make the nasal route an ideal alternative to
parenteral administration. Transnasal systemic drug delivery has become
a popular topic (Parr, 1983; Su, 1986) and was the subject of a recently
published Symposium held at Rutgers University in New Jersey (Chien, 1985).
The message from this meeting was that nasal drug delivery is indeed a
viable alternative with significant therapeutic and kinetic advantages,
especially for hormones. However, problems of bioavailability, reproducibility of plasma levels and effect on nasal pathology, i.e., local
toxicity, remain to be solved.

Although the biotechnology industry has prompted a resurgence of
interest in non-parenteral, non-oral delivery systems. a number of
therapeutic proteins predate recombinant DNA technology. Of these,
insulin is clearly the most widely prescribed. Attempts to utilize non-
parenteral routes of insulin administration are nearly as old as insulin
therapy itself. As early as 1922, Woodyatt reported studies which
examined the efficacy of insulin delivery by intranasal, oral, rectal,
and vaginal routes. This early work and that of others up to the 1960's
met with little success. (Heubner et al, 1924; Gansslen et al, 1925;
Collens and Goldzieher, 1932; Major, 1936; Hankiss and Hadhazy, 1958.)
These studies did serve to illustrate, however, the major problems of
intranasal delivery which are: (1) low bioavailability, (2) unreliable
dosing, and (3) acute local toxicity of formulations using permeation
enhancers. As discussed above, these remain the major challenges.

Recent work has focused on the use of a variety of surfactants as
permeation enhancers. These include non-ionic polyoxyethylene ethers
(Hirai et al, 1978, 1981; Salzman et al, 1985) and bile salts (Pontiroli
et al, 1982; Moses et al, 1983; Gordon et al, 1985). A strong correlation
was shown by Hirai (1981) between insulin uptake and membrane lysis for
the non-ionic surfactants. In spite of this correlation, Salzman and co-
workers (1985) used one of these, Laureth 9, in a study in type I diabetics for 3 months. This study demonstrated that one dose of subcutaneous
ultralente insulin and pre-meal nasal administration was effective in
controlling blood glucose concentration and was tolerated by most
patients. The mechanism of action of bile salts is not known. However,
it is thought to involve both solubilization of insulin, and direct
effects of the surfactant on cell membranes perhaps involving reverse
micelle formation (Gordon et al, 1985). In the presence of zinc ions,
insulin forms stable hexamers which aggregate (Blundell et al, 1972;
Jeffery et al, 1970). The addition of bile salts is thought to result in
formation of mixed micelles of bile salts and insulin as insulin monomers
(Gordon et al 1985). When sprayed into the nasal passages, a high transmembrane concentration gradient of soluble insulin monomers would serve to
drive insulin transport across the mucosal barrier.

Although recent clinical studies have indicated that formulations of
insulin with bile salts could provide reasonable efficacy of transport and
reproducible dosing (Pontiroli et al, 1982; Moses et al, 1983), a number
of concerns remain regarding the local toxicity and irritation of these
compounds. There are many reports in the literature indicating that
derivatives of cholic acid break down mucous membrane structure (Martin
et al, 1976), accelerate phospholipid and protein release from membranes
(Whitmore et al, 1979), and damage intestinal mucosa (Kimura et al, 1981),
liposomal membranes (Schubert et al, 1983) and isolated hepatocytes
(Scholmerich et al, 1984). Furthermore, O'Leary et al (1984) demonstrated
severe epithelial hyperplasia in a dog pancreas perfusion model using
sodium deoxycholate. Because insulin therapy involves multiple daily
administrations for life, the issue of irritation and local toxic effects
are serious ones which have led all workers to suggest a need for
alternative adjuvants.

Nazlin[R] - Transnasal Insulin Delivery

Nazlin[R] (Trademark of California Biotechnology, Inc.) is the brand
name of transnasal formulations of insulin with enhancers which are
derivatives of fusidic acid. These formulations were conceived following
a meeting between Dr. Martin Carey, a physician and physical chemist who
has worked for many years with bile salts and bile salt analogues, and
Drs. Jeffery Flier and Alan Moses, two diabetes specialists interested in
transnasal delivery of insulin. Sodium fusidate, a fungal metabolite
isolated from the fermentation products of Fusidium coccineum, was
originally developed by Leo Pharmaceuticals as an antibiotic in the
1960's. Interest in this molecule was stimulated by the obvious structural similarity of this steroid to the bile acids, e.g., cholic acid.
Figure 1 shows the chemical configuration and perspective structural
formulas of fusidic and cholic acids. Although the conventional chemical
representations resemble one another, their stereochemical configurations
are fundamentally different. The micellar properties of sodium fusidate
have been reported (Carey and Small, 1971) as well as the solution
properties of taurine and glycine conjugates of fusidic acid (Carey and
Small, 1973). Table 1 lists some of chemical properties of the preferred
adjuvant for nasal insulin administration, sodium taurodihydrofusidate
(STDHF). This compound has a critical micellar concentration (CMC) in
the same range as the bile salts, and is an anion at all pH's which might
be considered for an intranasal formulation, i.e., greater than 3. STDHF

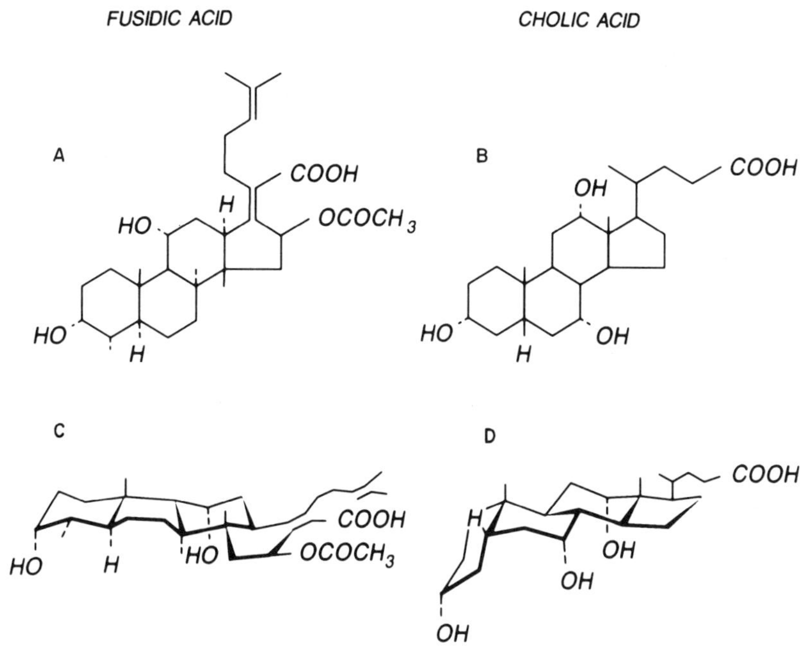

FUSIDIC ACID   CHOLIC ACID

Fig. 1. Fusidic and cholic acids: a, b, conventional chemical
configuration; c, d, perspective structural formulas.

forms micelles with an aggregation number of approximately 10. Quasi-
elastic light scattering of a 1%(w/v) solution of STDHF in sodium
phosphate buffer (20 mm, ph 7.4) indicates a unimodal particle size
distribution. The hydrodynamic radius (R_h) of these particles is 28A.
Addition of insulin to a concentration of 1% (w/v) results in an increase
in the particle size to 39.7A. This is consistent with the formation of
an expanded mixed micelle of insulin/STDHF (M. Carey, personal communication). These data show that STDHF and bile salts interact with insulin
in solution in a similar manner. As discussed above, solubilization of
insulin into monomers may play a large role in enhancing transport of
insulin across mucous membranes.

Table 1. Colloidal-Chemical properties of STDHF

Emperical Formula	$C_{33}H_{54}NO_8SNa$
Molecular Weight	625.88
CMC (0.01M Na^+	2.47 mM
CMT (1% soln)	0°C
pKa (1% soln)	2.35
Sol of 2.5% soln in NaCl	Sol 0.3M, insol 0.6M
Aggregation Number	10
Rh (1% Soln)	28.2A
Rh (1% Soln + 1% insulin)	39.7A

213

Since irritation and local toxicity are the primary reasons for searching for a better enhancer, the membranolytic potential of STDHF was assessed using the lysis of rabbit erythrocytes essentially as described by Hirai and co-workers (1981). Table 2 shows the relative hemolytic activity expressed as the reciprocal of the concentration of surfactant required to yield half maximal lysis. Laureth 9 is clearly the most lytic surfactant tested, in agreement with the data of Hirai et al, (1981). Both STDHF and sodium glycodihydrofusidate are far less lytic on a (w/v)% basis than the bile salts. Since the average molecular weight of STDHF and SGDHF is roughly twice that of sodium glycocholate and sodium deoxycholate, STDHF is nearly 5 times less lytic on a molar basis than the bile salts. These data suggest that these compounds are potentially less toxic enhancers of insulin transport.

Table 2. Effect of Surfactants on Erythrocyte Hemolysis

Surfactant	Hemolysis (ml/mg)[a]
Polyoxyetheylene 9 lauryl ether	>20.00
Sodium glycocholate	2.50
Sodium deoxycholate	1.11
Sodium taurodihydrofusidate	0.25
Sodium glycodihydrofusidate	<0.10

[a]Hemolysis is expressed as the recipricol of the concentration which resulted in half-maximal hemolysis.

Insulin Absorption in Sheep

In an attempt to assess the efficacy of STDHF as an enhancer of insulin absorption via the nasal route, a series of experiments were carried out using sheep as a model system. The data shown in Fig. 2 demonstrate the effect of varying the concentration of STDHF in formulations containing insulin at 1% (w/v). The intranasal (IN) dose was 1U/kg. Each point is the area under the curve (AUC) of a serum insulin vs time plot (out to 60 min.). These data show a sharp increase in insulin absorption at a STDHF concentration of 0.5% (w/v). Since the CMC of STDHF (in the absence of insulin) is approximately 0.15% (w/v), enhanced uptake seems to require micelle formation. The absorption seems to plateau between 0.5 and 1.0% (w/v) but increases at 2.0%. This increase at the higher concentration may be due to a lytic effect of STDHF on membranes.

The effect of adjusting insulin dose over the range 0.25 to 1.0 U/kg is shown in Fig. 3. In all these experiments, STDHF concentration was 1% (w/v) and changes IN dosing were achieved by varying the volume administered. Fig. 3A shows the kinetics of insulin absorption for the three doses. Insulin is absorbed rapidly, reaching peak serum levels at 10-15 minutes. These kinetics are highly reproducible and are similar to those reported by others in other species and in man (Hirai et al, 1978, 1981; Moses et al, 1983). The high transient serum insulin levels achieved after nasal administration mimic the kinetic pattern of pancreatic insulin secretion and represents a significant potential therapeutic advantage over conventional parenteral administration of insulin. Subcutaneously administered insulin results in a much delayed onset of serum insulin and a prolonged elevated blood level with high variability in both the peak

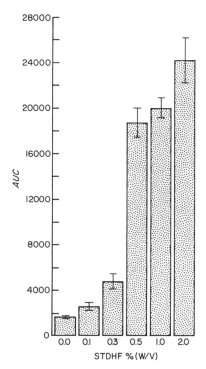

Fig. 2.   Area under serum insulin vs time plots as a function of
          STDHF concentration in IN formulations.   Each data point
          is the mean ± SEM of at least 4 sheep.   Insulin dose was
          1U/kg.

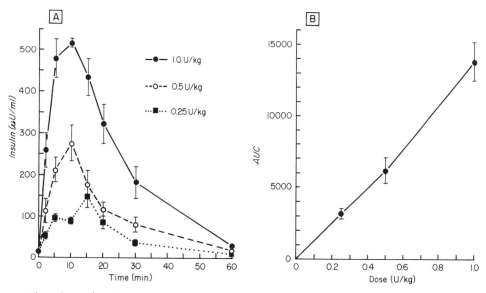

Fig. 3.   A) Kinetics of insulin absorption following IN dosing of
          insulin in 1% (w/v) solutions of STDHF.   Insulin doses
          were 0.25, 0.50, and 1.0 U/kg.   B) Plot of AUC vs dose
          (U/kg) from A showing linear dose response.

response and time of peak (Galloway et al, 1981).   Fig. 3B shows the approx.
linear relationship between AUC and insulin dose (U/kg) over this range.

Given the non-linear STDHF concentration relationship to AUC, it was of interest to determine the effect of adjusting the molar ratio of STDHF to insulin. The data of Fig. 4 are the AUC's as a function of STDHF/insulin over the range 1 to 20. These ratios were achieved using STDHF concentrations of either 0.5, 1.0, or 2.0% (w/v) and insulin concentrations of 1,2, or 3% (w/v). Thus the STDHF concentration was always well above the CMC. The insulin dose was held constant at 1U/kg. The data show a sharp rise with a plateau at a ratio of 5. This has significant implications regarding the probable molecular interaction of STDHF and insulin required for enhanced permeation of the mucosal barrier. A major unanswered question at present is what is the relative transport of STDHF and insulin into blood? Experiments are currently underway in an attempt to answer that question. The data of Fig. 4 establish that transnasal formulations of STDHF and insulin should be designed such that the molar ratio is equal to or greater than 5.

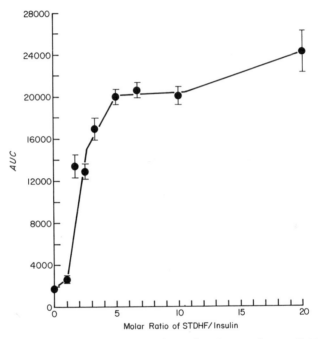

Fig. 4. The relationship between insulin absorption and the molar ratio of STDHF : insulin. Data are the mean ± SEM for at least 4 sheep. Insulin dose was 1U/kg.

These data demonstrated that STDHF is useful as an enhancer of transnasal insulin uptake. The questions of relative bioavailability and reproducibility of dosing were addressed by comparing intravenous (IV) and intranasal (IN) dosing as shown in Fig. 5. IV dosing was at 0.1 U/kg and IN at 1.0 U/kg. These data show intersheep variability from IV dosing to be higher than IN. The coefficients of variation being 14 and 32% for IN and IV, respectively. This reproducibility is far superior to that of conventional therapy (Galloway et al, 1981). The data of Fig. 5 also allows for calculation of percentage bioavailability based on the assumption that the AUC for IV dosing represents 100% bioavailability. When the average AUC's from Fig. 5 are used, the bioavailability is 14.2%. However, when bioavailability for individual sheep are averaged, the value ± SEM is 16.4 ± 0.7%. The bioavailability of subcutaneously (SC) administered insulin is approximately 50% (Galloway et al, 1981). Thus, a

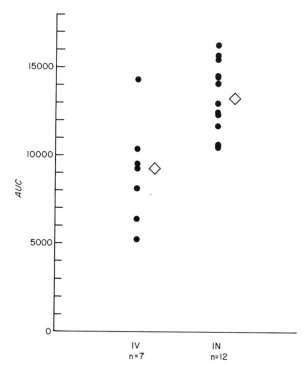

Fig. 5. Reproducibility of insulin absorption. IV dose was
0.1 U/kg, n=7.   IN dose 1.0 U/kg, n=12.

simplistic analysis would suggest a requirement for three times greater
dosing IN compared to SC. However, due to the great difference in
kinetics of insulin absorption by the two routes, this is certainly an
overestimate of the IN dose required. It can be argued that the peak
dose of serum insulin required to blunt meal induced hyperglycemia can be
more efficiently administered intranasally, as a pulse. This mimics the
normal pancreatic response. Although the absolute bioavailability of IN
insulin may never equal parenteral dosing, the therapeutic doses may be
much closer. If one assumes only one third of the SC administered
insulin is effectively utilized in blunting meal-related hyperglycemia,
then intranasal and SC insulin <u>therapeutic</u> doses become cost-equivalent.

Safety and Toxicity Studies

Although the data discussed in the preceding show that an effective
STDHF formulation exists, insulin administration is a long-term, multiple
daily therapy, and safety and toxicity issues are of paramount
concern. Formulations of insulin and STDHF have been assessed for safety
in a number of model systems. The LD_{50} (IV) is 150 mg/kg in rats and
mice. The IN dose of STDHF in a formulation for human use is approximately 33 μg/kg. The oral LD_{50} was greater than 1g/kg, consistent with
the poor oral absorption of this compound seen in dogs (Leo Pharmaceutical study). STDHF is not mutagenic as judged by the Ames <u>Salmonella</u>
mammalian microsome test, the L5178Y mouse lymphoma cells assay and
analysis of DNA repair synthesis in rat hepatocytes. Formulations of
STDHF are non-irritating to rabbit skin, eye and nasal cavities as
assessed in acute tests. Furthermore, thirty day intranasal toxicity
studies involving 3 administrations per day in both rats and dogs at
doses up to 10% (w/v) STDHF failed to show any local or systemic lesions
associated with the enhancer. Thus by all criteria assessed to date,

STDHF formulations with insulin (Nazlin[R]) have been shown to be safe and well suited for nasal administration of insulin.

Conclusions

Insulin is a unique therapeutic protein. It is the only protein presently self-administered by injection by millions of individuals. Currently evolving data suggests that tight control of blood glucose profiles may retard or alleviate some of the long term complications of diabetes. Tight control is very difficult to maintain, given presently available therapeutic approaches. The major limitation is the kinetic pattern of subcutaneously administered insulin which cannot reproduce the pattern seen in normal man. Transnasal administration of insulin does allow for a proper kinetic pattern, has been used to control blood glucose levels in man (Pontrioli et al, 1982; Moses et al, 1983; Salzman et al, 1985), and offers hope for a major change in available therapy. Nazlin[R] nasal insulin appears to be a safe, efficacious means of administering insulin with several advantages over previous adjuvant systems, including lowered local toxicity and rapid systemic clearance. The experiments described here using a sheep model have provided critical information which has been utilized to optimize formulations of insulin for use in human clinical trials. Preliminary data from these trials confirm Nazlin to be a reliable form of insulin delivery. Expanded clinical trials are continuing. Further research into the use of STDHF and other related surfactants with a variety of therapeutic peptides and proteins is ongoing. Investigations of use of these permeation enhancers to deliver drugs across other mucosal membranes, i.e., rectal, vaginal and buccal, are clearly indicated. The results to date demonstrate that transnasal delivery of therapeutic proteins and peptides will become a reality in the near future.

ACKNOWLEDGEMENTS

The author is grateful to Drs. Martin Carey, Jeffery Flier, and Alan Moses for valuable discussions and Ms. Amy Loffredo for technical assistance with the hemolysis experiments.

REFERENCE

Blundell, T.L., Cutfield, J.F., Cutfield, S.M., Dodson, E.J.; Dodson, G.G.; Hodgkin, D.C. and Mercola, D.A., 1972, Three dimensional atomic structure of insulin and its relationship to activity, Diabetes, 21:492.

Carey, M.C. and Small, D.M.; 1971, Micellar properties of sodium fusidate, a steroid antibiotic structurally resembling the bile salts, J. Lipid Res., 12:604.

Carey, M.C. and Small, D.M.; 1973 Solution properties of taurine and glycine conjugates of fusidic acid and its derivatives, Biochim et Biophys. Acta 305:51.

Chien, Y.W., 1985 "Transnasal Systemic Medications: Fundamentals, Developmental Concepts and Biomedical Assessments" Elsevier-Amsterdam.

Collens, W.S. and Goldzieher, 1932, Absorption of insulin by nasal mucous membrane, Proc. Soc. Exp. Bio. Med., 29:756.

Galloway, J.A.; Spradlin, C.T.; Nelson, R.L.; Wentworth, S.M.; Davidson, J.A. and Swarner, J.L. 1981, Factors influencing the absorption, serum insulin concentration, and blood glucose responses after injections of regular insulin and various insulin mixtures. Diabetes Care 3:366.

Gansslen M. 1925. Ueber inhalation van insulin Klin Schnschr 4:71

Gordon, G.S.; Moses, A.C.; Silver, R.D.; Flier, J.S. and Carey, M.C. 1985, Nasal absorption of insulin: enhancement by hydrophobic bile salts, Proc. Natl. Acad. Sci. USA 82:7419.

Hankiss, J. and Hadhazy, C.S., 1958, Resorption von insulin and asthmolysin von der nasenschleimhaut, Acta. Med. Acad. Sci-Hung. 12:107.

Heubner, W.; de Jough, S.E.; and Laquer, E., 1924, Ueber inhalation von insulin, Klin Schnshr. 3:2342.

Hirai, S.; Ikenaga, T. and Matsuzawa, T., 1978, Nasal Absorption of insulin in dogs, Diabetes 27:296.

Hirai, S.; Yashiki, T.; and Mima, H., 1981, Mechanisms for the enhancement of the nasal absorption of insulin by surfactants, Int. J. Pharm. 9:173.

Jeffery, P.D., Milthorpe, B.K. and Nichol, L.W., 1976, Polymerization pattern of insulin at ph 7.0, Biochemistry 15:4460.

Kimura, T.; Imamura, H.; Hasegawa, K.; and Yoshida, A., 1982 Mechanisims of toxicities of some detergents added to a diet and of the ameliorating effect of dietary fiber in the rat. J. Nut. Sci Vitaminol, 28:483.

Major, R.H., 1936, The intranasal application of insulin, experimental and clinical experiences, Am. J.M. Sci, 192:257.

Martin, G.P., and Marriott, C., 1981, Membrane damage by bile salts: the protective function of phospholipids, J. Pharm. Pharmacol 31:754.

Moses, A.C.; Gordon, G.S.; Carey, M.C. and Flier, J.S., 1983, Insulin administered intranasally as an insulin-bile salt aerosol: effectiveness and reproducibility in normal and diabetic subjects, Diabetes, 32:1040.

O'Leary, J.F.; Borner, J.w., Runge, W.J. Dehner, L.P. and Goodale, R.L., 1984, Hyperplasia of pancreatic duct epithelium produced by exposure to sodium deoxycholate, Am. J. Surg. 147:72.

Parr, G.D., 1983, Nasal delivery of drugs, Pharm. Int. Aug:202.

Pontiroli, A.E.; Alberetto, M.; Secchi, A.S.; Dossi, G.; Bosi, I. and Pozza, G. 1982, Insulin given intranasally induces hypoglycemia in normal and diabetic subjects, <u>Brit. Med. J.</u> 284:303.

Salzman, R.; Manson, J.E., Griffing, G.T.; Kimmerle, R.; Ruderman, N.; McCall, A.; Stoltz, E.I.; Mullin, C.; Small D.; Armstrong, J. and Melby, J.C., 1985, Intranasal aerosolized insulin: mixed meal studies and long-term use in type I diabetes <u>N. Engl. J. Med.</u> 312:1078.

Scholmerich, J.; Becher, M.S.; Schmidt, K.; Schubert, R.; Kremer, B.; Feldhaus, S. and Gerok, W., 1984, Influence of hydroxylation and conjugation of bile salts on their membrane damaging properties - studies on isolated hepatoyates and lipid membrane vesicles, <u>Hepatology</u> 4:661.

Schubert, R.; Jaroni, H.; Schoelmerich, J. and Schmidt, K.H., 1983, Studies on the mechanism of bile salt-induced liposomal membrane damage, <u>Digestion</u>, 28:181.

Su, K.S.E.; 1986, Intranasal delivery of peptides and proteins, <u>Pharm. Int.</u>, 7:8.

Whitmore, D.A., Bookes, L.G. and Wheeler, K.P. 1979, Relative effects of different surfactants on intestinal absorption and the release of proteins and phospholipids from the tissue, <u>J. Pharm. Pharmacol</u> 31:277.

Woodyatt, R.T., 1922, The clinical use of insulin, <u>J. Metab. Res.</u>, 2:793.

NASAL ABSORPTION OF ENKEPHALINS IN RATS

Kenneth S. E. Su,
Kristina M. Campanale,
Laurane G. Mendelsohn,
Gail A. Kerchner, and
Christian L. Gries

Pharmaceutical Research Department, Division of CNS and
Endocrine Research, and Toxicology Division, Lilly Research
Laboratories, Eli Lilly and Company, Indianapolis, Indiana
46285, U.S.A.

INTRODUCTION

In recent years, the possibility that the intranasal administration
route might be useful for many compounds which are not absorbed orally has
received a great deal of attention. For instance, the β-blocker
propranolol (Hussain et al, 1979, 1980 a,b), the contraceptive agent
progesterone (David et al, 1981; Hussain et al, 1981) and the anti-
arrhythmic compound clofilium tosylate (Su et al, 1984) have been shown to
be effectively absorbed via the intranasal route when compared to oral
administration. These compounds undergo extensive degradation due to
first-pass hepatic metabolism which can be minimized after nasal administration. For drugs which are poorly absorbed by the oral route such as
sulbenicillin, cefazolin, and cephacetrile, it was demonstrated that the
percent dose excreted in urine after nasal administration was nearly
one-half of that after intramuscular administration (Hirai et al, 1981).
The absorption of low molecular weight polypeptides, luteinising hormone-
releasing hormone (LH-RH) and its analogues used as a contraceptive agent,
was evaluated by the nasal route (Fink et al, 1974; Berquist et al, 1979;
Gennser and Liedholm, 1974; London et al, 1973; Anik et al, 1984).
Although the absorption efficiency by the nasal route was lower than the
I.V. route for these polypeptides, the absorption was reproducible, and
the advantage of non-parenteral route for such a compound was an important
factor. Research has also been carried out on the nasal absorption of
high molecular weight polypeptides such as insulin (Moses et al, 1983;
Hirai et al, 1978, 1981 a,b), interferon (Greenberg et al, 1978; Harmon
et al, 1976; 1977; Johnson et al, 1976) and growth hormone releasing
factor (Evans et al, 1983).

More recently, analogues of the naturally occurring enkephalins have been evaluated for their analgesic activity (Frederickson, 1970; Motta, 1980; Gesellchen et al, 1979, 1980; Leander and Wood, 1982). These polypeptides have to be administered parenterally to have measurable activity. This paper describes (1) the nasal absorption of analogues of enkephalin, (2) the effect of surfactant sodium glycocholate on nasal absorption, and (3) the histological examination of the nasal mucosa of rats after nasal administration of enkpehalins.

EXPERIMENTAL

Materials - Two polypeptides were chosen for the nasal absorption studies: (1) [3H]-Tyr*-D-Ala-Gly-L-Phe-D-Leu-OH[1] ([3H]DADLE), molecular weight = 569.7 and (2) metkephamid[2], Tyr-D-Ala-Gly-Phe-N-Me-Met-NH$_2$·CH$_3$COOH, molecular weight = 660.78. These two pentapeptides, tyrosine[3], Tyr-D-Ala-Gly (TDAG)[4], unlabeled DADLE[5] and PCS liquid scintillation fluid[6] were used as received. Distilled deionized water was used for preparation of the HPLC mobile phase. All other reagents were analytical grade. Stock solutions of DADLE and metkephamid were prepared fresh daily.

Equipment - For the assay of [3H]-DADLE, the high-performance liquid chromatography (HPLC) analyses were performed using a gradient liquid chromatography system[7] with variable UV wavelength absorbance detector[8]. The system consisted of two solvent delivery pumps[9], a guard column packed with pellicular ODS media[10], a 250 x 4.6-mm reverse phase C-18 Spheri-5 μm column[11], and an OmniScribe linear recorder[12].

For the assay of metkephamid, the HPLC system consisted of a solvent delivery pump[13], a guard column packed with pellicular ODS packing[14], a 250 x 4.6-mm reverse phase C-18 5-6 μm column[15], a recorder[16], a power supply[17], and a fluorescent detector[18].

Sample Preparation and Analysis - The relative absorption of [3H]-DADLE, expressed as total radioactive equivalents absorbed by the intranasal and subcutaneous routes, was measured as previously reported (Su et al, 1984). For the quantitative analyses of absorption of [3H]-DADLE, the procedure is described as follows. Serum samples from treated rats were stored at -20°C overnight and thawed just prior to HPLC analysis. The [3H]-DADLE stock solution and serum samples were chromatographed on a C-18 reverse phase HPLC column for separation and identification of

---

[1]New England Nuclear, Boston, MA.
[2]Synthesized by Lilly Research Laboratories, Indpls., IN.
[3]Ajinomota Company, Tokyo, Japan.
[4]Synthesized by Lilly Research Laboratories, Indpls., IN.
[5]Synthesized by Lilly Research Laboratories, Indpls., IN.
[6]Amersham, Arlington Heights, IL.
[7]Beckman Instruments, Inc., Fullerton, CA.
[8]Model LDC Spectromonitor III, Laboratory Data Control, Riviera Beach, FL.
[9]Beckman Instruments, Inc., Fullerton, CA.
[10]Whatman, Inc., Clifton, NJ.
[11]Brownlee Labs, Inc., Santa Clara, CA.
[12]Texas Instruments, Austin, TX.
[13]Altex Model 110A, Rainin Instrument Co., Inc., Emeryville, CA.
[14]Brownlee Labs, Inc., Santa Clara, CA.
[15]Zorbax ODS, DuPont Instruments, Wilmington, DE.
[16]Linear Instruments Corp., Irvine, CA.
[17]Model 150 Xenon Power Supply, Perkin Elmer, Norwalk, CT.
[18]Model 650-10S, Perkin Elmer, Norwalk, CT.

tritiated water, tyrosine, TDAG, and DADLE. A 95 µl sample was injected onto the column. A linear gradient of 0 - 12% of acetonitrile in 0.1 M $(NH_4)_2SO_4$, pH 4.0, was run for 12 minutes and followed by a 12 to 30% acetonitrile gradient over the next 5 minutes. A 30% acetonitrile isocratic elution was continued for an additional 10 minutes. The absorption of standards and serum samples was monitored at 210 nm. Thirty fractions of 1 ml each were collected from a chromatographed serum sample and counted for 5 minutes in 10 ml PCS scintillation fluid in a β-counter. [^{3}H] metabolites were identified and quantitated by their coelution with unlabeled standards. The standard retention time is 3 min. for water, 8 min. for tyrosine, 14 min. for TDAG, and 24 min. for DADLE. Tritiated water elutes in the void volume. [^{3}H] metabolites were expressed as percent of total serum radioactivity.

For the serum analyses of metkephamid, the procedure was described as follows. Samples from treated rats were kept on ice during the studies. To 200 µl of each serum sample was added 100 µl of NaF-EDTA solution containing 0.215 mmole of EDTA-disodium salt and 16.0 mmole of NaF. The serum samples were then stored at -20°C overnight and thawed just prior to HPLC analysis. One milliliter of acetone was added to the thawed mixture. The samples were capped, vortexed and allowed to stand for 10 minutes. After centrifuging at 2000 rpm for 10 minutes, as much as possible of the supernatant was transferred to another tube and the precipitate was discarded. To the supernatant was added 300 mg of NaCl and the samples were further vortexed. The resulting solution was extracted twice with 1 ml of ethyl acetate. The organic phases were combined and evaporated at 25°C under nitrogen. To the dried residue, 300 µl of 0.2 M Na_2HPO_4 (pH 8.0) and 100 µl of 0.03% Fluram[1] (fluorescamine) in acetone were added. After adequate mixing, a 50 µl sample was injected onto the column. The fluorescence of the sample was determined by HPLC with a fluorescence detector. The maximum excitation wavelength was 390 nm and maximum emission was 470 nm. The mobile phase consisted of 45% acetonitrile-55% 0.1 M ammonium formate buffer (pH 4.0). The flow rate was set at 1.5 ml/min. Metkephamid was identified and quantitated with a standard curve. The retention time of metkephamid in the chromatogram was 9 minutes. The minimum detectable concentration was 50 ng/ml; pentobarbital, used as the anesthetic agent, did not interfere with the assay. Baseline corrections were made using a blank of serum containing no metkephamid. The solvent was routinely degassed prior to use by applying a vacuum.

Absorption Studies in Animals - For intravenous, nasal, and oral administrations, the procedure was carried out as described in the literature (3,6). The peptides were dissolved in saline just prior to administration to the animals. For subcutaneous administration, the drug solution was administered by bolus injection under the skin surface of the back. Absorption into blood was determined by measuring the area under the concentration vs. time curve (AUC) within the studied time period. The AUC was calculated by the trapezoidal method under a linear scale. The biological elimination half-life was estimated from the terminal phase after administration. Statistical evaluation used Student's t-test.

Histological Examination of Nasal Mucosa in Rats - After the absorption studies, the rats were killed, beheaded, and the nasal passages were flushed with 10% buffered formalin. After fixation, the heads were decalcified and four cross-sections of the nasal cavity of each rat were stained and examined (Su et al, 1984).

---

[1]Sigma Chemical Company, St. Louis, MO.

RESULTS AND DISCUSSION

[³H]-DADLE - It is well known that surfactants can influence drug absorption and membrane transport, and that surfactants may also reduce proteolytic enzyme activity (Hirai et al, 1981). A number of publications reported that a conjugated bile salt, sodium glycocholate, enhanced the nasal absorption of polypeptides (Hirai et al, 1978, 1984; Moses et al, 1983).

The nasal absorption of an enkephalin analogue (DADLE), in the absence and presence of sodium glycocholate as a promoting agent, is shown in Figure 1 and Table 1. The radioactivity levels in the blood after nasal and subcutaneous administrations of [³H]-DADLE reflect the combined levels of the parent polypeptides and its metabolites. It was assumed that the elimination half-life of [³H]-DADLE was of the same magnitude following nasal and subcutaneous administrations. In addition, for the purpose of comparing the relative absorption of these two administration routes, the AUC was integrated from 0 to 300 minutes. As shown in Table I, in the absence of sodium glycocholate, a nasal absorption of about 59% of the sub-

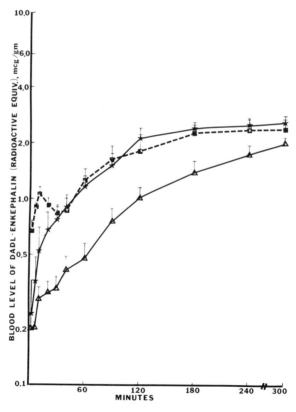

Figure 1: Total radioactivity equivalents of [³H]-DADLE blood levels in rats after various routes of administration of a dose of 2 mg/kg (n = 3-4). Key (✳) subcutaneous administration; (ᐃ) intranasal administration; (■) intranasal administration in the presence of 1% sodium glycocholate.

224

cutaneous dose was found based on the total amount of labeled compound appearing in the blood. However, in the presence of 1% sodium glycocholate in the formulation, the nasal absorption was enhanced to about 94% of the subcutaneous dose.

In an attempt to quantitate the polypeptides detected in the blood, whether present as the parent molecule or its metabolites, an HPLC analysis was then conducted. The intravenous administration route was used as the control in the study. The nasal formulation contained 1% sodium glycocholate since the formulation showed a good absorption in the previous study (ref. Table 1). The relative concentrations of intact [^{3}H]-DADLE and its tritiated metabolites, TDAG, tyrosine, and water expressed as a percentage of total tritium were determined for serum samples following nasal (Figure 2) or intravenous (Figure 3) administrations. The results represent the average of determinations in three animals. The elimination of [^{3}H]-DADLE from the serum of rats after nasal and I.V. administrations exhibited triphasic kinetics. The rapid redistribution phase after nasal administration was characterized by a 14.8 minute half-life followed by a second slower phase with an elimination half-life of 26.3 minutes. The third phase was characterized by an elimination half-life of 86.4 minutes. In contrast, the elimination half-life of [^{3}H]-DADLE from the serum of rats following intravenous administration was 3.06 minutes, 9.86 minutes, and 80.3 minutes for the three phases, respectively. The rapid elimination half-life following I.V. administration was also reflected in the degradation scheme. The rate of [^{3}H]-DADLE degradation to [^{3}H]-tyrosine and [^{3}H]-H_2O was much more rapid following intravenous administration than nasal administration. Only 20% of the total tritium remained as intact [^{3}H]-DADLE 12 minutes after I.V. vs. 33 minutes after nasal administration.

Table 1. Comparison of Blood Levels of Total Radioactivity Equivalents of [^{3}H]-DADLE in Rats After Various Routes of Administration of a 2 mg/kg Dose[a]

(Expressed as Mcg Equivalents of ^{3}H/g of Blood)

Route of Administration	n	AUC[b]	Relative Absorption[c]
Subcutaneous [^{3}H]-DADLE in saline	3	590.4 ± 41.4	-
Intranasal [^{3}H]-DADLE in saline	3	348.1 ± 48.3	59.0%
[^{3}H]-DADLE in saline plus 1% sodium glycocholate	4	555.9 ± 85.1	94.1%

[a]Expressed as microgram equivalents of tritium in blood; the dose volume was maintained at 0.1·mL. [b]AUC: μg·min/g, mean ± SEM. [c](AUC)$_{intranasal}$ (AUC)$_{sc}$ x 100%.

As shown in Figure 2, the peak concentration of intact [³H]-DADLE at the initial 1 minute sample time point was 74.2% (± 5.3%) after nasal administration. This peak percentage represented 0.63 µg/ml of [³H]-DADLE serum concentration. At 20 minutes, approximately equal percentages of the label were distributed among tritiated water (29.6 ± 8.3), tyrosine (33.6 ± 2.8), and DADLE (34.7 ± 7.79), respectively. At 60 minutes, about 80% of the total tritium was [³H]-H$_2$O, 13% was [³H]-tyrosine, and only 5.7% remained as intact [³H]-DADLE. Only trace concentrations of tripeptides were detected. The peak [³H]-DADLE serum concentration was 68.60 ± 9.49% at one minute following I.V. administration (Figure 3). This represented 3.37 µg/ml of DADLE serum concentration. Therefore, at the peak time of one minute, there was a 5.4-fold higher serum DADLE concentration in the I.V. compared to animals administered nasal solutions. However, the AUC was 19.60 ± 2.54 µg·min/ml in the I.V. study and 18.24 ± 8.15 µg·min/ml in the nasal study. The larger standard error, when comparing µg·min/ml to the expression of data as percent of total tritium, reflected individual variations in the absolute amount absorbed by each animal. The metabolism of this peptide, however, was similar in all three animals as can be seen by the smaller standard error in the normalized data (i.e. Figures 2 and 3). The bioavailability of [³H]-DADLE following nasal administration was approximately 93% of the I.V. dose; the difference in the extent of absorption was not statistically significant.

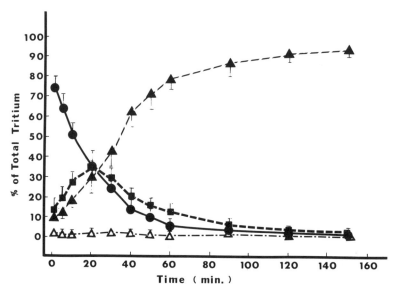

Figure 2: Absorption and distribution of [³H]-DADLE in rat serum following intranasal administration of a 2 mg/kg dose in the presence of 1% sodium glycocholate (n = 3). Key: (●) DADLE; (■) Tyrosine; (▲) H$_2$O; (△) TDAG.

Metkephamid - The absorption kinetics of metkephamid in the serum of rats by various administration routes is shown in Figure 4. The elimination of metkephamid from the serum of rats after I.V., nasal and s.c. administrations exhibited biphasic kinetics. The redistribution phase of the nasal administration was characterized by a 61.4 min. half-life followed by a terminal phase with an elimination half-life of 34.9 minutes. In contrast, the elimination half-life of metkephamid in the serum following I.V. administration was 6.3 minutes and 18.7 minutes for the two

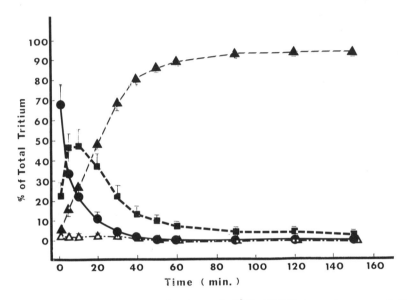

Figure 3: Absorption and distribution of [^{3}H]-DADLE in rat serum following intravenous administration of dose 2 mg/kg (n = 3). Key: (●) DADLE: (■) Tyrosine; (▲) H$_2$O; (△) TDAG.

phases, respectively. No metkephamid could be detected in the serum following oral administration. The nasal and subcutaneous administrations of metkephamid resulted in much higher serum levels of this peptide than the levels obtained by the oral administration. As shown in Table II, the AUC of metkephamid following nasal administration was about equivalent to the I.V. dose, whereas after S.C. administration the corresponding levels were found to be 91% of the I.V. dose. The difference in the extent of absorption was statistically insignificant (p > 0.1).

Table 2. Comparison of Metkephamid Serum Levels in Rats After Various Routes of Administration of a 25-mg/kg Dose[a]

Route of Administration	n	AUC[b]	Bioavailability %[c]
Intravenous	3	186.71 ± 34.74	-
Subcutaneous	3	169.14[d] ± 30.47	90.6
Intranasal	4	190.38[e] ± 65.33	101.9
Oral	3	0[f]	0

[a]Metkephamid (lot No. H37P73099) was dissolved in saline, and the volume was maintained at 0.1 mL. [b]AUC: $\mu g \cdot min/mL$, mean ± SEM, integrated from 0 to ∞. [c]$(AUC)_{sc, nasal, po}/(AUC)_{iv}$ × 100%. [d]$p > 0.1$, compared to nasal and intravenous. [e]$p > 0.1$, compared to intravenous. [f]No compound detected.

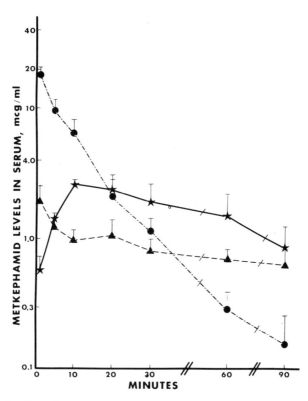

Figure 4: Metkephamid in rat serum after various routes of administration of a 25 mg/kg dose (n = 3-4). Key: (●) intravenous administration; (▲) subcutaneous administration; (*) intranasal administration. No compound was detected after oral administration.

The influence of surfactant on the nasal absorption of metkephamid was also studied. The difference in serum levels following nasal administration of metkephamid, in the presence or absence of 1% sodium glycocholate in the formulation (the AUC is 144.24 ± 4.77 µg·min/ml vs. 190.38 ± 65.33 µg·min/ml, respectively, calculated from 0 to ∞) was statistically insignificant (p > 0.1). The data indicate that there is no need to incorporate a surfactant to enhance the absorption of metkephamid, as compared to the other pentapeptide (ref. to Table 1). This observation is consistent with the reported data that metkephamid is a more stable analogue and less susceptible to enzymatic degradation (Gesellchen et al, 1980).

The effect of peptide dose on the nasal absorption is shown in Table 3. The area under the curve of serum metkephamid levels vs. time increased with dose. A linear relationship between the dose and the AUC was observed between 12.5 mg/kg and 50.0 mg/kg, with a correlation coefficient of 0.950. The extent of absorption under the AUC per unit dose remained relatively constant. Thus, the amount of metkephamid absorbed nasally was directly proportional to the dose administered according to the law of diffusion.

Table 3.   Effect of Dose on the Nasal Absorption of
Metkephamid in Rats[a]

Route of Administration	n	AUC[b]	Mean Sp AUC[c]	Bioavailability, %
Intravenous				
25 mg/kg	3	186.71 ± 34.74	7.47	-
Intranasal				
50 mg/kg	3	273.40 ± 35.57	5.47[d]	73.2
25 mg/kg	4	190.38 ± 65.33	7.61[d]	101.9
12.5 mg/kg	3	60.51 ± 15.57	4.84[d]	64.8

[a]Metkephamid (lot No. H37P73099) was dissolved in saline, and the volume was maintained at 0.1 mL.   [b]AUC: µg·min/mL, mean ± SEM, integrated from 0 to ∞.   [c]Mean specific AUC: (µg·min/mL)/(mg/kg) = mean AUC/administered dose.   [d]p > 0.1, comparison between various doses of nasal administration.

Histology - It is well known that the mucosal surface area of the nasal cavity is large. The vascular bed of the nasal mucosa is responsible for the rapid passage of fluid and dissolved materials from the mucosa to the systemic circulation (Proctor and Andersen, 1982). The possibility that nasal absorption of any compound could be attributable to damage to the mucosa was considered during the investigation. To avoid any possible physical damage to the epithilium of the nasal mucosa, the drug solution was carefully delivered as previously reported (Su et al, 1984). However, histopathological studies were conducted to ascertain the integrity of the mucosa. Typical microscopic specimens of exposed rat nasal mucosa are shown in Figures 5-6. The untreated control had naturally-occurring acute rhinitis characterized by purulent luminal debris and submucosal inflammation. This lesion was of bacterial or mycoplasmal origin. All treated rats had various amounts of luminal debris formed of proteinaceous fluid, sloughed mucosal cells, and neutrophils and various degrees of submucosal inflammation. Mucosal necrosis, a feature not present in the

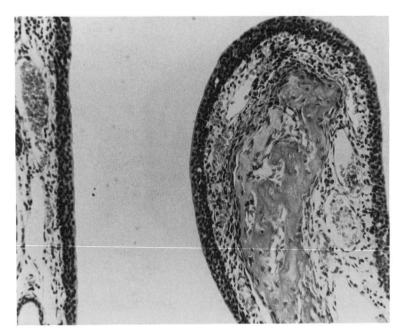

Figure 5: Nasal mucosa of untreated control rat.

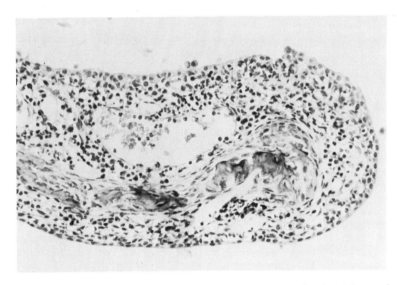

Figure 6: Nasal mucosa of rat exposed to 25 mg metkaphemid per kg for five hours.

untreated rats, also occurred. The necrosis was usually mild and characterized by occasional partly detached, eosinophilic mucosal cells with pyknotic nuclei. In some instances it was more severe and focal areas of mucosal loss were present.

The presence of sodium glycocholate had no consistent effect on the reactions, which were, in general, of mild to moderate severity. Considering the five-hour contact time, the degree of irritation produced was slight and probably repairable.

In summary, data from our laboratory has demonstrated that enkephalins can be absorbed into the systemic circulation through the nasal mucosa. The onset of absorption was rapid and serum levels after nasal administration were similar to those following I.V. administration. A good bioavailability for the two enkephalins studied was observed when compared to the I.V. dose. The data reveal that polypeptide absorption across the nasal membranes is a reasonable approach. A nasal delivery system could be an extremely useful route of systemic administration for proteins and polypeptides which are, in general, poorly absorbed across the gastrointestinal mucosa.

(This article was reproduced by permission of the copyright owner Journal of Pharmaceutical Sciences)

REFERENCES

Anik, S. T., McRae, G., Nerenberg, C., Worden, A., Foreman, J., Hwang, J. Y., Kushinsky, S., Jones, R. E., and Vickery, B., 1984, J. Pharm. Sci., 73:684.
Berquist, C., Nillius, S. J., and Wide, L., 1979, Lancet, 2:215.
David, G. F. X., Puri, C. P., and Anand Kuman, T. C., 1981, Experimentia, 37:533.
Evans, W. W., Borges, J. L. C., Kaiser, D. L., Vance, M. L., Sellers, R. P., MacLeod, R. M., Vale, W., Rivier, J., and Thorner, M. O., 1983, J. Clin. Endocr. Metab., 57:1081.
Fink, G., Gennser, G., Liedholm, P., Thorell, J., and Mulder, J., 1974, J. Endocr., 63:351.
R. C. A. Frederickson, Life Sci., 21, 23 (1970).
Gennser, G., and Liedholm, P., 1974, Lancet, 1:865.
Gesellchen, P. D., Tafur, S., and Shields, J. E., 1979, "Peptides: Structure and Biological Function, Proc. of the Sixth American Peptide Symp.", E. Gross and J. Neienhofer, Eds., Pierce Chemical Co., Rockfold, Ill., pp. 117-120.
Gesellchen, P. D., Parli, C. J., and Frederickson, R. C. A., 1980, "Peptides: Synthesis-Structure-Function, Proc. of the Seventh Ameri. Peptide Symp.", D. H. Rich and E. Gross, Eds., Pierce Chem. Co., Rockfold, Ill., pp. 637-640.
Greenberg, S. B., Harmon, M. W., Johnson, P. E., and Couch, R. B., 1978, Antimicro. Agents and Chemot., 14:596.
Harmon, M. W., Greenberg, S. B., and Couch, R. B., 1976, Proc. Soc. Exp. Biol. Med., 152:598.
Harmon, M. W., Greenberg, S. R., Johnson, P. E., and Couch, R. B., 1977, Infect. Immun., 16:480.
Hirai, S., Yashiki, T., Matsuzawa, T., and Mima, H., 1981, Int. J. Pharm., 7:317.
Hirai, S., Ikenaga, T., and Matsuzawa, T., 1978, ibid., 27:296.
Hirai, S., Yashiki, T., and Mima, H., 1981a, Int. J. Pharm., 9:165.
Hirai, S., Yashiki, T., and Mima, H., 1981b, ibid., 9:173.

Hussain, A., Hirai, S., and Bawarshi, R., 1979, J. Pharm. Sci., 68:1196.
Hussain, A., Foster, T., Hirai, S., Kashihara, T., Batenhorst, R., and Jones, M., 1980a, ibid., 69:1240.
Hussain, A., Hirai, S., and Bawarshi, R., 1980b, ibid., 69:1411.
Hussain, A., Hirai, S., and Bawarshi, R., 1981, J. Pharm. Sci., 70:466.
Johnson, P. E., Greenberg, S. B., Harmon, M. W., Alford, B. R., and Couch, R. B., 1976, J. Clin. Microbiol., 4:106.
Leander J. D., and Wood, C. R., Peptides, 3:771.
London, D. R., Butt, W. R., Lynch, S. S., Marshell, J. C. Owusu, S., Robinson, W. R., and Stephenson, J. M., 1973, J. Clin. Endocrinol. Metab., 37:829.
Moses, A. C., Gordon, G. S., Carey, M. C., and Flier, J. S., 1983, Diabetes, 32:1040.
Motta, M., 1980, "The Endocrine Functions of the Brain", Chap 12, pp. 233-270, Raven Press, New York, N.Y.
Proctor D. F., and Andersen, I. B., 1982, "The Nose: Upper Airway Physiology and the Atmospheric Environment", Chap. 2 and 3, pp. 23-69, Elsevier Biomedical Press, Amsterdam, Netherlands.
Su, K. S. E., Campanale, K. M., and Gries, C. L., 1984, ibid., 73:1251.

ACKNOWLEDGEMENTS

Presented to the Basic Pharmaceutical Section, A.Ph.A. Academy of Pharmaceutical Sciences 37th National Meeting, Philadelphia, PA, October 1984. The authors thank Dr. J. C. Parli and Ms. M. K. Frohnauer for providing assay methodology of metkephamid, Dr. P. D. Gesellchen and Mr. R. T. Shuman for supplying peptides, and Ms. A. Simpson for her assistance in preparing the manuscript.

INTRANASAL DELIVERY OF THE PEPTIDE, SALMON CALCITONIN

Musetta Hanson, G. Gazdick, J. Cahill, and M. Augustine

Pharmacy Research and Development
Rorer Group, Inc.
Tuckahoe, New York 10707

INTRODUCTION

Calcitonin is a polypeptide hormone normally secreted by the parafollicular cells of mammalian thyroid glands and by the ultimobronchial gland of birds and fish. The linear sequence of 32 amino acids found in the calcitonin of salmon origin has been synthesized. This synthetic salmon calcitonin (sCT) is currently formulated as a sterile solution for subcutaneous injection in the treatment of Paget's disease, hypercalcemia, and osteoporosis. Paget's disease is a disorder characterized by abnormal bone formation and resorption while hypercalcemia is an elevated serum calcium level, and osteoporosis is a loss of bone mass with increased fractures. Treatment calls for daily subcutaneous injections of salmon calcitonin over an extended period. The necessity of this daily injection is bothersome and inconvenient to patients. However, because the drug is a polypeptide subject to digestive degradation, it can not be given orally. Therefore, an alternate route of administration, such as intranasally, is attractive.

The nasal mucosa has been studied in a limited way as a route for the administration of drugs. Hussain (1979) showed that propranolol was readily absorbed across the nasal mucosa of rats but inefficiently and variably absorbed when given as an oral dose. This observation was confirmed in both dogs and man (Hussain, et al., 1980). Of even more interest are those references to absorption of peptides across the nasal mucosa. Hendricks et al (1960) compared the intranasal vs. intravenous effects of oxytocin and found the intranasal absorption to be only a fraction of the intravenous. Potashnik, et al., (1977) reported nasal absorption of synthetic gonadotropin-releasing hormone, but 25 times the amount of peptide used in the I.V. dose was required. Other authors have shown varying nasal absorption of secreton (B'hend, et al., 1973), ACTH Felber, et al., 1969; Keenan, et al., 1971; Smith, et al., 1952), H-releasing hormone (London, et al, 1973) and natural contraceptive steroids (Hussain, et al., 1978). Human calcitonin, delivered as nasal spray, had pharmacologic effect (Ziegler, et al., 1981). These drugs had been delivered in a variety of ways including snuff, drops, nebulized spray, and had been formulated with viscosity enhancers such as natural gum and methylcellulose.

Nasal absorption of insulin was measured in dogs when administered by nebulizer spray. The extent and duration of response was pH dependent

233

and greatest at acid pH. Use of surfactants (saponin, glycocholate, or BL-9) allowed the response even at neutral pH. The intranasal dosage needed was 3 to 4 times the I.V. dose to obtain the same effect (Hirai, et al, 1978). Hirai, et al., (1981) noted the use of surfactants enhanced of nasal absorption of insulin in rats. Surfactants used included various nonionic, anionic, and amphoteric surfactants, including bile salts and saponin. Ether-type surfactants with an hydrophilic lipophilic balance (HLB) value between 8 and 14 were most effective. Bile salts had a similar effect on absorption and were thought to possibly inhibit nasal mucosa proteolytic enzymes. In addition, bile salts were less irritative to the mucosa than the other surfactants (Hirai, et al., 1981).

Therefore, this study was undertaken to determine if salmon calcitonin could be absorbed through the nasal mucosa; if this absorption could be enhanced by the addition of other excipients; and if a formulation could be achieved that was stable and effective upon intranasal delivery.

Methods and Materials

In general, salmon calcitonin, sufficient to provide a dose of 1-10 U/kg body weight in 50 microliters, was dissolved in the vehicle (buffer or 1% gelatin solution) and other excipients such as surfactants were added as specified. These formulations were then tested using the following rat bioassay, which is a modification of the method of Hirai, et al, (1981).

Male rats weighting 150-250 g were weighed and anesthetized with sodium pentobarbital, 50 mg/kg, by intraperitoneal injection. Once anesthetized, the nasopalatine process was occluded with glue. The animals were randomly placed into groups of 5-7 rats. Supplemental pentobarbital anesthesia was administered as necessary throughout the study.

Prior to administration of the test material, blood was collected by cardiac puncture using a 25G 5/8 needle. Fifty (50) microliters of the salmon calcitonin-containing surfactant solution was then instilled into the nasal septum using polyethylene tubing (PE 20, Peterson Technics, Monmouth Junction, NJ) connected to a 1 ml syringe; the tubing was inserted about 1 cm into the nasal septum. One and three hours after nasal instillation blood was again collected by cardiac puncture.

Blood samples were allowed to clot at room temperature and were then refrigerated for 30-60 minutes to provide maximum clot retraction. The samples were centrifuged at 4°C, 5000 rpm for 10 minutes (Beckman Model J2-21) Centrifuge, Beckman Instruments, Palo Alto, CA). Serum calcium was quantitated using a Calcette (Model 4008, Precision Systems, Sudbury, MA).

Serum Calcium values at 0, 1 and 3 hours were expressed as the mean. In addition, the absolute change and the percent change from the pretreatment (0 time) value at 1 and 3 hours was also calculated. Statistical analysis consisted of comparison of the serum calcium values at 0 and 1 hour, 0 and 3 hours, and 1 and 3 hours using a t-test.

The effect of various molecules on inhibition of nasal proteolytic enzymes was studied in two ways. First, purified porcine Kidney Leucine Aminopeptidase from Sigma Chemical (St. Louis) was used. And in the second, an extract of rat nasal tissue was prepared by dissecting out the nasal septum, homogenizing it in phosphate buffered saline, pH 7.4, and centrifuging at 9000 g. The supernatant was stored at -60°C. The enzyme were shown to degrade salmon calcitonin by measuring loss of peptide after incubation with the enzyme using an isocratic reverse phase HPLC method.

The inhibition of these enzymes was also measured by a standard enzymatic assay using a substrate for aminopeptidases. Aminopeptidases catalyse the following reaction (1) which is then coupled to reaction (2) and reaction (3) to produce a blue color that can be read spectrophotometrically at 580 nm.

1. Leucyl ß Naphthylamide + H_2O $\xrightarrow{\text{AP}}$ Leucine + ß Naphthylamide

2. ß Naphthylamide + $NaNO_2$ $\xleftarrow{\text{H+}}$ Diazo reagent

3. Diazo reagent + N(1-Naphthyl)Ethylenediamine $\longrightarrow$ Blue Azo Dye

The amount of absorbance at 580 nm is proportional to the level of enzyme activity. The reagents used for this assay are those in Sigma Chemical Company's LAP Kit 251 AW.

Results

The initial screening experiments were done using a 1.0% gelatin solution at pH 3.6 or acetate buffer at pH 4.0 as the vehicle for calcitonin without the vehicle effecting absorption. It was found that some salmon calcitonin was absorbed even without any agents added to enhance absorption. The absorption was measured by looking for a drop in serum calcium at 1 and 3 hours after dosing, indicating calcitonin action. While there is some assay variability, this method is useful to screen the enhancement of absorption of various excipients. An indication of enhancement is a sustained calcium drop at three hours or a parallel calcium drop at one and three hours when less calcitonin is administered.

Figure 1 shows that when a rat is injected subcutaneously with 10 U/kg body weight of sCT, a maximal 25-30% drop in serum calcium is seen within one hour and is sustained for 5-8 hours before returning to baseline. However, when the sCT is delivered intranasally, 2 U/kg produces no response, 5 U/kg produces a minimal 7% decrease at one hour with return to baseline, and 10 U/kg results in a one hour drop of 17% and a return to baseline by 3 hours. While this data is encouraging because it says that sCT is being absorbed intranasally, it also means that a much higher dose than that given parenterally will be needed to get the same physiological response.

When surfactants of various types are added to the formulation, an enhancement of absorption of the peptide is seen. Figure 2 shows the effect of a representative from each of the classes of surfactants after administration intranasally of 10 U/kg of sCT. The maximum decrease in serum calcium at one hour of 25-30% is seen with all surfactants and the effect is prolonged to different degrees at 3 hours. This increased and prolonged drop of serum calcium levels with surfactant suggested that the dose of sCT could be reduced and still remain effective.

In Figure 3, it can be seen that the maximal drop of serum calcium (30%) at one hour can be achieved with a dose of 3 U/kg in the presence of surfactants and again some prolongation at 3 hours is observed.

This physiological response to sCT with surfactant was proportional to the concentration of surfactant used. Figure 4 shows a plot of the 3 hour serum calcium drops as a function of surfactant concentration. As the concentration increases, the prolongation of calcium drop increases, suggesting that more sCT is absorbed with increasing surfactant.

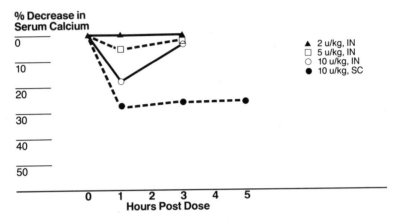

Fig. 1.   Decrease in Serum Calcium As a Function of Dose and Route of Administration of Calcitonin

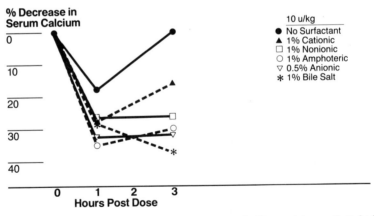

Fig. 2.   Effect of Surfactants on Intranasal Absorption of Calcitonin

236

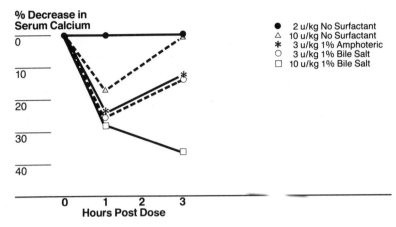

Fig. 3.   Effect of Surfactants on Intranasal Absorption of Calcitonin

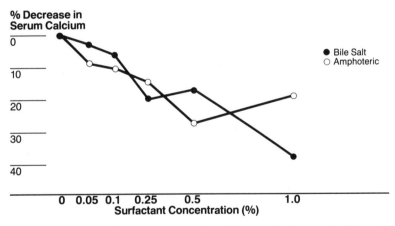

Fig. 4.   Effect of Surfactant Concentration on Intranasal Absorption of
Calcitonin (10 μ/kg) at 3 Hours Post Dose

In order to determine if inhibition of delivery site proteases might be a mechanism by which molecules exert an absorption promoting effect, studies were done using both a purified procine kidney leucine aminopeptidase and an extract of rat nasal mucosa. It was first shown that salmon calcitonin as a substrate is degraded by both pure leucine aminopeptidase and by the rat nasal extract. Then the effect of various molecules on these proteolytic enzymes was determined using leucine-ß-naphthylamide as the substrate. The selected potential inhibitor was incubated with the enzyme and substrate for one hour at 37°C and the reaction then stopped. After appropriate color development, the percent of activity remaining was calculated by dividing by the level found in a control tube with no inhibitor. Figure 5 shows the amount of purified leucine aminopeptidase activity remaining with increasing levels of various surfactants. The bile salt inhibits at much lower concentrations than the nonionic or amphoteric do. The effect of this same bile salt on the proteolytic activity of the rat nasal extract is shown in Figure 6. Here higher levels of bile salt are needed to inhibit the proteolytic activity but this is likely due to a more dilute enzyme concentration. Also, the line has two slopes suggesting that a second proteolytic enzyme not inhibited by the bile salt at the same rate may be present.

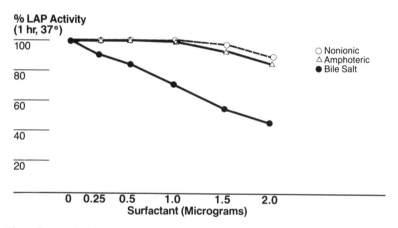

Fig. 5. Inhibition of Leucine Amino Peptidase by Surfactants

To see if correlation exists between the in vitro rat nasal extract inhibition and the in vivo test, well known protease inhibitors, were tested in both. In the in vitro test, the enzyme was rat nasal extract and the substrate leucine-ß-napthylamide. The percent inhibition was determined by subtracting the percent of remaining activity from 100%. The in vivo assay was as described previously. Figure 7 shows that in general if a molecule inhibits the rat nasal extract's proteolytic activity, it also enhances the serum calcium drop seen in vivo at 1-2 hours and often prolongs this drop. The fact that some molecules do not show this correlation has not been explained and may mean that more than one

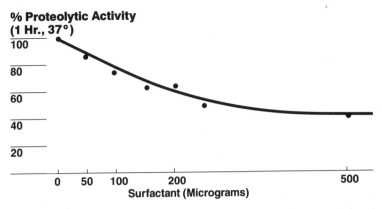

Fig. 6.   Inhibition of Rat Nasal Mucosal Proteolytic Activity by an
Absorption Promoter

mechanism is responsible for absorption promotion.   Characterization of the
enzymes present in the rat mucosal extract remains to be done.

Compound	In Vitro % Inhibition	In Vivo	
		Max. % CA^{++} Drop	Time Max.
None	0	18	2
Bile Salt	68	30	3
FA Deriv.	82	30	3
Aprotinin	0	30	4
Kallikrein Inh. I	80	29	2
RG-I	56	26	2
Bestatin	79	13	1
Fusidic Acid	50	19	2
Chymostatin	37	18	2
Benzamidine	0	25	2
Chymotrypsin Inh. II	0	17	2
Trypsin Inh. III-0	0	18	2
Anti Pain	18	18	2
Leupeptin	0	19	2

Fig. 7.   Correlation of In Vitro Inhibition of Proteolytic Activity
with In Vivo Enhancement of sCT Absorption Intranasally

A major concern of incorporating surfactants into intranasal formulations that might be delivered daily is their effect on the nasal tissue. A number of safety studies were done on selected formulations, including a study that called for 21 day repeated dosing, twice a day in both rats and rabbits. At the end of the 21 day period, the animals were sacrificed and histological evaluation of the nasal mucosa was made. No mortality, change in body weight, hemotology, or clinical chemistry had been observed during the study. Furthermore, no changes in the histology of the mucosa could be detected.

Before testing in humans could begin, a suitable delivery system had to be found. The precompression pump was chosen for further study because it delivers a metered dose, formulation problems using aerosols could be avoided, and the drug is delivered as a fine mist over a larger area of the nasal mucosa than drops would allow. Several different pumps were evaluated for the consistency of delivery, spray pattern, and particle size. By doing repeated spraying and weighing of a statistically significant number of pumps, it was determined that all pumps deliver within 5-10% the labeled volume delivered, that an additional 5% varibility is the result of operator differences, that the larger volume pumps are more consistent than the smaller volume pumps, and that heating some of the pumps above 40°C will begin to effect their consistency of delivery.

Once the delivery method was chosen, a selected formulation was tested clinically in twenty normal volunteers. In a two way crossover, patients were given a single dose of 400U sCT (consisting of two actuations pre nostril) of either a formulation of sCT without promoter or sCT with a surfactant promoter. The actual blood levels of sCT were measured using a radioimmune assay for sCT. Figure 8 shows the average picograms of sCT of all twenty patients plotted versus time after dosing. Without promoter, only trace amounts of sCT appear in the plasma. However, with promoter significant levels of sCT are found in the plasma with the AUC being 10 times that without promoter. The formulation was also evaluated with repeat dosing for safety and tolerance and found to be well tolerated.

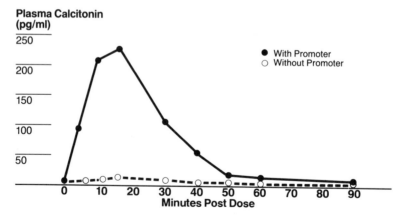

Fig. 8. Plasma Levels of Intranasally Delivered Calcitonin in Normal Volunteers

Conclusions

Using the rat as a animal model, it has been shown that salmon calcitonin can be absorbed intranasally. Furthermore, the biological response (drop in serum calcium) could be increased by inclusion of various surfactant type molecules in the formulation but using lower doses of peptide, suggesting enhancement of absorption. When commonly known inhibitors of proteolytic enzymes were evaluated in an in vitro assay using an extract of rat nasal mucosa as a proteolytic enzyme and were assayed in vivo in the rat, generally good correlation of inhibitory properties and enhancement of absorption were found. This suggests that inhibition of nasal proteases and protection of the peptide at the delivery site may be one mechanism by which absorption is promoted.

Precompression pumps were evaluated and found to reproducibly deliver the drug within ± 15%.

The use of an absorption promoter in one formulation has been used successfully in humans producing a 10 fold increase in serum calcitonin levels over the control without promoter.

References

B'hend, P., Hadron, B., Haldeman, B., Klebb, M., and Luthi, H., 1973, Stimulation of pancreatic secretion in man by secretin snuff, Lancet, i:510.

Felber, J., Aubert, M., and Deguillaume, R., 1969, Administration by nasal spray of an 18 amino acid synthetic polypeptide with corticotrophic action, Experimentia, 25:1195.

Hendrick, C. and Gabel, R., 1960, Use of intranasal oxytocin in obsterics, Am. J. Obstet. Gynec., 79:780.

Hirai, S., Ikenaga, T., and Matsuzana, T., 1978, Nasal absorption of insulin in dogs, Diabetes, 27:296.

Hirai, S., Yashiki, T., and Mima, H., 1978, Effect of surfactants on the nasal absorption of insulin in rats, Int. J. Pharm., 9:165.

Hirai, S., Yashiki, T. and Mina, H., 1978, Mechanism for the enhancement of the nasal absorption of insulin by surfactants, Int. J. Pharm., 9:173.

Hussain, A., Hirai, S., and Bawarshi, R., 1979, Nasal absorption of propranolol in rats, J. Pharm. Sci., 68:1196.

Hussain, A., Foster, T., Hirai, S., Kashihara, T., Batenhorst, R., and Jones, M., 1980, Nasal absorption of propranolol in humans, J. Pharm. Sci., 69:1240.

Hussain, A., Hirai, S., and Bawarshi, R., 1980, Nasal absorption of propranolol from different dosage forms by rats and dogs, J. Pharm. Sci., 69:1411.

Hussain, A., Hirai, S., and Bawarshi, R., 1981, Nasal absorption of natural contraceptive steroids in rats - progesterone absorption, J. Pharm. Sci., 70:466.

Keenan, J., Thompson, J., Chamberlain, M. and Bessir, G., 1971, Prolonged corticotrophic action of a synthetic substituted 1-18 ACTH, Brit. Med. J., 3:742.

London, D., Butt, W., and Marshall, J., 1973, Intranasal LH-releasing harmone, Lancet, i:1258.

Potashnik, G., Ben-Adereth, N., Lunenfeld, B., and Rote, C., 1977, Nasal application of synthetic gonadotropin-releasing hormone in men, Fertil. Steril., 28:650.

Smith, R., 1952, Nasal administration of ACTH: observation of effectiveness measured by blood eosinopenic response, Endocrine Soc. Abst., 12:958.

Ziegler, R., Holz, G., Steribl, W., and Raue, F., 1978, Nasal application of calcitonin in Paget's disease of bone, Acta Endroc. Suppl., 215:54.

METABOLIC EFFECTS OF INTRANASALLY ADMINISTERED INSULIN AND GLUCAGON IN MAN

A. E. Pontiroli, M. Alberetto, A. Calderara, E. Pajetta, and G. Pozza

Istituto Scientifico Ospedale San Raffaele, Cattedra di Clinica Medica, Universita' di Milano
Milano, Italy

INTRODUCTION

After isolation, chemical characterization and purification, several polypeptide hormones, i.e. insulin, glucagon, vasopressin and its analogues. LHRH and its derivatives. ACTH, calcitonin. growth hormone. gonadotropins, are currently employed in clinical practice. These hormones are administered parenterally, either by the subcutaneous. the intramuscular, the intravenous or the intraperitoneal route and by means of syringes or pumps. Some of these hormones require continuous or prolonged treatments in several chronic diseases, and this can cause severe reactions and may reduce the compliance of patients during the course of the disease. For these reasons, alternative routes of administration of peptidic hormones have been investigated. Oral administration has been tried for many of them but the gastrointestinal proteolytic digestion remains a limiting factor for most of them, with the noticeable exception of dDAVP (Pontiroli et al., 1985).
The mucosa of the respiratory system is able to absorb some inhaled materials such as vasopressin and dDAVP now widely employed for the treatment of diabetes insipidus, and LHRH and its analogues, employed both in experimental endocrinology and in the management of prostatic cancer (Pontiroli et al.,1985).
We have previously shown that insulin, administered as nasal drops, is effectively absorbed and lowers blood glucose levels in normal and in diabetic subjects (Pontiroli et al., 1982). Similar results were obtained by Moses et al., and Salzman et al. showed that intranasal insulin is as effective as subcutaneously injected insulin in controlling glucose metabolism in type 1 (insulin-dependent) diabetic patients (Moses et al., 1983; Salzman et al., 1985).
Intranasally administered glugagon, on the other hand, has been shown to enhance blood glucose levels (Pontiroli et al., 1983). and this might be beneficial for the management of hypoglycaemic crises, whatever their etiology, which are currently managed by means of glucose (p.o. or i.v.) or by glucagon (i.m.).
The aim of our studies was to investigate the effectiveness and bioavailability of different formulations of insulin and glucagon administered intranasally.

MATERIALS AND METHODS

The protocols of the studies were approved by the ethical committee of Istituto Scientifico San Raffaele. We performed two series of studies to evaluate the bioavailability and metabolic effects of insulin and glucagon administered intranasally.

28 healthy volunteers, chosen among medical students or physicians of Istituto Scientifico San Raffaele, were studied. They were aged 22-28 years, were free from endocrine and metabolic diseases and of normal body weight. All subjects were studied at 08.00 a.m. after an overnight fast and no smoking. 15 of them received insulin and 13 of them received glucagon. Venous blood glucose concentrations were determined by a glucose-oxidase method. Serum insulin (IRI) and plasma glucagon (IRG) levels were determined by radioimmunoassay. Statistical analysis were carried out by means of Student t test for paired or unpaired data as appropriate.

Studies with Insulin Intranasally

Study 1. Regular porcine insulin (Actrapid MC 40 UI/ml) was mixed with sodium glycocholate 1% w/v, used as a surfactant, at doses of 0.9 UI/Kg b.w. and it was administered as intranasal drops, subjects being asked to take a deep breath.

Study 2. According to a double-blind cross-over design, two different experiments were performed with 4 normal subjects with a one week interval between two consecutive experiments: in the first one regular porcine insulin (Actrapid MC 40 UI/ml) and in the second one regular human insulin (Actrapid HM 40 UI/ml) were used as in study 1.

Study 3. According to a latin square design, 5 healthy subjects underwent two different experiments with a one week interval between the tests: regular insulin (more concentrated) was mixed in one experiment with 9-lauryl-ether 0.8% w/v: in the other, insulin was mixed with an other surfactant, and under both circumstances insulin was administered as a spray solution at doses of 0.5 UI/Kg b.w.

Studies with Glucagon Intranasally

Study 1. Commercially available porcine glucagon, 1 mg, from Novo (Copenhagen, Denmark) was mixed with sodium glycocholate 1% w/v as surfactant and administered in drops to 7 subjects and in a spray formulation to 6 subjects. 4 subjects received only sodium glycocholate 1% as drops while 3 subjects received glucagon alone, 1 mg, as spray. 4 subjects received glucagon, 1 mg, intra venously and 5 subjects received glucagon, 1 mg, intramuscularly.

Study 2. According to a latin square design, 3 different experiments were performed with 5 normal subjects with a one week interval between two consecutive tests: in the first experiment, glucagon, 1 mg, plus sodium glycocholate 1% was administered as a spray solution; in the second one, glucagon, 1 mg, plus 9-lauryl-ether 0.8% was administered as a spray solution; in the third experiment, glucagon 1 mg, premixed with sodium glycocholate 1% was employed as inhaled powder.

Sodium glycocholate was purchased from Calbiochem, La Jolla, California; 9-lauryl-ether from Sigma, St.Louis, Missouri; Actrapid HM was a gift from Novo Industri, Copenhagen, Denmark.

RESULTS

Nasal Insulin

Study 1. Insulin in drops significantly raised serum IRI levels

244

and significantly decreased blood glucose levels. The increase of IRI levels lasted about 40 min, and the decrease of BG levels lasted about 60 min (fig.1.1).

Study 2. Human and porcine insulin administered in drops showed the same metabolic effects (fig. 1.2).

Study 3. The new spray device showed maximum metabolic effects, serum insulin levels being significantly higher and blood glucose levels being lower than in studies 1 and 2 (fig. 1.3).

When the surfactant was 9-lauryl-ether, serum insulin levels were lower than with the new device, but higher than with drops: also the fall of blood glucose levels was intermediate between drops and the new spray device. The potency ratio, calculated as metabolic effect divided by the dose of insulin administered, was maximal with the new spray device, intermediate with 9-lauryl-ether, and minimal with drops.

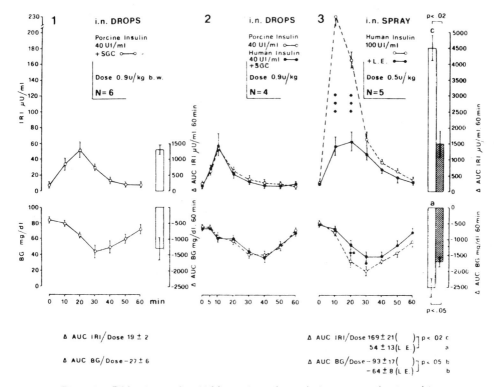

Δ AUC IRI/Dose 19 ± 2

Δ AUC BG/Dose –27 ± 6

Δ AUC IRI/Dose 169 ± 21 ( ) ⌉ p< 02 c
              54 ± 13 (L E) ⌋   a

Δ AUC BG/Dose –93 ± 17 ( ) ⌉ p< 05 b
            –64 ± 8 (L E) ⌋   b

Fig. 1. Effect of different formulations of insulin, administered intranasally to normal subjects, on serum insulin (IRI, μU/ml, upper part of the graphs) and on blood glucose (BG, mg/dl, lower part of the graphs) levels. In graphs 1 and 3, also areas under the curves (Δ AUC IRI μU/ml. 60 min and Δ AUC BG mg/dl. 60 min) are represented as columns. Potency ratio of different formulations (ΔAUC IRI/dose and ΔAUC BG/dose) are indicated on the bottom of graphs 1 and 3. Means ± SEM. N= number of subjects tested. All formulations were administered at time 0 min. *= p<0.05; **= p<0.02; ***= p<0.001 vs corresponding values; a= p<0.05; b= p<0.01; c= p<0.001 vs the AUCs and the AUCs/doses indicated in graph 1. SGC= sodium glycocholate; L.E.= 9-lauryl-ether.

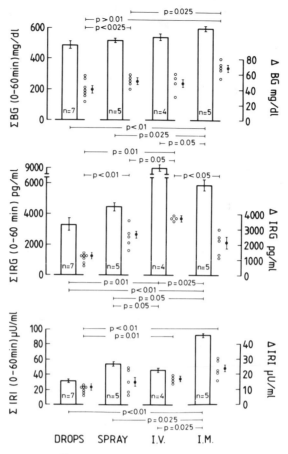

Fig. 2. Sums ($\sum$ 0-60 min) of BG, IRG and IRI values
(columns) and net peak increases (Δ) of BG,
IRG and IRI (individual points) observed after
administration of drops and spray solutions
containing glucagon 1 mg plus Na-glycocholate
15.0 mg and after intravenous and
intramuscular injection of glucagon, 1 mg.
Data are expressed as means ± SEM;
only significant differences are shown.

Intranasal Glucagon

Study 1. Glucagon in drops with sodium glycocholate 1% w/v significantly rose plasma IRG levels and BG levels. The surfactant alone was
ineffective, as glucagon alone. Spray solution was more effective than
drops: plasma IRG and BG levels were more elevated with the former form
of administration. I.v. glucagon showed highest plasma IRG levels, but BG
levels were not different from those obtained with spray solution, while
BG levels were higher with i.m. administration (fig. 2).

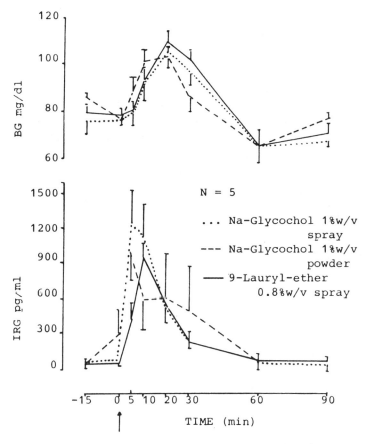

Fig. 3. Effect of different formulations of glucagon, administered intranasally, on blood glucose (BG mg/dl) and on plasma glucagon (IRG, pg/ml) levels in four normal subjects. N= 4; Means ± SEM.

Study 2. The different formulations employed showed superimposable metabolic effect in terms of BG and IRG levels (fig. 3).

DISCUSSION

In agreement with previous reports by ourselves and by others (Pontiroli et al., 1982; Moses et al., Salwman et al., 1985; Pontiroli et al., 1983) the efficacy of glucagon and of insulin, administered intranasally, is of the same order of magnitude of traditional parenteral routes of administration. The aim of these studies was to compare different formulations of glucagon and of insulin, administered intranasally. The new spray formulation employed for insulin was more effective than drops or spray formulation using 9-lauryl-ether as a surfactant, while human and porcine insulin, administered intranasally as drops, showed the same metabolic effects, as already claimed by other authors who compared the two insulins for traditional routes of adminstrations (i.v., i.m., s.c.) (Owens et al., 1981). With drops the potency ratio was about 1:9 compared to i.v. insulin. With the new spray formulation, metabolic effects are more evident and quicker than with any other formulation reported so far. Although subject to improvement, this formulation is worth to be tried as it is in diabetic patients. Following our previous studies, we have confirmed here that glucagon is absorbed through the nasal mucosa and enhances blood glucose levels. The effect we observed in our studies is probably tapered by the concomitant stimulation of insulin release (Pontiroli et al., 1983), so that even higher effects might be anticipated in patients with insulin-dependent diabetes mellitus. The effect was more marked with spray formulations than with the use of drops and was not different when spray solutions or dry powder were employed.

ACKNOWLEDGEMENTS

The authors whish to acknowledge all the physicians and students who volunteered for the experiments performed in these studies.

REFERENCES

Moses A. C., Gordon G. S., Carey M. C., and Flier J. S., 1983, Insulin administered intranasally as an insulin-bile salt aerosol. Effectiveness and reproducibility in normal and diabetic subjects, Diabetes, 32: 1040.

Owens D. S., Hayes T. M., Jones M. K., Heding L. G., Albert G. M., Horne P. D., and Burrin J. M., 1981, Comparative study of subcutaneous, intramuscular and intravenous administration of human insulin, Lancet, ii: 118.

Pontiroli A. E., Alberetto M., and Pozza G., 1983, Intranasal glucagon raises blood glucose concentrations in healthy volunteers., Br. Med. J., 287: 462.

Pontiroli A. E., Alberetto M., Secchi A., Dossi G., Bosi I., and Pozza G., 1982, Insulin given intranasally induces hypoglycaemia in normal and diabetic subjects., Br. Med. J., 284: 303.

Pontiroli A. E., Secchi A., and Alberetto M., 1985, Alternative routes of peptide hormones administration, In: "Special topics in endocrinology and metabolism." Eds P. P. Foa' and M. P. Cohen. Inc. A. R. Liss., New York, 7: 77.

Salzman R., Manson J. E., Griffing G. T., Rimmerle R., Ruderman R., MacCall A., Stoltz E. I., Mullin C., Small D., Armstrong J., and Melby J.C., 1985, Intranasal aerosolized insulin., New. Engl. J. Med., 312: 1078.

HUMAN CALCITONIN ADMINISTERED BY THE NASAL ROUTE: BIOAVAILABILITY OF DIFFERENT FORMULATIONS AND EFFICACY IN POST-MENOPAUSAL OSTEOPOROSIS

A. E. Pontiroli, M. Alberetto, A. Calderara, E. Pajetta,
V. Manganelli, L. Tessari, and G. Pozza
Istituto Scientifico Ospedale San Raffaele. Clinica Medica
and Clinica Ortopedica, Universita' di Milano,
Milano, Italy

INTRODUCTION

After its discovery by Copp et al. in 1962, calcitonin has been employed in the management of several bone diseases, for instance post-menopausal osteoporosis and Paget's disease. Treatment of the above disease requires i.m. or s.c. administrations daily or on alternate days for prolonged periods, and this can reduce patient compliance during the course of the disease (Stevenson et al., 1981).
This has led to the search for alternative routes of administration of calcitonin.
In 1979 the intranasal administration of human synthetic calcitonin has been attempted in Paget's disease (Ziegler et al., 1979). In that study the clinical efficacy was short-lived, disappearing over prolonged administration.
In a previous study (Pontiroli et al., 1985) we have shown that human calcitonin, administered to normal subjects intranasally as drops mixed with sodium glycocholate as a surfactant, is absorbed through the nasal mucosa, yielding plasma calcitonin concentrations similar to those obtained with intravenous administration. The efficacy of synthetic salmon calcitonin administered intranasally was shown by Reginster et al. (1985) in 5 patients with Paget's disease, over a 6 months period.
The first aim of this study was to evaluate the bioavailability of different formulations of human calcitonin intranasally administered to normal volunteers; the second aim was to investigate the efficacy of repeated administration of calcitonin intranasally in women affected by post menopausal osteoporosis.

MATERIALS AND METHODS

First Study

10 healthy subjects aged 20-30 years without bone or endocrine diseases volunteered for this study.
In 6 subjects calcitonin was given intravenously and intranasally according to a randomized cross-over design. Two tests were performed in each subject with a one week interval, after an overnight fast and abstention from smoking.
100 U human calcitonin (Cibacalcin, Ciba Geigy) was administered

intravenously or intranasally as drops containing also 15 mg sodium glycocholate as a surfactant (total volume 0.5 ml).
200 U human calcitonin plus sodium glycocholate 15 mg was administered to four subjects on a separate occasion.
Following a randomized design the last 4 subjects received, with a one week interval, 2 different formulations: a) human calcitonin 100 U plus sodium glycocholate 15 mg as a spray solution; b) placebo plus 15 mg sodium glycocholate as a spray solution.
Blood samples were drawn every 30 minutes during 180 minutes to evaluate serum calcium and plasma calcitonin levels.
Plasma calcitonin was determined by RIA, using kits from Biomedica (Saluggia, Italy); serum calcium was determined by colorimetric method by the Hitachi 737 (Boehringer Biochemia Robin, Milano, Italy).

Second Study

6 osteoporotic out-patients, aged 45-70, were admitted to the trial. Osteoporotic patients with fractures and secondary osteoporosis were excluded.
Each patient received, on alternate days, 100 U human calcitonin (Cibacalcin, Ciba Geigy), mixed with 15 mg sodium glycocholate as a surfactant, as spray solution; the study lasted 2 months.
The following variables were evaluated:
clinical history and laboratory data (alkaline phosphatase, serum Ca and P, urinary Ca, P, hydroxyproline and c-AMP, plus plasma immunoreactive calcitonin and serum creatinine levels) at the start of study and after 7, 15, 30 and 60 days; bone mineral content (BMC) at the start of study and after 60 days; pain score (by the visual analogic scale) at each visit.
4 patients completed the trial, 1 patient dropped-out after 15 days for poor compliance and 1 patient dropped-out after 1 month because of a road accident with multiple bone fractures.

RESULTS

First Study

100 U human calcitonin lowered serum calcium concentrations in the same way whether given intranasally as drops or intraveously, though plasma calcitonin concentrations were higher after i.v. than after i.n. administration.
200 U human calcitonin elicited higher plasma calcitonin concentrations than 100 U, but did not further decrease serum calcium levels. The effect of calcitonin, as a spray solution, is slightly but not significantly higher than drops. Sodium glycocholate, used alone, had no effect. 5 subjects experienced nausea and facial flush, one also vomiting. The last 4 subjects had no side effects (fig. 1).

Second Study

In the four patients completing the study the following data were observed: serum alkaline phosphatase, as well as serum Ca and P were unchanged; urinary P, Ca and hydroxyproline increased over the whole period; urinary cAMP levels showed an initial increase up to the first month and then they returned to pretreatment levels; pain score decreased since the first control after 15 days and remained low throughout the entire period; BMC was unchanged. No patient complained of any side effect (fig. 2).

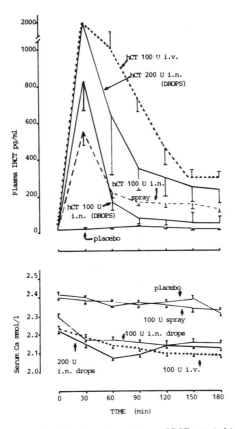

Fig. 1. Plasma calcitonin levels (IRCT pg/ml) and serum
calcium levels (s-Ca mmol/l) following i.v.
calcitonin (100 U), i.n. calcitonin (100 U plus
sodium glycocholate 15 mg as drops or as spray or
200 U plus sodium glycocholate 15 mg as drops) and
i.n. sodium glycocholate alone. Means ± SEM.

DISCUSSION

Bioavailability data from this study performed with healthy
volunteers indicate that intranasal administration of calcitonin causes
plasma calcitonin levels of the same order of magnitude, as i.v.
administration. The endocrine effects of 100 U, are almost doubled when a
dose of 200 U is used; on the other hand, placebo was at all
ineffective, while spray solutions were slightly more effective than
drops.
Anyhow, we decided to use spray solutions for the long-term trial
involving women affected by post-menopausal osteoporosis. At this stage,
we have only preliminary results, which however indicate that: 1) the

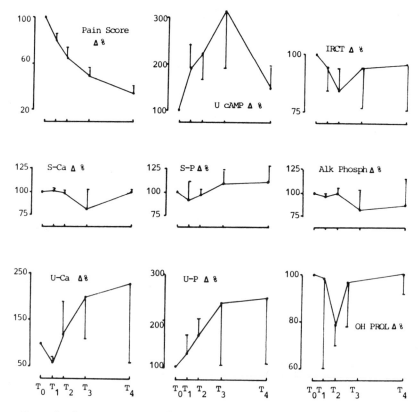

Fig. 2. Percent changes (Δ%) of pain score and of laboratory variables during a 60 days administration of calcitonin (100 U plus sodium glycocholate 15 mg as spray solution) to 6 women with post-menopausal osteoporosis. Means ± SEM.
IRCT= Calcitonin; Alk.Phosph.= Alkaline Phosphatase
S-Ca= Serum Calcium; S-P= Serum Phosphorus;
U-Ca= Urinary Calcium; U-P= Urinary Phosphorus;
OH-PROL= Hydroxyproline.
T0= Start; T1= 1 week; T2= 2 weeks; T3= 1 month;
T4= 2 months.

analgesic effect of intranasal calcitonin is prompt and long-lasting; 2) metabolic effects (i.e. changes in variables chosen) are similar to those observed after traditional parenteral routes of administration (Austin et al., 1981); 3) a 2 months course of treatment is probably unnecessarily long (c-AMP levels increase only up to 1 month and decrease thereafter) (Heersche et al., 1974); 4) patients' drug compliance was satisfactory; 5) the fact that the analgesic effect was accompanied by metabolic changes is against a mere placebo effect.
Although controlled studies are required, our impression is that intranasal administration of human calcitonin represents an effective and safe form of treatment of post-menopausal osteoporosis.

REFERENCES

Austin L. A., and Heat H., 1981, Calcitonin., New Engl. Med. J., 304: 269.
Copp D. H., Cameron B. A., Cheney B. A., Davidson A. G. F., and Henze K.

G., 1962, Evidence for calcitonin : a new hormone from the parathyroid that lowers blood calcium, Endocrinology, 70: 638.

Heerse J. N. M., Marcus R., and Aurbach G. D., 1974, Calcitonin and formation of 3'5'-AMP in bone and kidney., Endocrinology, 94: 241.

Pontiroli A. E., Alberetto M., and Pozza G., 1985, Intranasal calcitonin and plasma calcium concentrations in normal subjects., Brit. Med. Journal, 290:1390.

Reginster J. Y., Albert A., and Franchimont P., 1985, Salmon calcitonin nasal spray in Paget's disease of bone. Calcified Tissue International, 37: 577.

Ziegler R., Holz G., Raue F., and Streibl W., 1979, Nasal application of human calcitonin in Paget's disease of bone., Mol. Endocrinol., 1: 293.

ROUTES OF ADMINISTRATION FOR POLAR COMPOUNDS OF MODERATE MOLECULAR WEIGHT

WITH PARTICULAR REFERENCE TO ANALOGUES OF SOMATOSTATIN

Colin McMartin and Gill Peters

Horsham Research Centre
CIBA-GEIGY Pharmaceuticals,
Horsham, West Sussex RH12 4AB

Introduction

Somatostatin (SS) is a 14-amino acid peptide with a cystine bridge forming a 12-amino acid ring. SS suppresses the release of many peptide hormones (eg: insulin; glucagon; growth hormone). Interest has centred on its potential use in acromegaly (growth hormone suppression) and diabetes (glucagon suppression). Because of its multiple actions it has been considered necessary to search for analogues with more specific properties.

Somatostatin has a very short half-life (McMartin and Purdon 1978, Peters 1982) and its effects in man are only clearly manifest after infusion (Bloom et al 1974). It is therefore essential either to develop methods for prolonged release or to prepare analogues - this time with the additional requirement of greater stability in vivo.

There is also a need for suitable means of administering peptides such as somatostatin and here again there has been interest in trying to discover compounds with superior absorption after oral and other non-parenteral routes of administration. Apart from the use of infusion little success has been achieved in the delivery of somatostatin. There has however been considerable progress in the discovery of analogues which not only have a longer circulating half-life but may have additional useful characteristics following sub-cutaneous, oral and intranasal administration.

Design And Properties Of Analogues

Initial work involved replacement of L by D amino acids and stabilisation of the sulphur bridge. Consideration of the results obtained by these means and also the results of NMR studies led scientists at Merck Sharpe and Dohme to propose a model in which the ring is stabilised by a hydrophobic bond making it effectively bicyclic. Using this model it has been possible to make several analogues of greatly reduced size (Hruby et al 1984). The analogues to which I will be mainly referring are a cyclic octapeptide of CIBA-GEIGY (SS8; cyclo[-Asn-Phe-Phe-D-Trp-Lys-Thr-Phe-Gaba-]) and a cyclic hexapeptide of Merck Sharpe and Dohme (SS6; cyclo[-Pro-Phe-D-Trp-Lys-Thr-Phe]). These analogues have a high proportion of hydrophobic aromatic amino-acids but nevertheless are

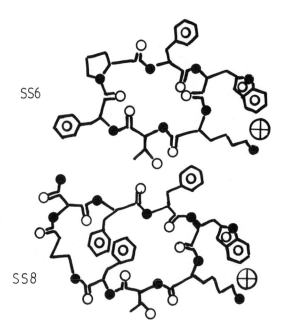

SS6

SS8

Diagram 1. Open circles oxygen, closed circles nitrogen

water soluble because of the hydrophilic peptide backbone and polar side-chains. Each peptide has a single positive charge at pH 7 (due to the amino group on lysine).

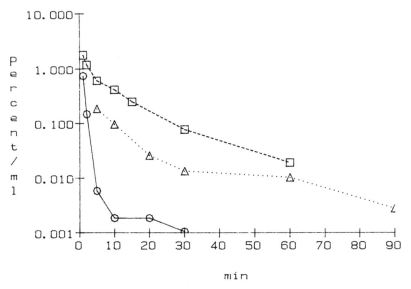

Fig 1. Plasma concentrations in the rat after i.v. dosage. Concentration of intact peptide was determined by HPLC and scintillation counting of tritium labelled peptides. Circles, somatostatin, 1.6mg/kg; triangles, SS8, 1.6mg/kg; squares. SS6 1.6mg/kg. For further details see Baker et al 1984.

As shown in Fig 1 the analogues have extended plasma half-lives (approx 5 min for SS8, Baker et al 1984) but nevertheless relatively short initial plasma half-lives more than offsets a possible loss in in vitro potency resulting from the structural alterations but is not sufficient to produce prolonged action unless large doses are used which will result in high blood levels at early times.

Sub-Cutaneous Administration

Although a non-parenteral route would be preferred, if injection cannot be avoided then an injected formulation will be more acceptable if it does not require frequent administration. The sub-cutaneous (sc) route is the most suitable since it permits self-administration. Compounds administered sc are normally resorbed within 30-60 minutes and this is true for larger molecules such as insulin (mwt 6000). However prolonged action of certain SS analogues has been observed after sc injection in man (Bloom et al 1978). We found that this could be explained by a depot effect observed with SS8 after sc injection (Baker et al 1984 and see Fig 2). The peptide leaves the site of injection slowly and the degree of prolongation depends on the size of the dose and at large doses the blood concentrations suggest that release from the site is approaching zero order. It seems possible therefore that analogues of this type will be suitable for sc administration without depot formulation. The mechanism responsible for the depot effect is not understood. Binding to tissues seems implausible since this would saturate at higher doses giving less of a depot effect the higher the dose. The peptides do have hydrophobic patches and it is possible that micelles form at higher concentrations. If the micelles could not leave the site due to size and high charge density this would result in the observed kinetics since rate of entry to the circulation would depend on the approximately constant free drug concentration at total concentrations above the critical micelle concentration.

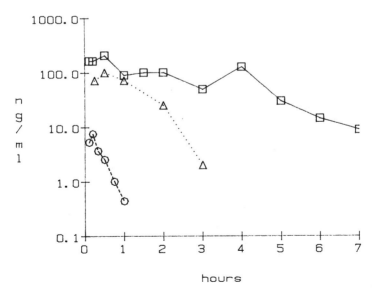

Fig 2. Plasma concentration of SS8 after sc administration in the rat. Concentration of intact SS8 was determined by HPLC and liquid scintillation counting. Squares, 1.6mg/kg; triangles 0.3mg/kg; circles 0.01mg/kg. For further details see Baker et al 1984.

The depot effect might be difficult to exploit in practical terms because the release rate is likely to be dependent on the physiochemical constitution of each type of molecule. It would therefore be necessary to select the compound or modify the formulation to achieve the therapeutically desirable rate of input into the circulation.

Oral Administration

The oral administration of peptides is complicated by the facts that many peptides are highly susceptible to peptidases of the gastrointestinal tract and also by the poor transport of polar molecules of greater than one or two hundred molecular weight across the intestinal wall. Exceptions to the latter rule normally involve active or facilitated transport.

We have investigated both aspects of the behaviour of somatostatin analogues. Somatostatin is stable in gastric juice but very rapidly degraded in the small intestine. SS8 is degraded more slowly in the small intestine (Allen et al 1984) and when large oral doses are administered low but highly variable levels of intact peptide can be found in the plasma for periods up to 8 hours (Fig 3). Detailed investigation of the mechanism of degradation of SS8 revealed that a single primary cleavage was introduced by tryptic enzymes after the lysine and this was followed by rapid secondary fragmentation of the linear product. It is clear therefore that modification of the lability of the Lys-Thr bond could lead to greater stability.

SS6, although it also contains a Lys-Thr bond, is much more stable than SS8. The orientation of the bond or the adjacent amino acid side chains may hinder effective interaction with trypsin (the cleavage rate of SS8 is already well below that for a typical tryptic substrate).

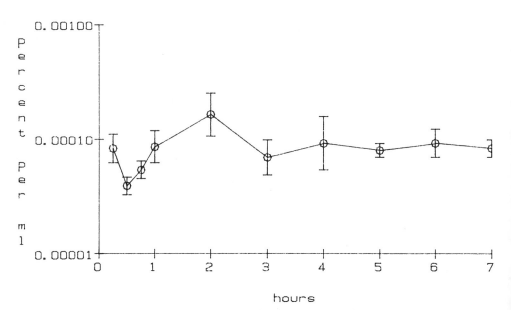

Fig 3. Plasma concentrations of SS8 after oral administration to the rat at a dose of 4mg/kg. Assay methods as in Fig 2.

In view of the greater stability of SS6 and reports of efficacy after oral administration to dogs (Veber et al 1981) we have carried out further investigation of resorption from rat intestine using an in situ perfused preparation with total portal blood collection (Peters and Sibbons 1984; Peters et al 1986a). For comparison insulin and horse radish peroxidase were also studied. The amount absorbed intact over a 1 hour period was small (0.35%) but was greater than uptake of insulin (0.05%) or the enzyme horse-radish peroxidase (less that 0.02%). The results were reproducible and the model was used to investigate the effect of the adjuvant sodium 5-methoxysalicylate. This was found to greatly enhance uptake of SS6, insulin and HRP to respective values of 8.09, 2.07, 0.82% at doses of 60mg but had much less effect at 32mg or less. Although the methoxysalicylate caused progressive damage to the mucosa over 1 hour the adjuvant effect peaked at 15-30 min for all three compounds. Therefore this effect may not be a direct result of damage. However the dose required is large and the effects on permeability and mucosal structure could be complex.

Nasal Absorption

The uptake of the peptide from the gut was disappointing and so for comparison nasal administration was tested (Peters et al 1986b, see Fig 4 and 5). The rat model of Hirai et al 1981 was used. This allows drugs to be administered quantitatively to the nasal cavity of anaesthetised rats. For comparison drug can be administered intravenously. Comparison of areas under the blood concentration time curve extrapolated to infinite time suggest nasal uptake of 73%. For comparison the protein horse radish peroxidase (mwt 35,000) was also tested. The uptake of HRP calculated in this way was 0.6%.

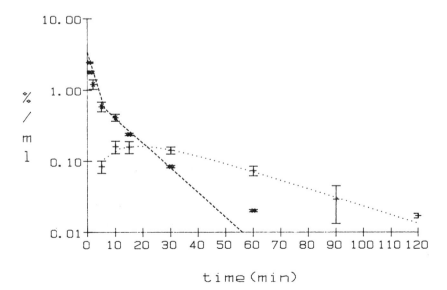

Fig 4. Plasma concentrations of intact SS6 after intravenous (dashes) and intranasal (dots) administration using the method of Hirai et al 1981.

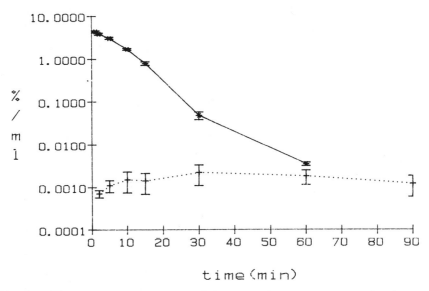

Fig 5. Plasma concentrations of horse-radish peroxidase (HRP) after intravenous (continuous) and intranasal (dashes) administration to the rat. The model of Hirai et al 1981 was used and HRP was assayed using an immunospecific assay described by Ambler and Peters 1984.

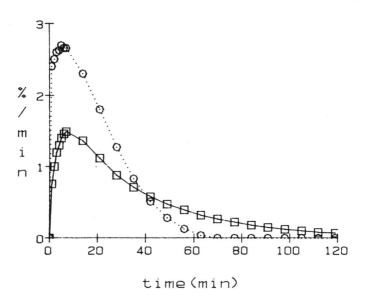

Fig 6. Input rates after intranasal administration to the rat of SS6 (from data of Fig 4) and sodium cromoglycate (from data of Fisher et al 1985). The input rates were obtained by numerical deconvolution of values obtained at one minute intervals from least-squares fitted biexponential functions (see Peters et al 1986b).

Numerical deconvolution of the SS6 results and of results for sodium cromoglycate (Fisher et al 1985) show a similar profile for the rate of entry to the systemic circulation with peak input rates being reached in about 10 minutes (Fig 6).

Nasal Absorption of other Molecules

A number of studies of nasal administration of peptides and of more conventional drugs have been published. In some cases the data does not permit calculation of extent of absorption but comparison of efficacy after nasal and parenteral administration can give an estimate of nasal bioavailability. These data have been collected and the effect of molecular weight on absorption is shown in Fig 7. The compounds include small molecules eg propranalol and TRH and also peptides such as LHRH and insulin (for more details see Peters et al 1986b). It can be seen that there is considerable departure from any simple curve of best fit but that there does seem to be a strong dependence on molecular weight.

Most compounds give peak plasma concentrations in less than 30 min. This finding is consistent with a model in which there is competition between drug transport into the circulation and removal from the site of absorption eg by mucociliary clearance. This situation can be modelled mathematically and if the mucosal transport is assumed to be related to molecular weight by a power law the least squares fit shown in Fig 7 is obtained. The coefficients obtained show that transport is inversely proportional to the square to the molecular weight. A similar relationship can be shown to apply to data produced by Nimmerfall and Rosenthaler 1980 (Peters et al 1986b) and this raises the possibility that mucus may be a major limiting barrier for nasal uptake of drugs.

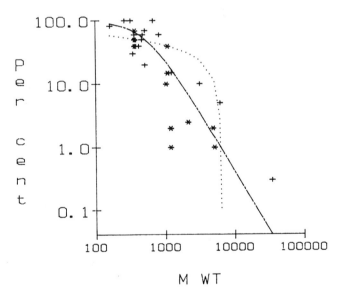

Fig 7. Bioavailability after nasal administration of 25 compounds for which published data is available on either biological effects or blood concentrations after both nasal and a non-parenteral mode of administration. Log absorption is plotted against log molecular weight. Asterisks show values obtained in man and the crosses values obtained in the rat. The dotted line shows predicted values for a uniform population of slits just wide enough to pass insulin using the formula given by Crone and Levitt 1984. The broken line shows
(continued next page)

Fig 7. (Continued)
the least squares fit of $100/(1 + a \times M^b)$, where M is the molecular weight. The best fit values are: $a = 9 \times 10^{-6}$, $b = 1.86$.

Conclusions

The oral route of administration for polar compounds intended for systemic applications would appear to be limited either to molecules which can take advantage of selective transport or to the development of a satisfactory adjuvant. Adjuvants however may be non-selective and it seems likely that mucosal damage may occur.

For potent molecules where a rapid onset of action is required the nasal route would appear to be indicated provided the molecule has a molecular weight of less than around 1000. This suggests that a useful strategy for peptides of moderate size is to develop small stable analogues. This leaves unsolved the problem of administration of larger peptides and proteins where there may be a limit to the reduction of size which is possible. For these molecules it is possible that the delivery problem will be solved either by the use of adjuvants (see Salzmann et al 1985 for details of a recent clinical study with insulin) or with systems which prolong the time of contact between peptide and the absorptive mucosa.

REFERENCES

Allen, M., McMartin, C., Peters, G.E. and Wade R., 1984, The mechanism of degradation of cyclo(-Asn-Phe-D-Trp-Lys-Thr-Phe-Gaba-) and the relative stabilities of this and other octapeptide somatostatin analogues in rat intestinal juice. Reg. Peptides, 10:29.

Ambler, L. and Peters, G.E., 1982, An Immunospecific Enzyme Assay for Horseradish Peroxidase. Anal. Biochem., 137:66.

Baker, J.R.J., Kemmenoe, B.H., McMartin, C. and Peters, G.E., 1984, Pharmacokinetics, distribution and elimination of a synthetic octapeptide analogue of somatostatin in the rat, Reg. Peptides, 9:213.

Bloom, S.R., Mortimer, C.H., Thorner, M.D., Besser, G.M., Hall, R., Gomez-Pan, A., Roy, V.M., Russell, R.C.G., Coy, D.H., Kastin, A.J. and Schally, A.V., 1974, Inhibition of gastrin and gastric-acid secretion by growth-hormone release-inhibiting hormone, Lancet ii:1106.

Bloom, S.R., Adrian, T.E., Barnes, A.J., Long, R.G., Hanley, J., Mallinson, C.N., Rivier, J.E. and Broen, M.R., 1978, New specific long-acting somatostatin analogues in treatment of pancreatic endocrine tumours, Gastroenterology 74:1013.

Crone, C. and Levitt, D.G., 1984, Capillary permeability to small solutes, Handbook of Physiol. 6:411.

Fisher, A.N., Brown, K., Davis, S.S., Parr, G.D. and Smith, D.A., 1985, The nasal absorption of sodium cromoglycate in the albino rat, J.Pharm. Pharmacol. 37:38.

Hirai, S., Yashiki, T., Matsuzawa, T. and Mima, H., 1981, Absorption of drugs from the nasal mucosa of rat. Int. J. Pharmacol. 7:317.

Hruby, V.J., Krstenasky, J.L. and Cody, W.L., 1984, Recent progress in the rational design of peptide hormones and neurotransmitters, Ann. Rep. Med. Chem. 19:303.

McMartin, C. and Purdon, G.E., 1978, Early fate of somatostatin in the circulation of the rat after intravenous injection, J. Endocr. 77:67.

Nimmerfall, F. and Rosenthaler, J., 1980, Significance of the goblet-cell mucin layer, the outermost luminal barrier to passage through the gut wall, Biochem. Biophys. Res. Comm. 94:960.

Peters, G.E., 1982, Distribution and metabolism of exogenous somatostatin in the rat, Reg. Peptides, 3:361.

Peters, G.E., Hutchinson, L.E.F., Hyde, R., McMartin, C., Metcalfe, S.B. and Sibbons, P.D., 1986a, The effects of sodium 5-methoxysalicylate on macromolecule absorption in a vascularly perfused rat gut preparation in vivo, in preparation.

Peters, G.E. and Sibbons, P.D., 1984, Macromolecule absorption in a vascularly perfused rat gut preparation in vivo, Second Eur. Cong. Biopharm. and Pharmacokin. 2:424.

Salzmann, R., Manson, J.E., Griffing, G.T., Kimmerle, R., Rudderman, N., McCall, A., Stolz, E.I., Mullin, C., Small, D., Armstrong, J. and Melby, J.C., 1985, Intranasal aerosolized insulin mixed-meal studies and long-term use in type 1 diabetes, New Eng. Med. J. 312:1078.

Veber, D.L. Freidinger, M.R., Schwenk, P.D., Palvedo, W.J.Jr., Holly, F.W., Strachan, R.G., Nutt, R.F., Arison, B.H., Homnick, C., Randall, W.C., Glitzer, M.S., Saperstein, R. and Hirschmann, R., 1981, A potent cyclin hexapeptide analogue of somatostatin, Nature, 292:55.

THE TRANSDERMAL ROUTE FOR THE DELIVERY OF PEPTIDES AND PROTEINS

B. W. Barry

Postgraduate School of Pharmacy
University of Bradford
Bradford BD7 1DP, U.K.

INTRODUCTION

Little work has been reported in the literature on the percutaneous delivery of peptides and proteins. This chapter therefore aims to survey the problems associated with the use of the intact skin as a pathway of entry of drugs into the systemic circulation, and to attempt to predict some of the difficulties likely to arise if the penetrants are peptides. However, at the outset we can deduce with some confidence that the efficient, controlled delivery of intact peptides and proteins to the systemic circulation via the transdermal route will prove to be the most challenging project to date in skin permeation technology.

ANATOMY AND PHYSIOLOGY OF HUMAN SKIN

Human skin consists of two distinct layers, the stratified, avascular cellular epidermis and an underlying dermis composed of connective tissue. A fatty, subcutaneous layer lies beneath the dermis. Hairy skin develops hair follicles and sebaceous glands, whereas glabrous integument of the palms and soles constructs an epidermis with a thick stratum corneum. The highly vascularized dermis also supports the eccrine and apocrine sweat glands which reach the skin surface through pores in the epidermis.

As far as drug permeation is concerned, the most important tissue in this complex membrane is the stratum corneum, which usually provides the rate-limiting step (slowest) in the penetration process. For polar peptides, we can assume that the horny layer will interpose a formidable barrier between topically applied material and viable, target tissue. On general body areas which we may plan to use for drug delivery, the horny layer provides 10-15 sheets of much flattened, keratinized dead cells stacked in a highly organised structure. The barrier may be less than 10µm thick when dry but on hydration it swells dramatically.

SKIN TRANSPORT

The transport mechanisms by which drugs may cross the intact skin are complex and still not well understood (for reviews, see Idson, 1971, 1975; Katz, 1973; Katz and Poulsen, 1971, 1972; Poulsen, 1973; Higuchi, 1977; Dugard, 1977; Scheuplein, 1978; Flynn, 1979; Chien, 1982; Schaefer et al, 1982; Barry, 1983; Bronaugh and Maibach, 1985). Material may enter the systemic circulation by the transepidermal route - across the stratum corneum (intracellular or intercellular) and the viable epidermis to be removed by the capillaries in the superficial dermis. Alternatively the transappendageal route provides pathways through the pilosebaceous unit (hair follicle and sebaceous gland) and the eccrine gland with subsequent removal by the capillaries (see Fig. 1). The relative importance of the various possible routes depends on many factors, including the chemical characteristics of the penetrant (for example, its solubility, partition coefficient, pK_a, molecular size, stability, binding affinity), the time scale of permeation (transient versus steady state diffusion), thickness and integrity of the membrane, density of follicles and sweat glands, skin hydration, metabolism and vehicle effects.

For large polar molecules such as peptides and proteins with their assumed very low diffusion coefficients through stratum corneum and their likewise low partition coefficients from aqueous media, we can predict that shunt diffusion through the appendages may be significant. Unless we somehow drastically increase the permeability of the horny layer (for example, by using penetration enhancers), these appendages, despite their low fractional areas and volumes, may provide the main entry route through the skin under both transient and steady state conditions. For polar materials permeating skin via the stratum corneum, it was considered for many years that the probable route was through the hydrated keratin within the corneocyte (Scheuplein, 1972). However, it now seems more likely that the polar regions of the intercellular lipid bilayers provide a significant route, as proposed by Elias (1981). Figure 2 illustrates these possible routes.

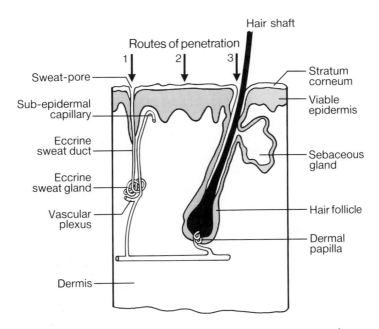

Figure 1. Potential routes of penetration: 1) via the sweat ducts; 2) across the continuous stratum corneum; or 3) through the hair follicles and sebaceous glands.

THEORETICAL ADVANTAGES OF THE TRANSDERMAL ROUTE

If we were able to formulate a satisfactory transdermal device for inserting polypeptides into the systemic circulation, what possible advantages would we secure over, for example, the oral route? (For general reviews which discuss the disadvantages of the traditional routes for drug delivery, see Wagner, 1975; Gibaldi and Perrier, 1975; Gibaldi, 1984). It is universally recognised that intestinal absorption of intact peptides and proteins is difficult, but it is not as widely known that significant quantities can cross the intestine. There is at least qualitative proof of this for dietary components as well as for biologically active peptides, such as luteinizing hormone releasing hormone (LHRH - a decapeptide), thyrotrophin releasing hormone (TRH - a modified tripeptide), vasopressin (a nonapeptide) and insulin (Gardner, 1984, 1985). There is now abundant evidence for the penetration of a variety of macromolecules and even particulate matter across the intestine of healthy adults. Thus, the gut is not the formidable physical barricade that once it was presumed to be. However, such gut passage is somewhat random, variable, inefficient and difficult to control, hence the interest in maximising any possible benefits of transdermal delivery.

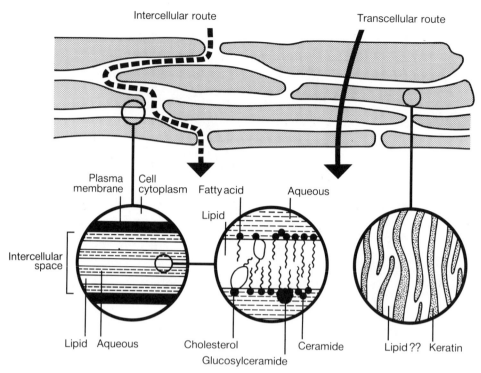

Figure 2. Diagram of possible permeation routes through the stratum corneum, together with idealised representation of intracellular keratin and intercellular bilayer lipids - not to scale. Note that the presence of significant amounts of intracellular lipid is now questionable and that the intercellular domain is probably of greater value than was once thought. (For further detail, see Barry, 1983 and Elias, 1981).

The first advantage to be considered is that transdermal input of a peptide could eliminate the variables that influence gastrointestinal absorption. These include the dramatic changes in pH as the peptide moves through the gut from the acid of the stomach to intestinal pH of up to 8, the changing food intake, the wide variations in stomach emptying times, intestinal motilities and transit times, and the presence of enzymes, human and bacterial.

Through skin, the peptide passes into the systemic circulation without first entering the portal system and traversing the liver. This pathway eliminates the "first pass" phenomenon by which the liver, the main metabolizing organ of the body for most drugs, may significantly reduce the amount of intact peptide getting through to the circulation. Enzymes present in the gut wall are also avoided. However, we should note that the skin itself is a highly active metabolic organ (see later).

If we arrange matters correctly, the transdermal input of a drug may provide controlled administration of the medicament and so display only one pharmacological effect from a chemical that, in a conventional dosage form, may well exhibit several effects, some of which may be toxic. Continuity of input raises the possibility of using drugs with short half-lives, thus also aiding patient compliance.

The percutaneous administration of drugs under such rate control could minimise pulse entry into the blood stream. Drug plasma peaks are particularly associated with undesirable side effects. However, it would be a more difficult matter if the aim was deliberately to provide controlled on/off action - skin membranes are intrinsically slow response systems with long lag times, at least in their normal intact state and when shunt diffusion via the appendages is negligible.

This route permits administration of drugs with low therapeutic indices i.e. those for which the clinical concentration in the plasma hovers close to the toxic level.

If the physician needs to terminate therapy, simple removal of a topical device would interrupt the delivery of the medicament. However, absorption of the drug into the circulation is not so readily aborted. The stratum corneum would be expected to continued to deliver molecules to the viable tissues for some time afterwards, at a declining rate as governed by the properties of the horny layer drug reservoir. This behaviour provides another example of the long response time of stratum corneum membranes.

PROBLEMS OF THE TRANSDERMAL ROUTE

In attempting to deliver peptides and proteins to central sites via a percutaneous absorption process, there will be many difficulties to be overcome, chemical, biological and technical. To examine just a representative few of these problems, it is instructive to accompany in the imagination a stream of peptide drug as it diffuses from a device on the surface of the skin through the cutis to the blood capillaries (Fig.3).

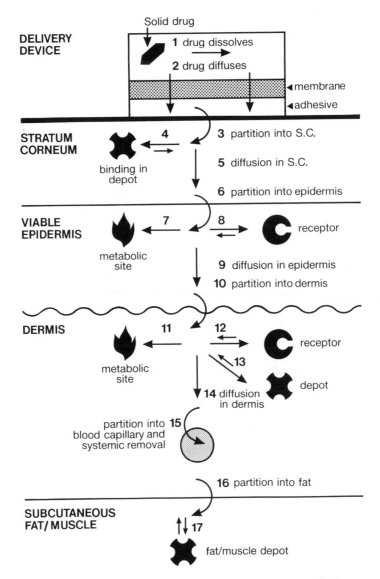

Figure 3. Some stages in percutaneous absorption of a peptide from a topical delivery device.

Drug in the Device

There are many traditional dermatological formulations, such as ointments, creams, gels, lotions and sprays, as well as the newer delivery devices with and without rate controlling membranes (the 'patches'). The formulator will need to produce a stable preparation of controlled chemical potential with the correct partition coefficient for ensuring that the drug will move into the skin (Barry, 1983). If the device contains a rate controlling membrane the flux across this barrier must be low enough that even the most impermeable skin acts as a sink. This is a rigorous restriction, but if it is not met, the individual patient's skin will control drug input, with all the consequences which flow from the great biological variability existing between people and from skin site to skin site. A possible solution to the difficulty posed by stratum corneum resistance is chemically to remove the barrier by incorporating penetration enhancers in the device. If this is done effectively, we also cope with patient variability in relation to horny layer permeability.

Drug at the Skin Surface

At the surface, the peptide may be exposed to degradative mechanisms arising from light, oxygen and bacteria. For example, skin microflora can degrade steroid esters and nitroglycerin (Brooks et al, 1982; Denyer et al, 1984, 1985). The application of occlusive devices over prolonged periods may change skin flora, macerate and irritate the skin and shut down sweat glands.

Drug in the Stratum Corneum

Interfacial effects are usually considered to be unimportant in skin diffusion processes, but for the peptide to move through the skin it must first partition into the stratum corneum and diffuse through this very impermeable barrier via the possible routes mentioned previously. The molecule will interact with many binding sites and may form a depot in the horny layer. The unbound molecules diffuse through the stratum corneum, meet a second interfacial barrier, and partition into the viable epidermis.

Drug in the Viable Epidermis

The epidermis is a rich source of enzymes which may have real activities in the range 80-90% of those in the liver, with oxidative, reductive, hydrolytic, and conjugative reactions all being evident (Wester and Noonan, 1980; Noonan and Wester, 1985; Barry, 1983; Schaeffer et al, 1982). The extreme dilution at which molecules cross the living epidermis lays them open to attack, although this is somewhat counterbalanced by the orders-of-magnitude greater diffusional speeds compared to those prevailing in the stratum corneum. Metabolism may alter the pharmacokinetics of permeation (Guy and Hadgraft, 1984), destroying active drug, generating active and inactive metabolites and activating prodrugs. It is in the epidermis that the drug first meets pharmacologic receptors as it diffuses to the epidermal/dermal boundary, there to partition into the dermis. (As both these viable tissues are mainly water, in the absence of different binding sites in close proximity at each interface, we expect the partition coefficient to approximate to unity.)

Drug in the Dermis

Within the dermis, additional receptor, metabolic and depot sites may intervene as peptides progress to a blood capillary, partition into the wall, then out into the blood, to be removed by the circulation while undergoing further chemical attack. The lymph system may also play a role in drug elimination. We know little about equilibration in the subepidermal environment and the pharmacokinetics which rule there.

Drug in the Subcutaneous Fat and Muscle

A fraction of the diffusant may partition into the subcutaneous fat and even the underlying muscle to form further depots, even though this may see unlikely at first sight (Marty et al, 1985).

Although the above treatment represents a simple unidirectional idealization of peptide transport through skin, in practice the situation would be further complicated. Such factors may be important as the nonhomogeneity of the various tissues; the presence of hair follicles and sweat glands; and the division of cells in the basal layer, their transport through the horny layer, and their surface loss. In addition, penetrants permeate the skin under dynamic conditions. Thus, the drug, the components of the vehicle, and occlusive hydration effects may progressively modify the skin barrier. Physiological materials, including sweat, sebum, and cellular debris, may pass into the formulated product and change its physicochemical characteristics. Emulsions may crack or invert when rubbed into the skin, and volatile solvents may evaporate. These processes will alter the chemical potential, possibly even leading to the formation of supersaturated solutions.

CONCLUDING REMARKS

At the present time, it seems highly unlikely that simple application to the

272

skin of a peptide in a vehicle will produce suitable clinical effects. One possible approach is to develop delivery devices which insert a suitable penetration enhancer into the stratum corneum, as well as the peptide. This would not be a simple matter, as it would include considerations such as the following;

1. The enhancer should be pharmacologically inert, affecting no receptor sites in the skin or body generally.

2. It should be nontoxic, nonirritating, and nonallergenic.

3. On application, the onset of enhancing-action should be immediate; the duration should be predictable and suitable (Azone, for example, which often appears to function well with polar penetrants, takes some hours to act).

4. When the material is removed from the skin, the tissue should immediately and fully recover its normal barrier properties - Azone appears to resist washing out from the horny layer.

5. The enhancer should be chemically and physically compatible with a range of drugs and adjuvants.

6. It should be cosmetically acceptable.

7. The enhancer should not increase entry of other vehicle components and environmental chemicals, nor should it encourage loss through the skin of endogenous material.

A patent has been published which claims skin enhancement of polypeptide permeation by using aliphatic monocarboxylic acids, monohydric alcohols and monoamides (Uda and Ameda, 1984). However, much of the experimental work was with tritiated species, detected by simple counting of total radioactivity, with all that this implies with respect to peptide stability, tritium exchange, and the validity of the data.

Another possibility would be to employ iontophoresis, a technique which has been used for a number of ionic drugs. Russian workers have achieved some success with amino acids (Ulashchik and Boitsov, 1977).

It may be possible to combine a penetration enhancer with iontophoresis to encourage transdermal peptide permeation. Whatever the means used, the task should provide a challenge to a multidisciplinary approach, although I imagine that most drug delivery groups will view the percutaneous route as one of last resort!

REFERENCES

Barry, B. W., 1983, "Dermatological Formulations: Percutaneous Absorption", Dekker, New York and Basel.

Bronough, R. L., and Maibach, H. I., 1985, "Percutaneous Absorption", Dekker, New York and Basel.

Brooks, F. L., Hugo, W. B., and Denyer, S. P., 1982, Transformation of betamethasone-17-valerate by skin microflora, J. Pharm Pharmacol., 34:61P.

Chien, Y. W., 1982, "Novel Drug Systems", Dekker, New York and Basel.

Denyer, S. P., Hugo, W. B., and O'Brien, M., 1984, Metabolism of glyceryl trinitrate by skin staphylococci, J. Pharm. Pharmacol., 36: 61P.

Denyer, S. P., Guy, R. H., Hadgraft, J., and Hugo, W. B., 1985, The microbial degradation of topically applied drugs, J.Pharm.Pharmacol., 37: 89.

Dugard, P. H., 1977, Skin permeability theory in relation to percutaneous absorption in toxicology, Adv. Mod. Toxicol., 4: 525.

Elias, P. M., 1981, Epidermal lipids, membranes, and keratinization, Int.J.Dermatol., 20: 1.

Flynn, G. L., 1979, Topical drug absorption and topical pharmaceutical systems, in: "Modern Pharmaceutics", G. S. Banker and C. T. Rhodes, eds., Dekker, New York and Basel.

Gardner, M. L. G., 1984, Intestinal assimilation of intact peptides and proteins from the diet - a neglected field? Biol.Rev., 59: 289.

Gardner, M. L. G., 1985, Production of pharmacologically active peptides from food in the gut, in: "Food and the Gut", J. O. Hunter and V. A. Jones, eds., Bailliere Tindall, London.

Gibaldi, M., 1984, "Biopharmaceutics and Clinical Pharmacokinetics", 3rd ed., Lea & Febiger, Philadelphia.

Gibaldi, M., and Perrier, D., 1975, "Pharmacokinetics", Dekker, New York and Basel.

Higuchi, T., 1977, Pro-drug, molecular structure and percutaneous delivery, in: "Design of Biopharmaceutical Properties Through Prodrugs and Analogs", B.Roche, ed., American Pharmaceutical Association, Washington.

Guy, R. H. and Hadgraft, J., 1984, Pharmacokinetics of percutaneous absorption and concurrent metabolism, Int.J.Pharm., 20: 43.

Idson, B., 1971, Percutaneous absorption, in: "Absorption Phenomena",
J. L. Rabinowitz and R. M. Myerson, eds., Wiley (Interscience), New York.

Idson, B., 1975, Percutaneous absorption, J.Pharm.Sci., 64: 901.

Katz, M., 1973, Design of topical drug products: pharmaceutics, in: "Drug Design",
E. J. Ariens, ed., Academic Press, New York.

Katz, M., and Poulsen, B. J., 1971, Absorption of drugs through the skin, in:
"Handbook of Experimental Pharmacology", Vol.28,Pt.1, B. B. Brodie and
J. Gillette, eds., Springer-Verlag, New York.

Marty, J.-P., Guy, R. H., and Maibach, H. I., 1985, Percutaneous penetration as a
method of delivery to muscle and other tissues, in: "Percutaneous
Absorption", R. L. Bronaugh and H. I. Maibach, eds., Dekker, New York and
Basel.

Noonan, P. K., and Wester, R. K., 1985, Cutaneous metabolism of xenobiotics, in:
"Percutaneous Absorption", R. L. Bronaugh and H. I. Maibach, eds., Dekker,
New York and Basel.

Poulsen, B. J., 1973, Design of topical drug products: biopharmaceutics In: "Drug
Design", E. J. Ariens, ed., Academic Press, New York.

Schaefer, H., Zesch, A., and Stuttgen, G., 1982, "Skin Permeability",
Springer-Verlag, New York.

Scheuplein, R. J., 1972, Properties of the skin as a membrane, Adv.Biol.Skin.,
12:125.

Scheuplein, R. J., 1978, The skin as a barrier, Skin permeation, Site variation in
diffusion and permeability, in: "The Physiology and Pathophysiology of the
Skin", A. Jarrett, ed., Academic Press, New York and London.

Uda, Y., and Yamada, M., 1984 European Patent 0 127 426 A1.

Ulashchik, V. S., and Boitsov, L. N., 1977, On the physiocochemical principles and
quantitative mechanisms of aminoacid electrophoresis,
Vopr.Kurortol.Fizioter.Lech.Fiz.Kul't., 4: 58.

Wagner, J.G., 1975, "Fundamentals of Clinical Pharmacokinetics", Drug
Intelligence Publications, Hamilton, Illinois.

Wester, R. C., and Noonan, P. K., 1980, Relevance of animal models for
percutaneous absorption, Int J. Pharm., 7: 99.

CONTROLLED-RELEASE AND LOCALIZED TARGETING OF INTERFERONS

Deborah A. Eppstein[1], Marjorie A. van der Pas[1],
Brian B. Schryver[1], Philip L. Felgner[1],
Carol A. Gloff[2], and Kenneth F. Soike[3]

[1]Institute of Bio-Organic Chemistry, Syntex Research, Palo
  Alto, CA 94304*
[2]Triton Bio-Sciences, Inc., Alameda, CA 94501
[3]Delta Regional Primate Center, Tulane University
  Covington, LA 70433

INTRODUCTION

Interferon's (α and β), produced both by recombinant DNA technology as well as purified from natural sources, have been shown to be efficacious in treating certain cancers and viral diseases. Studies with γ-interferon have more recently been undertaken, and thus definition of their clinical utility is not yet as well defined. The treatment schedules usually involve multiple injections of the interferon (IFN) over a period of several weeks to many months. Using such treatment regimens, the dose levels of the interferons needed to obtain efficacy can result in toxic side effects. For all these reasons, methods of increasing the ease of administration as well as the therapeutic ratio of interferons are warranted.

We have chosen the approach of developing bio-degradable sustained-release interferon preparations for systemic and/or localized treatment. We have utilized methods involving both liposomal-interferon preparations as well as poly(d,l-lactide-co-glycolide) polymer matrices. A discussion of the general considerations important in developing delivery systems for interferons is presented by Eppstein (1986). We have studied the in vitro properties and in vivo release kinetics of the interferon in sustained-

---

*This is Contribution #247 from the Institute of Bio-Organic Chemistry,
Syntex Research.

release formulations, and _in vivo_ efficacy studies in monkeys are in progress.

LIPOSOMAL-INTERFERON

Interferon (β or γ) was incorporated to high efficacy (100% for β, 50–100% for γ) into liposomes (lyophilization multilamellar vesicles, LMLV) prepared by hydrating lyophilized lipids with an aqueous solution of the interferon (Eppstein et al., 1985; Eppstein, 1986; Eppstein and Felgner, 1987). Conditions were optimized to obtain this high degree of incorporation of the protein: _e.g._, the lipids were lyophilized from the solvent (rather than using the traditional method of drying to a thin film) to obtain a fluffy powder which allowed maximal interaction of the aqueous solution with the lipid molecules; a high ratio of lipids to aqueous solution was employed for hydration (10–40 mM lipid); a low ionic strength buffer was employed; and the pH was chosen to optimize charge interactions between the lipids and the interferon.

We previously showed that interferon-γ had to leak out of a liposomal preparation before it could exert its biological effects, which are triggered subsequent to binding of the interferon to its specific cell-surface receptor (Eppstein et al., 1985). The same holds true for β-interferon as determined by antibody neutralization studies (unpublished results). The presence of serum and cells induces the leakage of the interferon from the liposome preparations, with the most "solid" vesicles (_i.e._, those made with phospholipids with saturated acyl chains) being the least leaky. Accordingly, liposome compositions can be prepared to control to different degrees the rate of release of the interferon after subcutaneous (SC) or intramuscular (IM) injection. Formulations of recombinant human interferon-β_{ser-17} (rHuIFN-β_{ser-17}, obtained from Triton Biosciences Inc., Alameda, CA) in LMLV consisting of diarachidoyl-phosphatidylchloline:dipalmitoylphosphatidylglycerol (DAPC:DPPG, 9:1) were able to retain the IFN at the site of IM or SC injection in mice, resulting in a slow release of the IFN from the vicinity of the injection site over a 1–2 week period. Thus 50% of the interferon was still retained after two days, 15% remained after 6 days, and 5% remained after 9 days. By contrast, free IFN was gone after one day (Eppstein, 1986; Eppstein and Felgner, 1987). When saturated phospholipids of progressively shorter acyl chain length (C18, C16, and C14) were employed, the duration of retention of the interferon was progressively reduced (unpublished results). Alternatively, when the unsaturated C18 phospholipids dioleoylphosphatidylcholine (DOPC) and dioleoylphosphatidyl gylcerol (DOPG) (7:3), were employed, the localized retention time of the interferon was comparable to that obtained with the saturated C14-phospholipids, dimyristoylphosphatidylcholine (DMPC): dimyristoylphosphatidylglycerol (DMPG) (7:3).

The efficacy of liposomal formulations of rHuIFN-β_{ser-17} was studied in a primate model of varicella zoster virus (VZV). African green monkeys were infected systemically with simian VZV, and 24 hr later interferon treatments were initiated. Initial results indicate that free rHuIFN-β_{ser-17}, given IM twice daily at 10^6 U/kg/dose for ten days (2 x 10^7 U/kg total dose), showed very good efficacy in suppressing the systemic VZV infection: treated monkeys had minimal viremia and rash and did not die. Placebo-treated controls showed extensive viremia and rash, and died 10-11 days post-infection. However, if the same total dose of IFN was given in only two or three injections (given on day 1 and day 6, or on days 1, 4, and 7 post-infection) instead of the 20 twice-daily injections, minimal to no efficacy was obtained. By contrast, if this same total amount of interferon was given on days 1 and 6, but in liposomal formulation (distearoylphosphatidylcholine (DSPC):DPPG, 9:1, 40 µmoles lipid/kg per dose), intermediate efficacy was obtained: death was prevented and viremia and rash were reduced, although not to the extent obtained with the 20 doses of free IFN (Soike, van der Pas, Gloff, and Eppstein, manuscript in preparation). Although liposomes have been reported to act as immunological adjuvants for some proteins (Allison and Gregoriadis, 1974), formation of neutralizing antibodies to the human β-IFN was not obtained in the monkeys one to four weeks after injection of the second dose of liposomal-IFN. These initial results suggest that liposomal formulations of IFN's can be obtained that will enhance the efficacy of an injection of IFN, most likely by providing a slow release of the IFN over several days. Optimization of the formulation will likely be necessary for specific applications (such as discussed below).

In several diseases of a circumscribed nature (e.g., herpes simplex viral infections, cervical papilloma viral infections), it could be beneficial to deliver an interferon to the site of infection via topical administration. For such an interferon treatment to begin to be efficacious, it must be able to penetrate through the stratum corneum or mucus membrane to reach the infected target cells. We have recently observed that liposomes prepared with a novel positively-charged fluid lipid, (S)-N-2,3-di[(Z)-9-octadecenyloxy] propyl-1-N,N,N-trimethyl ammonium chloride (DOTMA) (P. Felgner, D. Eppstein, G. Jones, R. Roman, unpublished results) could introduce a fluorescent phospholipid into the stratum corneum of the mouse (Eppstein and Felgner, 1987). The mechanism of this transfer may involve a fusion between the positively-charged DOTMA and the negatively-charged lipids of the stratum corneum. We are presently studying the applicability of using liposomes containing this novel positively-charged lipid, along with other bilayer perturbing agents, to facilitate topical and mucosal penetration of the various interferons.

BIODEGRADABLE POLYMER MATRICES

To achieve a controlled-release of an IFN over a longer time frame than was possible with liposomal-formulations, biodegradable polymers of poly ($\underline{d}$, $\underline{l}$-lactide-co-glycolide) (PLGA) were employed. Such polymers have been utilized in development of controlled-release systems for small peptide hormones such as luteinizing hormone-releasing hormone (LHRH) (Sanders et al., 1984), but their application to larger, more labile, polypeptides requires quite different formulation techniques in order to avoid protein denaturation.

We were able to prepare rHuIFN-β_{ser-17} in PLGA polymer matrices with 100% incorporation of IFN and full retention of biological activity by utilizing novel formulation techniques (Schryver, van der Pas, and Eppstein, manuscript in preparation). This involved first forming a micro-suspension of the protein in a solution of the polymer in an organic solvent (such as acetone), and then spraying the suspension, with rapid subsequent evaporation of the solvent, to form a thin film of the polymer containing the protein uniformly-dispersed throughout. This thin film could then be utilized to form an implant of desired size and shape (e.g., flat film, laminated film, or rolled cylindrical implant). The release profile of the IFN was determined over a three month period by quantitating the radio-activity remaining in a mouse at the site of SC implantation of a PLGA-IFN pellet or film (containing ^{125}I-rHuIFN-β_{ser-17}) (Eppstein, 1986). The release profile of the IFN was influenced both by the method of preparation as well as the geometry of the final implant.

Figure 1 shows a range of release profiles obtained over a two month time frame employing different formulation methods as well as different final implant geometries. With some formulations, a very "triphasic" release profile was obtained as has been observed with PLGA formulations of small peptides (Sanders et al., 1984). Such a triphasic release profile is believed to represent first an augmented initial release rate of peptide as a result of diffusion from the surface of the PLGA implant or microspheres, followed by a relatively latent period of minimal drug release while the polymer chains gradually are hydrolyzed to progressively shorter chain lengths, and then culminating with a high release rate when the polymer has

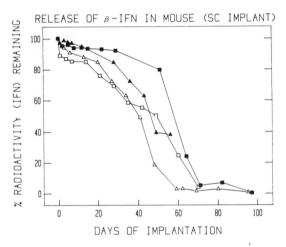

Figure 1.   Radioactivity from [^{125}I]rHuIFN-β_{ser-17} remaining in implants vs. duration of implantation in mice. Each point is an average of three implant values, determined on PLGA pellets plus immediately-surrounding tissue removed from mice at the times indicated. PLGA-interferon formulations were made as described above utilizing either acetone or methylene dichloride as the solvent for initial dissolution of the PLGA; where indicated, an inert reinforcement silk mesh was included. ■, Acetone method, rolled implant, no reinforcement; ▲, methylene dichloride method, rolled implant, no reinforcement; Δ, acetone method, flat film segment, with silk reinforcement; □, acetone method, flat film segment, no reinforcement.

become hydrolyzed to short enough chain lengths to become solubilized (Sanders et al., 1984). However, by varying parameters of implant geometry, in vivo release profiles of IFN could be obtained that were fairly linear over a 60-70 day period. Extraction of the IFN from implants retrieved up to five weeks after implantation in the mouse showed that the rHuIFN-β_{ser-17} retained remarkably good biological (antiviral) activity. In fact, the PLGA formulation appeared to significantly stabilize the IFN, such that only a 0.3 $\log_{10}$ loss in biological activity occurred after five weeks of implantation in the mouse, whereas over two $\log_{10}$'s of activity were lost when the same interferon (containing stabilizers) was incubated at 37°C in buffer in a test tube (Eppstein, 1986; Schryver, van der Pas, and Eppstein, manuscript in preparation).

Although sustained-release delivery systems have been shown to act as immunological adjuvants for certain proteins (Amkraut and Martins, 1984), no antibody formation (neutralizing or non-neutralizing) was detected in the mouse with this human interferon-PLGA formulation. As the actual daily dose of interferon protein can be quite low in a sustained-release system, this may help circumvent the unwanted formation of antibodies.

POTENTIAL MEDICAL APPLICATIONS

Of the three classes of IFNs, most extensive clinical testing has been conducted with α-IFN and hence more information is available on its clinical utility. In the cancer field, α-IFN systemic therapy has shown strikingly positive results against hairy cell leukemia (Quesada et al., 1984) as well as some efficacy against renal cell carcinoma (Quesada et al., 1985), and varying degrees of generally low-to-moderate efficacy against a range of other tumors (reviewed in Bonnem and Spiegel, 1984; and Borden, 1984). Based on these currently available anticancer results, one application where a long-acting sustained-release IFN preparation (such as a PLGA formulation) could be very beneficial is in the treatment of hairy cell leukemia, as the current efficacious treatment regimens require repeated IFN injections over a many-month period. β-IFN has shown efficacy in treating glioblastomas by continuous slow-infusion to the site of the tumor, and thus the potential likewise exists here for utilization of a sustained-release IFN formulation.

In the antiviral area, IFNs (α and β) have shown significant efficacy in treating venereal warts (condylomata acuminata) caused by papilloma viruses, but the dosing regimens involve multiple injections (daily or thrice weekly) of the IFN over a two to four week period (Schonfeld et al., 1984; Vance et al., 1986). Thus a formulation that resulted in a gradual and continuous delivery of the IFN over a two to four week period might eliminate the necessity of repeated injections. Similarly, another potential application for sustained release IFN is in the treatment of juvenile laryngeal papilloma virus infections. These benign tumors (caused by papilloma viruses) respond very well to repeated systemic injections of IFN-α, but recur once IFN treatment is stopped. Thus a two to three month sustained release preparation of IFN might prove very useful.

The utility of a sustained-release IFN formulation for the various diseases mentioned above, as well as for other potential applications that are identified as further clinical trials are completed, obviously will need to be tested experimentally to determine if indeed a sustained-release IFN formulation can achieve the desired results. Our initial findings of increased efficacy of a liposomal-IFN-β formulation vs. comparable IM injections of free β-IFN in a simian model of systemic varicella zoster virus infection suggest that, at least in some cases, sustained-release IFN can be efficacious.

REFERENCES

Allison, A.C. and Gregoriadis, G. (1974). Liposomes as immunological adjuvants. Nature 252: 252.

Amkraut, A.A., and Martins, A.B. (1984). Method for administering immunopotentiator. U.S. Patent #4,484,923.

Bonnem, E.M. and Spiegel, R.J. (1984). Interferon-α: current status and future promise. J. Biol. Resp. Mod. 3: 580-598.

Borden, E.C. (1984). Progress toward therapeutic application of inter-ferons, 1979-1983. Cancer, 54: 2770-2776.

Eppstein, D.A. (1986). Alternate delivery of interferons. In "Drug Targeting with Synthetic Systems," NATO ASI Conference, 1985, Ed. G. Gregoriadis, Plenum Pub. Co. (in press).

Eppstein, D.A. and Felgner, P.L. (1987). Applications of liposome formula-tions for antimicrobial/antiviral therapy, in "Liposomes as Drug Carrriers: Trends and Progress," Ed. G. Gregoriadis, John Wiley and Sons, LTD. (in press).

Eppstein, D.A., Marsh, Y.V., van der Pas, M.A., Felgner, P.L., and Schreiber, A.B. (1985). Biological activity of liposome-encapsulated murine interferon γ is mediated by a cell membrane receptor. Proc. Natl. Acad. Sci. USA 82: 3688-3692.

Quesada, J.R., Reuben, J., Manning, J.T., Hersh, E.M., and Gutterman, J.U. (1984). Alpha interferon for induction of remission in hairy-cell leukemia. N. Eng. J. Med. 310: 15-18.

Quesada, J.R., Rios, A., Swanson, D., Trown, P. and Gutterman, J.U. (1985). Antitumor activity of recombinant-derived interferon alpha in metastatic renal cell carcinoma. J. Clin. Oncol. 3: 1522-1528.

Sanders, L.M., Kent, J.S., McRae, G.I., Vickery, B.H., Tice, T.R., and Lewis, D.H. (1984). Controlled release of a luteinizing hormone-releasing hormone analog from poly (d,l-lactide-co-glycolide)-microspheres. J. Pharmaceut. Sci. 73: 1294-1297.

Schonfeld, A., Schattner, A., Crespi, M., Levavi, H., Shoham, J., Nitke, S., Wallach, D., Hahn, T., Yarden, O., Doerner, T., and Revel, M. (1984). Intramuscular human interferon-β injections in treatment of condylomata acuminata. Lancet 1: 1038-1042.

Vance, J.C., Bart, B.J., Hansen, R.C., Reichman, R.C., McEwen, C., Hatch, K.D., Berman, B., and Tanner, D.J. (1986). Intralesional recombinant alpha-2 interferon for the treatment of patients with condyloma acuminatum or verruca plantaris. Arch. Dermatol. 122: 272-277.

DELIVERY OF MACROPHAGE ACTIVATING FACTORS BY MEANS OF LIPOSOMES

F.H. Roerdink, T. Daemen, D. Regts, A. Veninga, O. de Boer and
G.L. Scherphof

Laboratory of Physiological Chemistry, University of Groningen
Medical School, Bloemsingel 10, 9712 KZ Groningen,
The Netherlands

INTRODUCTION

     Successful treatment of patients with cancer is often hampered by the
development of metastases (Fidler, 1985). Especially the biological
heterogeneity of metastatic tumor cells with respect to growth rate, ability
to metastasize, sensitivity to various cytotoxic drugs etc. is a tremendous
obstacle to complete eradication of tumor cells. Therefore, alternative
methods for the treatment of metastases are highly desirable. Activation of
the host mononuclear phagocyte system appears to be a promising approach
towards that purpose (Fidler, 1985). In vitro exposure of monocytes and
alveolar or peritoneal macrophages to a variety of macrophage activating
factors such as lymphokines (Kleinerman et al., 1983), γ-interferon (Varesio
et al., 1984) and muramyl dipeptide (MDP) (Lopez-Berestein et al., 1984;
Fidler et al., 1982) has been shown to render these cells tumoricidal. After
in vivo administration of free MDP, however, no enhancement of macrophage-
mediated cytotoxicity is achieved since the drug is rapidly excreted from
the body (Parant et al., 1979; Fogler et al., 1985). This circumstance calls
for the design of an efficient drug delivery system for these agents.
Studies on the use of liposomes as drug carriers have shown that these
phospholipid vesicles are predominantly taken up by cells of the mononuclear
phagocyte system (Roerdink et al., 1977; Ellens et al., 1981; Poste et al.,
1982). Encapsulation of the MDP within liposomes indeed greatly enhances the
ability of the drug to render mouse peritoneal and alveolar macrophages
tumoricidal in vivo (Poste et al., 1982). Fidler et al. (1984), for example,
achieved significant reduction of experimental lung metastases by the
systemic administration of MDP-containing liposomes into mice inoculated
with syngeneic B16 melanoma cells. Similar results were reported by Thombre
and Deodhar (1984) on the inhibition of liver metastases from murine colon
adenocarcinoma by liposome-encapsulated C-reactive protein or crude
lymphokines.
     Some recent observations suggest that the lipid composition and
structure of MDP-containing liposomes are important determinants for their
macrophage-activating potency. For example, studies by Schroit and Fidler
(1982) showed that MDP encapsulated in distearoylphosphatidylcholine/phos-
phatidylserine (DSPC/PS) liposomes induces a higher level of cytotoxicity
than MDP encapsulated in egg phosphatidylcholine/phosphatidylserine
(egg-PC/PS) liposomes. DSPC/PS liposomes may be more resistant to
intracellular degradation than liposomes containing egg-PC, thus producing a
sustained activation of the macrophages by virtue of a relatively slow

285

intracellular release of the MDP after uptake by the macrophages.

We are searching for optimal conditions for drug delivery to liver macrophages (Kupffer cells) by means of liposomes. The reason for choosing this cell type is two-fold. Firstly, these cells play a dominant role in the uptake of intravenously injected liposomes. Secondly, the liver is a major site of metastases originating from e.g. primary colorectal tumors (Wood, 1984). Activation of liver macrophages to tumorcytotoxicity by means of liposome-encapsulated macrophage activating factors might offer an attractive therapeutic approach as an alternative to or in combination with conventional chemotherapy, since the latter alone or in combination with surgery generally can provide only a poor prognosis to patients with hepatic metastases.

In the first part of the present paper we will describe and discuss experiments in which we attempted to modulate the rates of uptake and intracellular degradation of liposomes by liver macrophages by varying liposomal parameters such as surface charge, size, number of lamellae, cholesterol content and "fluidity" of liposomal membranes.

In the second part of this paper we demonstrate that isolated liver macrophages can be rendered cytostatic and cytolytic against tumor cells by incubating the cells with MDP and that encapsulation of MDP in liposomes substantially enhances the MDP-induced cytotoxicity.

Basic aspects of liposome-macrophage interactions

As outlined above, after intravenous injection liposomes are taken up mainly by cells of the mononuclear phagocyte system especially macrophages in the liver and spleen (Roerdink et al., 1981; 1984; 1984). Uptake occurs by way of endocytosis, thus causing the liposomes to end up in the lysosomal compartment of the cells (Dijkstra et al., 1984; 1984). There the vesicles are subjected to the hydrolytic action of lysosomal phospholipases. Lipid degradation products are partly released by the cells, partly utilized for synthesis of endogenous (phospho)lipid (Dijkstra et al., 1985; Scherphof et al., 1985). As a result of the intralysosomal degradation liposome-encapsulated drugs, when resistant to the intralysosomal environment, are released intracellularly and could become available to exert their action.

Rate of uptake by liver and spleen macrophages is determined, at least in part, by the size of the vesicles: large-size multilamellar vesicles (MLV, 100-400 nm diameter) are taken up much more rapidly than small unilamellar vesicles (SUV, 25-40 nm diameter) (Roerdink et al., 1984). The preferential uptake of MLV by macrophages in addition to the relatively high entrapped aqueous volume (MLV; approx. 3 1/mol of lipid vs SUV, approx. 0.3 1/mol of lipid) renders this liposome type an attractive candidate to serve as a drug carrier to macrophages.

Uptake and intracellular processing of liposomes by macrophages is also strongly dependent on the lipid composition. Table 1 shows the relative rates of uptake of neutral and charged SUV by cultured liver macrophages with sphingomyelin or phosphatidylcholine as the main phospholipid. Neutral vesicles consisting of sphingomyelin/cholesterol display a very low affinity for the cells while substitution of sphingomyelin by phosphatidylcholine slightly increases the uptake. Incorporation of the positively charged stearylamine further increases the uptake while negatively charged phosphatidylserine-containing vesicles are taken up even more efficiently.

These results are compatible with the extremely long half life in blood of neutral sphingomyelin/cholesterol SUV (Spanjer, 1985). Incorporation of phosphatidylserine increases the blood elimination and concurrently stimulates the uptake of the vesicles by liver and spleen macrophages (Spanjer, 1985). Apparently, introduction of negative charge (phosphatidylserine) increases the affinity of the liposomes for the macrophages.

Negatively charged phosphatidylserine liposomes are not only rapidly

Table 1. Effect of surface charge on the uptake of
          cholesteryl-[^{14}C]oleate-labeled liposomes
          by cultured liver macrophages.

Liposome composition	Molar ratio	Uptake (nmol lipid/mg protein)
SM/CHOL	5/5	1.1
SM/CHOL/SA	4/5/1	3.8
SM/CHOL/PS	4/5/1	15.3
PC/CHOL	5/5	1.8
PC/CHOL/SA	4/5/1	5.4
PC/CHOL/PS	4/5/1	28.8

Liver macrophages were isolated by pronase digestion
of the liver and purified by centrifugal elutriation
as described before (Dijkstra et al., 1984). The cells
(1.9 x 10^6) were cultured in monolayer and incubated
with SUV (70 nmol lipid) of various lipid compositions
at 37°C for 3 h in the absence of serum. Liposome
composition: sphingomyelin (SM) or egg phosphatidylcholine (PC)/cholesterol (CHOL)/stearylamine (SA) or
phosphatidylserine (PS).

Table 2. Effect of surface charge on the intracellular
          degradation of [^{14}C]sphingomyelin-labeled
          liposomes by cultured liver macrophages.

Liposome composition	Time of degradation(min)	% of hydrolysis of cell-associated ^{14}C-SM
^{14}C-SM:CHOL:PS	0	9.8
(4 : 5 : 1)	60	29.5
	120	42.0
^{14}C-SM:CHOL:SA	0	1.6
(4 : 5 : 1)	60	5.5
	120	6.1

[^{14}C]sphingomyelin-labeled phosphatidylserine and
stearylamine SUV were incubated with cultured liver
macrophages (300 nmol and 375 nmol lipid per 5.1 x 10^6
cells respectively) in the presence of 10 mM NH$_4$Cl at
37°C. After 120 min SUV were removed from the medium
and the cells were incubated for another 30 min in the
presence of NH$_4$Cl. After 150 min (indicated as zero
time) the medium was replaced by an NH$_4$Cl-free medium
and at 60 and 120 min the relative amount of label in
the chloroform-soluble cell extract associated with
sphingomyelin was determined.
Abbreviations: SM = sphingomyelin; CHOL = cholesterol;
SA = stearylamine; PS = phosphatidylserine.

287

phagocytozed by the macrophages, but are also efficiently degraded once taken up by the cells. These results are shown in Table 2. Appropriate amounts of [^{14}C]sphingomyelin-labeled phosphatidylserine and stearylamine liposomes were incubated with Kupffer cells so as to obtain comparable extents of liposome uptake by the cells. Ammonium chloride was present in the medium to prevent liposomal degradation during the uptake period by inhibiting lysosomal enzyme activity. After the liposomes were removed from the medium the cells were incubated for another 30 min in the presence of NH$_4$Cl to allow liposome-containing endosomes to fuse with primary lysosomes.

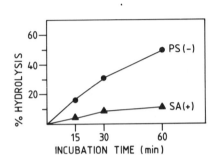

Fig. 1. Effect of surface charge on the degradation of [^{14}C]sphingomyelin-labeled liposomes by lysosomal sphingomyelinase. SUV containing phosphatidylserine or stearylamine were incubated at pH 4.8 with lysosomal fractions from rat liver. Lysosomal sphingomyelinase activity was measured at 37° in 0.5 ml medium containing 50 mM Na-acetate, pH 4.8, 50 nmol [^{14}C]sphingomyelin-labeled SUV and 100 µg of lysosomal protein. The reaction was stopped by adding 3 ml methanol/chloroform (2:1 v/v) and the lipids were extracted. Sphingomyelinase activity was expressed as the percentage of [^{14}C]-choline released into the water-soluble fraction. Liposome compositon: SM/CHOL/PS or SM/CHOL/SA = 4:5:1. See for abbreviations legend to Table 2.

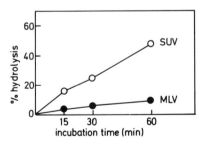

Fig. 2. Effect of liposomal structure on the degradation of [^{14}C]sphingo-myelin-labeled liposomes by lysosomal sphingomyelinase. SUV and MLV of identical lipid composition (PC/CHOL/PS = 4:5:1) were incubated at pH 4.8 with lysosomal fractions isolated from rat liver. See for further experimental details legend to Fig. 1.

288

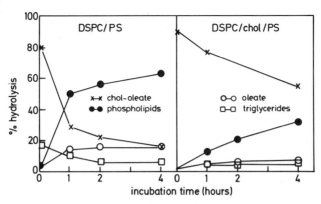

Fig. 3. Effect of cholesterol content on the intracellular degradation of
cholesteryl-[^{14}C]oleate-labeled liposomes by cultured liver
macrophages. Liver macrophages in maintenance culture were incubated
with cholesteryl-[^{14}C]oleate-labeled MLV (liposome composition:
DSPC/PS = 7:3 and DSPC/CHOL/PS = 4:5:1) at 37°C for 1 h in the
presence of 10 mM NH$_4$Cl. 80 nmol vesicle lipid was added to 2.5 x
10^6 macrophages. After 1 h the liposomes were removed and the cells
were incubated for another 0.5 h in the presence of NH$_4$Cl. After 1.5
h (indicated as zero time) the medium was replaced by an NH$_4$Cl-free
medium. At times indicated the cells were extracted with chloroform/
methanol and the extracts were chromatographed on thin-layer plates
with petroleum ether (40/60) : diethylether : formic acid =
60:40:1.5 as a solvent. The amounts of label in the relevant spots
were determined and expressed as percent of total chloroform-soluble
radioactivity in the cells. Abbreviations: DSPC = distearoylphosphatidylcholine; CHOL = cholesterol; PS = phosphatidylserine.

From the results shown in Table 2 it is clear that negatively charged
phosphatidylserine vesicles are degraded much faster than the positively
charged stearylamine-containing liposomes. Apparently, positive charge
renders the vesicles unfavourable substrates for lysosomal sphingomyelinase
activity. Similar observations were obtained by Wilschut et al. (1976) with
positively charged dimyristoyl phosphatidylcholine vesicles as substrates
for phospholipase A$_2$ activity.

The difference in susceptibility to lysosomal degradation of the two
liposome preparations could also be demonstrated by incubating [^{14}C]-
sphingomyelin-labeled liposomes at pH 4.8 with lysosomal fractions isolated
from rat liver homogenates (Fig. 1): phosphatidylserine vesicles are much
more sensitive to lysosomal sphingomyelinase than the stearylamine vesicles.
In the same system we found that SUV are degraded substantially faster than
MLV of identical lipid composition (Fig. 2). Apparently, the susceptibility
of the liposomes to lysosomal enzymes is also influenced by liposomal
parameters such as bilayer curvature and/or number of lamellae.

Liposomal lipid degradation is also dependent on the cholesterol
content of the vesicles: cholesterol-containing liposomes are degraded much
more slowly by cultured liver macrophages than cholesterol-free liposomes.
These results are shown in Fig. 3. Negatively charged distearoylphosphatidylcholine (DSPC) MLV, with or without cholesterol, labeled with
cholesteryl-[^{14}C]oleate, were incubated with cultured liver macrophages in

289

monolayer. After endocytosis of the vesicles the liposomal cholesteryl-$[^{14}C]$
-oleate is susceptible to intralysosomal esterase activity resulting in the
liberation of the labeled oleate from the cholesterol moiety. The $[^{14}C]$-
oleate is partly released by the cells and partly incorporated into cellular
phospholipids and triglycerides. As is clear from the data shown in Fig. 3
the cholesterol-containing DSPC liposomes are more resistant to lysosomal
esterase activity than the cholesterol-free DSPC vesicles. At the same time
efficient incorporation of the liberated $[^{14}C]$oleate into cellular phospholipids is observed, whereas there is only marginal fatty acid
incorporation into triglycerides. Cholesterol is known to condense lipid
membranes thereby impeding penetration of enzymes or other (lipo)proteins
into the lipid bilayers (Op den Kamp et al., 1975), resulting in an
increased intracellular stability of liposomes. We believe that the results
presented in this section are relevant to the application of liposomes as a
drug delivery system of e.g. macrophage activating factors. By manipulating
the size and the lipid composition of the vesicles, rates of uptake and/or
intracellular degradation can be influenced, which, in turn, will determine
the rate of intracellular release of the drug and thereby, conceivably, its
therapeutic effect.

Activation of liver macrophages by liposome-encapsulated muramyl dipeptide
(MDP)
    As an extension of our investigations on uptake and processing of
liposomes by liver macrophages we initiated a study on the activation of rat

Table 3. Potentiation of tumoricidal activity of rat
         liver macrophages by muramyl dipeptide (MDP)
         in liposomes.

Macrophage treatment[a]	Liposomal lipid (mM)	MDP (µg/ml)	% cytotoxicity[b]
free MDP	–	50	31
	–	25	31
	–	12.5	30
MDP-liposomes	0.375	0.375	54
(1 µg MDP/µmol	0.250	0.250	57
lipid)	0.050	0.050	38

[a]Rat liver macrophages were isolated by pronase
perfusion of the liver and purified by centrifugal
elutriation. 25×10^4 cells were incubated with
medium (RPMI) containing 10% heat-inactivated fetal
calf serum (FCS), free MDP or MDP encapsulated in
liposomes (MLV, lipid composition: PC/PS/CHOL, molar
ratio 4:1:5). After 4 h ^{3}H-thymidine labeled B16
melanoma cells were added per well. After a 48-h
coculture period cytotoxicity was assayed by measuring
the release of ^{3}H-label from the melanoma cells into
the medium.
[b]Percent cytotoxicity was calculated according to the
formule: $100 \times (A-B)/(C-B)$, in which A = radioactivity in supernatant of tumor cells co-cultured
with treated macrophages, B = radioactivity in supernatant of tumor cells co-cultured with control macrophages and C = radioactivity in the total amount of
tumor cells added per well.

liver macrophages to tumor cytotoxicity by means of liposome-encapsulated immunomodulators. As mentioned in the introduction Thombre and Deodhar (1984) were able to inhibit the development of liver metastases from an experimental colon adenocarcinoma in mice by the systemic administration of liposome-entrapped lymphokines. The therapeutic effect was supposed to be mediated by the activation of liver macrophages.

We exposed cultured rat liver macrophages to free, non-encapsulated MDP at concentration of 50 µg/ml. After 4 h [^{3}H]-thymidine-labeled xenogeneic murine B16 melanoma cells were added to the macrophages and cocultured for another 48 h. Macrophage-mediated cytotoxicity was assayed by measuring the release of ^{3}H-label from the melanoma cells into the medium. At the applied ratio of rat liver macrophages to tumor cells (25:1) no spontaneous cytotoxicity was observed. In Table 3 it is shown that the percentage of cytotoxicity induced by free MDP (12.5-50 µg/ml) reaches a maximal level of approx. 30%. With liposome-entrapped MDP, on the other hand, as little as 0.050 µg MDP per ml was sufficient to obtain this level of cytotoxicity. The results also show that entrapment of the drug within liposomes significantly increases its cytolytic potency. Whereas free MDP induced cytolysis to a

Table 4. Effect of liposome-encapsulated MDP on macrophage cytolytic and cytostatic activity.

Macrophage treatment[a]	Liposomal lipid (mM)	Cytolysis[b] dpm ± SD released in supernatant	Cytostasis[c] dpm ± SD incorporated
MDP-liposomes	1	1306 ± 3(56)	121 ± 16(99)
(1 µg MDP/µmol	0.25	929 ± 64(31)	962 ± 21(89)
lipid			
control liposomes	1	485 ± 42(1)	9367 ± 56(0)
	0.25	439 ± 11(0)	9092 ± 868(0)
medium		463 ± 43	9105 ± 572
none, B16 cells alone		420 ± 21	8668 ± 556

[a]Per well 25 x 10^4 liver macrophages were incubated with medium, control liposomes or liposomes containing 1 µg MDP/µmol liposomal lipid.
[b]After 4 h, 10^4 ^{3}H-thymidine-labeled melanoma cells were added per well. After another 48 h, ^{3}H-release into the supernatant was determined in triplicate experiments. In parentheses, % of cytolysis (see legend to Table 3).
[c]After a 4-h incubation with control and MDP-containing liposomes 10^4 melanoma cells were added per well. After 24 h of cocultivation ^{3}H-thymidine was added to the cells for another 24 h. At this time the cultures were washed and the cells were lysed with 0.5 M NaOH. Incorporation of ^{3}H-thymidine into the DNA of the tumor cells was measured by determining the radioactivity of the lysate. Inhibition of tumor cell proliferation was calculated as follows: % inhibition = $100(1-\frac{x}{y})$, in which x = dpm in tumor cells cocultured with test macrophages and y = dpm in tumor cells cocultured with control macrophages (% of cytostasis in parentheses). Incorporation of ^{3}H-thymidine in control or activated liver macrophages, cultured alone without tumor cells, was negligible (not shown).

maximal level of approx. 30%, incubation of the macrophages with 0.250-0.375 μg of liposomal MDP per ml resulted in a maximal level of 50-60%.

The difference in potency to induce tumor cytotoxicity between free and liposomal MDP may be due to a number of factors such as rate of internalization, intracellular processing and/or compartmentalization of the MDP. The results published by Mehta et al. (1982; 1984) suggest that most of the target sites for MDP are localized intracellularly and that relatively high intracellular levels of MDP are required for activation. Apparently, high intracellular MDP concentrations are achieved by encapsulating the drug within liposomes rather than by incubating the cells with free MDP.

Table 4 shows that, besides causing tumor cell lysis, activated liver macrophages also strongly inhibit tumor cell proliferation. Tumor cell lysis induced by liposomal MDP ranged from 31-56%, as determined by the amount of ^{3}H-label, released from damaged tumor cells. In the remaining tumor cells DNA replication was strongly inhibited as determined by the decrease in the amount of ^{3}H-thymidine incorporated after a 24-h coculture period; inhibition of DNA synthesis as a combined result of tumor cell lysis and tumor cell stasis was 89-99%. Control liposomes, without MDP, did not induce any significant cytolysis or cytostasis.

Interestingly, we also noticed that enhancement of tumorcytotoxicity by a fixed amount of liposome-entrapped MDP increases by increasing the amount of lipid in which it is encapsulated (Daemen et al., 1986). Apparently, application of a larger amount of encapsulating lipid slows down the rate of intracellular release of the drug after uptake by the liver macrophages, thus allowing prolonged exposure of intracellular target sites of MDP.

We are currently investigating whether liposomes which by virtue of their structure (multilamellar vs unilamellar) or their lipid composition (e.g. cholesterol content) are only slowly degraded by lysosomal phospholipases, are more effective in rendering liver macrophages cytotoxic. Slow intracellular degradation of the liposomes may result in a prolongation of the period of sustained release of the immunomodulators within the macrophages, thus increasing the level and duration of tumor cytotoxicity.

ACKNOWLEDGEMENTS

The authors wish to thank CIBA GEIGY for generous supply of MDP, Bert Dontje and Jan Wijbenga for skilful technical assistance and Rinske Kuperus for preparing the manuscript. These investigators were supported in part by the Dutch Foundation for Cancer Research, the Koningin Wilhelmina Fonds.

REFERENCES

Daemen, T., Veninga, A., Scherphof, G., and Roerdink F., 1986, The activation of Kupffer cells to tumorcytotoxicity with immunomodulators encapsulated in liposomes, in: "Cells of the hepatic sinusoid", A. Kirn, D. L. Knook and E. Wisse, eds., The Kupffer Cell Foundation, The Netherlands.

Dijkstra, J., van Galen, W. J. M., Hulstaert, C. E., Kalicharan, D., Roerdink, F. H., and Scherphof, G. L., 1984, Interaction of liposomes with Kupffer cells in vitro, Exp. Cell Res., 150:161.

Dijkstra, J., van Galen, M., and Scherphof, G., 1984, Effects of ammonium-chloride and chloroquine on endocytic uptake of liposomes by Kupffer cells in vitro, Biochim. Biophys. Acta, 804:58.

Dijkstra, J., van Galen, M., Regts, J., and Scherphof, G., 1985, Uptake and processing of liposomal phospholipids by Kupffer cells in vitro. Eur. J. Biochem., 148:391.

Ellens, H., Morselt, H., and Scherphof, G., 1981, In vivo fate of large unilamellar sphingomyelin/cholesterol liposomes after intraperitoneal and intravenous injection into rats. Biochim. Biophys. Acta, 674:10.

Fidler, I. J., 1985, Macrophages and metastases. A biological approach to cancer therapy: presidential address, Cancer Res., 45:4714.

Fidler, I. J., Barnes, Z., Fogler, W.E., Kirsh, R., Bugelski, P., and Poste, G., 1982, Involvement of macrophages in the eradication of established metastases following intravenous injection of liposomes containing macrophage activators. Cancer Res., 42:496.

Fidler, I. J., Sone, S., Fogler, W.E., and Barnes, Z.L., 1984, Eradication of spontaneous metastases and activation of alveolar macrophages by intravenous injection of liposomes containing muramyl dipeptide, Proc. Natl. Acad. Sci. USA, 78:1680.

Fogler, W.E., Wade, R., Brundish, D.E., and Fidler, I. J., 1985, Distribution and fate of free and liposome-encapsulated ^{3}H nor-muramyl dipeptide and ^{3}H muramyl tripeptide phosphatidyl ethanolamine in mice, J. Immunol., 135:1372.

Kleinerman, E.A., Schroit, A.J., Fogler, W.E., and Fidler, I. J., 1983, Tumoricidal activity of human monocytes activated in vitro by free and liposome-encapsulated human lymphokines. J. Clin. Invest., 72:304.

Lopez-Berestein, G., Mehta, K., Mehta, R., Juliano, R.L., and Hersh, E.M., 1983, The activation of human monocytes by liposome-encapsulated muramyl dipeptide analogues, J. Immunol., 130:1500.

Mehta, K., Lopez-Berestein, G., Hersh, E.M., Juliano, R. L., 1982, Uptake of liposomes and liposome-encapsulated muramyl dipeptide by human peripheral blood monocytes, J. Reticuloendoth. Soc. 32:155.

Mehta, K., Juliano, R.L., and Lopez-Berestein, G., 1984, Stimulation of macrophage protease secretion via liposomal delivery of muramyl dipeptide derivatives to intracellular sites, Immunol., 51:517.

Op den Kamp, J. A. F., Kauerz, M. Th., and van Deenen, L. L. M., 1975, Action of pancreatic phospholipase A_2 on phosphatidylcholine bilayers in different physical states, Biochim. Biophys. Acta, 406:169.

Parant, M., Parant, F., Chedid, L., Yapo, A., Petit, J.F., and Lederer, E., 1979, Fate of synthetic immunoadjuvant, muramyl dipeptide (^{14}C-labeled) in the mouse, Int. J. Immunopharmacol., 1:35.

Poste, G., Bucana, C., Raz, A., Bugelski, P., Kirsh, R., Fidler, I. J., 1982, Analysis of the fate of systemically administered liposomes and implications for their use in drug delivery, Cancer Res. 42-1412.

Poste, G., Bucana, C., and Fidler, I. J., 1982, Stimulation of host response against metastatic tumours by liposome-encapsulated immunomodulators, in: "Targeting of drugs", G. Gregoriadis, J. Senior, and A. Trouet, eds., Plenum, New York.

Roerdink, F. H., Wisse, E., Morselt, H. W. M., van der Meulen, J., and Scherphof, G.L., 1977, Cellular distribution of intravenously injected protein-containing liposomes in the rat liver, in: "Kupffer cells and other liver sinusoidal cells", E. Wisse, and D. L. Knook, eds., Elsevier, Amsterdam.

Roerdink, F., Dijkstra, J., Hartman, G., Bolscher, B., and Scherphof, G., 1981, The involvement of parenchymal, Kupffer and endothelial liver cells in the hepatic uptake of intravenously injected liposomes. Effects of lanthanum and gadolinium salts, Biochim. Biophys. Acta, 677:79.

Roerdink, F. H., Dijkstra, J., Spanjer, H. H., Scherphof, G. L., 1984, In vivo and in vitro interactions of liposomes with hepatocytes and Kupffer cells, Biochem. Soc. Trans., 12:335.

Roerdink, F. H., Regts, J., van Leeuwen, B., and Scherphof, G., 1984, Intrahepatic phospholipid vesicles in rats, Biochim. Biophys. Acta, 770:195.

Scherphof, G. L., Dijkstra, J., Spanjer, H.H., Derksen, J. T. P., and Roerdink, F. H., 1985, Uptake and intracellular processing of targeted and non-targeted liposomes by rat Kupffer cells in vivo and in vitro, Ann. N. Y. Acad. Sci., 446:368.

Schroit, A. J., and Fidler, I. J., 1982, Effect of liposome structure and
    lipid composition on the activation of the tumoricidal properties of
    macrophages by liposomes containing muramyl dipeptide, Cancer Res.,
    42:161.
Spanjer, H. H., 1985, Targeting of liposomes to liver cells in vivo, Ph.D.
    Thesis, State University Groningen.
Thombre, P. S., and Deodhar, S. D., 1984, Inhibition of liver metastases in
    murine colon adenocarcinoma by liposomes containing human C-reactive
    protein or crude lymphokines, Cancer Immunol. Immunother., 16:145.
Varesio, L., Blasi, E., Thurman, G. B., Talmadge, G. E.,
    Wiltrout, R. H., and Herberman, R. B., 1984, Potent activation of
    mouse macrophages by recombinant Interferon., Cancer Res., 44:4465.
Wilschut, J. C., Regts, J., Westenberg, H., and Scherphof, G., 1976, Hy-
    drolysis of phosphatidylcholine liposomes by phospolipases A$_2$. Ef-
    fects of the local anesthetic dibucanine, Biochim, Biophys. Acta,
    433:20.
Wood, C. B., 1984, Natural history of liver metastasis, in: "Liver meta-
    stasis, basic aspects, detection amd management, C. J. H. van de
    Velde and P. H. Sugarbaker, eds., Martinus Nijhoff Publ.

ACTIVATORS OF PLASMINOGEN

Alice K. Robison and Burton E. Sobel

Cardiovascular Division
Washington University School of Medicine
St. Louis, Missouri, U.S.A.

INTRODUCTION

Fluidity of the blood without hemorrhage is maintained by the physiological equilibrium between the coagulation and fibrinolytic systems, each of which is comprised of intrinsic and extrinsic components. Activators of fibrinogen are compounds whose teleological function is the dissolution of fibrin clots which could potentially upset this hemostatic balance if left undisturbed.

Dissolution of fibrin clots, or fibrinolysis, occurs after the plasma protein plasminogen, which is inert, is converted to its active analog plasmin. This is accomplished by cleavage of a single Arg-Val bond, a reaction catalyzed by physiologic plasminogen activators such as tissue type plasminogen activator, t-PA, and urokinase, u-PA. Plasminogen also can be activated to plasmin by a bacterial protein, streptokinase, or SK. In this instance the activation can occur because the catalytic center of plasminogen is exposed following a conformational change accompanying its binding to streptokinase. Two plasminogen activators, u-PA, and SK are used clinically in pharmacological amounts for dissolution of fibrin clots. Some closely related compounds such as single chain u-PA and anisoylated plasminogen:streptokinase activator complexes (APSAC) as well as t-PA are currently under investigation in clinical trials. Primary uses of all of the agents focus on treatment or prophylaxis of acute myocardial infarction (AMI) and pulmonary emboli such as deep vein thrombosis (DVT).

This presentation will focus on the use of plasminogen activators in acute myocardial infarction in patients, concentrating on clinical experience with regulatory agency-approved methods of drug delivery. Additional information will be provided with reference to clinical research experience with t-PA and APSAC, the two preparations showing the most promise as thrombolytic agents because of their "clot selectivity". The final portion of my presentation will concern our laboratory research designed to deliver t-PA to animals by intramuscular injection with the aid of absorption-enhancing agents.

THE SYSTEMIC LYTIC STATE

The conventional plasminogen activators, streptokinase and urokinase, activate circulating plasminogen and fibrin clot-associated plasminogen equally well. Because of this, plasmin is generated in the intravascular compartment where it can initiate proteolytic attack on other plasma proteins, including fibrinogen, coagulation factors V and VIII and of course plasminogen itself. The primary plasmin inhibitor, α_2-antiplasmin, binds to circulating plasmin; when circulating plasmin levels exceed those of α_2-antiplasmin, the inhibitor is consumed. Additionally, fibrinogen degradation products accumulate; these have anticoagulant and antiplatelet properties. Collectively these plasmin-dependent phenomena are referred to as a "systemic lytic state." They predispose the patient to bleeding. The systemic lytic state occurs whenever SK and UK are used in doses sufficiently high for fibrin clot lysis, regardless of whether they delivered intravenously or via the intracoronary route.

TISSUE-TYPE PLASMINOGEN ACTIVATOR, t-PA

The attractiveness of t-PA lies in its relative fibrin clot selectivity. t-PA has a much higher affinity for plasminogen bound to fibrin clots than for circulating plasminogen. Thus, in the setting of evolving acute myocardial infarction t-PA lyses coronary thrombi without inducing a systemic lytic state. The "clot selectivity" occurs with either intravenous or intracoronary administration.

t-PA is found in bodily fluids and in extracts of tissues and organs of various mammals and birds. Broadly speaking the highest specific activity (in units/g tissue) of intrinsic t-PA is found in humans followed by pigs and dogs. The relative amount of t-PA in human organs is greatest in uterus, followed by the prostate, lung, ovary, muscle, heart, spleen, and liver (Rijken et al, 1981). In addition to its presence in mammalian organs and blood vessels, t-PA is produced and secreted into the growth medium of several types of cells in culture. An example of a high producer is the human Bowes melanoma cell line. t-PA was originally purified from conditioned medium of this cell line by Rijken and Collen (1981) who produced it in pharmacological amounts initially for study of thrombolysis for use in dogs and later for use in patients. Subsequently the t-PA gene for this cell line was cloned in E. coli (Pennica et al, 1983) and in a mammalian cell line (Browne et al, 1985; Pennica, personal communication). Expression of t-PA cDNA in mammalian cells enabled Genentech Inc., South San Francisco, to produce the recombinant DNA t-PA (rt-PA) now being used in clinical trials.

t-PA is a serine protease. Its only known physiological substrate is plasminogen. After cleaving plasminogen to plasmin at the Arg_{560}-Val_{561} bond, t-PA is in turn subject to cleavage by plasmin into two disulfide connected chains, A and B, originating from the amino and carboxy terminus respectively. Both single and two chain t-PA possess full biological activity.

In the carboxy terminal portion of its A chain, t-PA contains two kringles, or triple disulfide loops of approximately 82 amino acids. These kringles are present also in prothrombin, plasminogen and urokinase. Kringles are potential fibrin binding sites for t-PA (Ny et al, 1984). The amino portion of its A chain contains a domain homologous with the fibrin-binding finger domains of fibronectin. It also contains a domain homologous with epidermal growth factor.

The B chain contains the reactive site of the molecule, which consists of a Ser-His-Asp charge relay system. It bears extensive homology with B chains of other serine proteases such as urokinase, plasmin and thrombin.

In experiments in vitro the reaction between t-PA and plasminogen is much less effective in the absence of fibrin than in its presence. Depending on the concentration of reagents and on the assay system used, the presence of fibrin results in a 100 to 1000 fold stimulation of the catalytic efficiency of t-PA.

Results with Animals Given t-PA

t-PA lyses fibrin clots in coronary arteries when it is given by either the intracoronary (i.c.) or intravenous (i.v.) route. In animals and in patients successful lysis is no more common after i.c. compared with an i.v. delivery although the dose required may be higher for intravenous administration. It appears that lysis occurs more rapidly when the dose is higher. The incidence may be dependent on the interval between fibrin clot formation (which probably coincides with the onset of ischemia) and initiation of treatment with fibrinolytic agents. Older clots tend to be more highly organized, and may therefore be more resistant to lysis.

In experiments done by our group (Bergmann et al, 1983) successful coronary thrombolysis was demonstrated with t-PA. Closed-chest anesthetized dogs were subjected to coronary artery thrombosis by placement of a thrombogenic copper coil in the left anterior descending artery. Thrombus formation and cessation of blood flow distal to the insult occurred within 7-10 min. t-PA was administered one to two hours later. A solution of t-PA purified from melanoma cells by Désiré Collen was infused intravenously at a dose of 500 IU/kg/min. Clot lysis occurred within 10 min and was not accompanied by a systemic lytic state as judged by the maintenance of initial plasma levels of fibrinogen, plasminogen, and α_2-antiplasmin. Nutritive myocardial blood flow and regional myocardial metabolism were restored within 90 min of clot lysis as determined by quantification of uptake of $H_2^{15}O$ and ^{11}C-palmitate by positron emission tomography.

After recombinant t-PA (rt-PA) became available from Genentech, Inc., we extended our work to dogs with coronary thrombi induced with a copper coil (Van de Werf et al, 1984). One hour following coronary occlusion induced by the thrombogenic copper coil, rt-PA was administered by i.v. infusion at a rate of 1000 IU/kg/min (10 μg/kg/min). Angiographically documented recanalization was achieved in each of 9 dogs in 13.7 ± 1.9 min (mean ± SEM) without the generation of a systemic lytic state. Lysis occurred with a mean plasma concentration of 1 μg/ml. In this study t-PA was compared with intravenous urokinase, which resulted in reperfusion in only 7 of 10 dogs and a longer interval prior to reperfusion (19.3 ± 2.2 min). Thrombolysis with urokinase was accompanied by marked defibrinogenation in four of these seven dogs indicating the presence of a systemic lytic state.

t-PA has been shown to lyse coronary thrombi in dogs in a dose-dependent fashion (Gold et al, 1984) following i.v. administration of 5 to 25 μg/kg/min. It appears to exhibit dose-dependent qualities in patients as well (Tiefenbrunn et al, 1985). A dose-response relationship is not always evident however, perhaps because of the variable amount of time elapsing between coronary artery occlusion and time of treatment, and the variable extent and loci of naturally-occurring clots in patients.

In experiments in vitro, at least three groups of workers (Brommer, 1984; Zamarron et al, 1984; and Fox et al, 1985) have shown that t-PA incorporated into a nascent clot is more effective in eliciting clot lysis than t-PA applied to the surface of a preformed clot. Fox et al in our laboratory extended these in vitro observations to demonstrate that the presence of t-PA in a dog's circulation inhibited or delayed copper coil-induced thrombus formation in a dose-dependent fashion. In our study, t-PA administered by i.v. infusion at a rate of 3.75 - 10 μg/kg/min completely prevented angiographically-visible thrombus formation, whereas at a rate of 1-2 μg/kg/min it delayed thrombus formation by 18 min. After cessation of the t-PA infusion, t-PA plasma levels decreased. Thrombus formation occurred only when mean t-PA plasma levels had declined to 85-91 ng/ml.

t-PA in Patients

The first study in which t-PA was administered to patients with evolving acute myocardial infarction was performed in 1985 as a joint study involving Professor Désiré Collen and colleagues at the University of Leuven and Professor Burton Sobel and colleagues at Washington University in St. Louis (Van de Werf et al, 1984). They administered t-PA harvested from Bowes melanoma conditioned medium to seven men with angiographically-documented coronary artery occlusions. The administered dose was 20,000 to 40,000 IU/min for 30 to 60 min, given intravenously or intracoronarily. Lysis was documented in 6 of 7 patients 19 to 50 min after the onset of the t-PA infusion. In one patient a clot refractory to t-PA was refractory also to a subsequent dose of i.v. streptokinase. None of the patients given t-PA alone manifested signs of a systemic lytic state. However, after administration of streptokinase two patients exhibited abrupt decreases in plasma fibrinogen, plasminogen and α_2-antiplasmin levels.

The favorable results of this initial small scale clinical study and those of studies with animals led to a multicenter double blind randomized clinical trial sponsored by Genentech, Inc. (Collen et al, 1984). rt-PA was administered intravenously over 60 min to patients at Washington University, Johns Hopkins, Massachusetts General Hospital and the University of Leuven. Doses of 0.5 mg/kg elicited recanalization in 75% of the 45 patients studied. Fibrinogenolysis was modest or absent.

The next clinical trial, called Thrombolysis in Myocardial Infarction (TIMI) and sponsored by the U.S. National Heart, Lung and Blood Institute, compared i.v. t-PA in doses similar to those used in the Genentech-sponsored trial with i.v. streptokinase (1.5 million units given over 60 min) (TIMI, 1985). Recanalization rates were 66% for t-PA, in accord with previous results, versus 36% for streptokinase. Several additional phases of TIMI have followed, using higher doses and durations of infusion and using single chain t-PA; results are qualitatively similar to those in the initial phase.

Another double blind multicenter trial, the European Cooperative Trial, was conducted to directly compare rt-PA and streptokinase (European Cooperative Study Group, 1985). Results from patients given i.v. rt-PA at 0.75 mg/kg over a 90 min period were compared with those from patients treated with i.v. streptokinase given 1.5 million units over 60 min. Recanalization rates with t-PA were 70% in contrast to 55% for patients given streptokinase. Laboratory criteria confirmed the relative safety of t-PA over streptokinase which was previously observed in the TIMI trial and in the original Genentech trial.

To summarize the existing clinical trial experience with patients:
1. Lysis occurs consistently when plasma t-PA levels are 1 μg/ml or greater and often with lower levels;
2. Lysis of angiographically confirmed coronary artery clots treated with t-PA occurs in 65-70% of patients;

3. Treatment with lytic doses of t-PA is associated with at most a modest decline of plasma fibringen, plasminogen and α_2-anti-plasmin. A systemic lytic state is usually not encountered;
4. Higher recanalization rates are achieved with t-PA than with conventional activators of the fibrinolytic system; and
5. Risks of reocclusion are no greater than those encountered with conventional activators.

ANISOYLATED-PLASMINOGEN:STREPTOKINASE ACTIVATOR COMPLEX, APSAC

As stated repeatedly, clinical and animal use of the conventional plasminogen activators, streptokinase and urokinase, in doses sufficient for lysis of coronary artery occlusions, results in a systemic lytic state; that is, depletion from the circulation of fibrinogen, plasminogen and α_2-antiplasmin. The systemic lytic state occurs independent of the mode of administration (i.c. or i.v.). A second generation class of streptokinase compounds was developed by scientists at Beecham Research Laboratories in the UK (Smith et al, 1981) in order to minimize the hemostatic abnormalities by providing some clot selectivity. The agent showing the most promise in the treatment of coronary artery thrombosis is BRL 26921, or p-anisoylated plasminogen:streptokinase activator complex, also called APSAC.

Streptokinase, a 45000-47000 dalton protein produced by strains of Lancefield group C β-hemolytic streptococci, was the first activator of fibrinolysis to be used clinically. Because of its ready availability, ease of preparation and relatively low cost, it has been used for thrombolysis for many years. Its use in patients has been limited by its antigenicity in addition to its systemic lytic effects.

SK is not a serine protease and it lacks the kringle structures present in t-PA. SK activates the fibrinolytic system indirectly forming stoichiometric complexes with plasminogen, plasmin or plasmin B-chain. A proteolytic site is exposed in these complexes which converts other plasminogen molecules to plasmin. Because SK lacks fibrin clot selectivity (presumably due to the absence of kringles and their putative fibrin binding sites), it attacks circulating plasminogen, leading to the systemic lytic state.

APSAC was synthesized in 1981 by Smith and coworkers (Smith et al, 1981) at Beecham, who sought an agent with 1) enhanced efficiency (over SK) due to evasion of inhibitor systems; 2) sustained release pharmaco-kinetics, leading to simplified administration and easier clinical control; 3) reduction in systemic toxicity attributable to hyperplasminaemia; and 4) protection against autolytic degradation. APSAC consists of a strepto-kinase moiety bound to human plasminogen which has its active center blocked by p-anisic acid (4-methoxybenzoic acid). The complex is inert as a plasminogen activator until deacylation occurs in plasma. Acylation apparently does not interfere with the ability of the plasminogen moiety of APSAC to bind to fibrin.

Results of Experiments with Animals Given APSAC

The deacylation half-life in vitro is 40 min at 37° at pH 7.4. In rabbits and human subjects (Dupe et al, 1985) the plasma clearance half life is 60 - 75 min as opposed to approximately 15 min for SK or SK-plasmin complex. Presumably the measured clearance half-life reflects contri-butions from both unaltered ASPAC and its deacylated derivatives.

ASPAC can be delivered by bolus injection since it is inactive until deacylated. In rabbit and dog experiments its administration produced dose-related clot lysis from 40 to 280 µg/kg while avoiding significant systemic effects (Smith et al, 1982; Matsuo et al, 1981; Dupe et al, 1984).

In 1981 Matsuo, Collen and Verstraete (Matsuo et al, 1981) reported that incubation of a human blood clot in citrated rabbit plasma containing APSAC was accompanied by a marked degree of thrombolysis without significant activation of the fibrinolytic system. However, when the rabbit plasma was replaced by citrated human plasma the discrimination between thrombolysis and systemic activation of the fibrinolytic system was lost. This in vitro result presaged actual clinical experience with APSAC.

APSAC in Patients

Similar doses of APSAC (in terms of streptokinase equivalents) are needed for thrombolysis compared with streptokinase alone. Therefore, in general, initial clinical trial findings have indicated that APSAC administration to humans in lytic doses, either as a single bolus injection, repeated bolus injections or short-term infusion, has resulted in some systemic activation of the fibrinolytic system. Its use is also accompanied by an anamestic rise in streptokinase antibody production and a delayed mild febrile reaction. APSAC has been an effective fibrinolytic agent with demonstrated recanalization rates of 60 -100% in several small scale studies conducted to date. The first report that APSAC is less "selectively" thrombolytic in patients than in animals came from Walker's group in Glasgow (Walker et al, 1983, 1984). They found that 5 to 25 mg of APSAC given i.v. or i.c. to patients with acute myocardial infarction resulted in a dose-related increase in fibrinogenolysis and other indicators of systemic activation. They also observed quenching of fibrinogenolysis in patients having high titers of anti-streptokinase antibodies.

Kasper and associates in Mainz (1984) reported a 74% reperfusion rate within 42 ± 37 min following i.c. administration of 5 to 20 mg APSAC to 23 patients with acute myocardial infarction. They observed plasminemia in most patients and bleeding complications in two patients.

Been and colleagues in Glasgow (1985) observed patency in all 16 patients receiving 30 mg APSAC by i.v. infusion and in only 2 of 16 patients receiving placebo. They reported less systemic defibrinogenation than an equivalent dose of streptokinase.

Hoffmann and coworkers in the Netherlands (1985) used a short i.v. infusion to deliver 30 mg of APSAC to myocardial infarction patients. They found that a substantial degree of systemic fibrinogenolysis in 12-13 patients was accompanied by a therapeutic efficiency of 85%. They concluded that the incidence of bleeding problems and reocclusion rates were not essentially different from streptokinase therapy.

The most recent clinical study of which we are aware is that of Marder et al in New York (1986) who found a dose-related reperfusion rate following a slow bolus injection. Using the top dose of 30 mg, reperfusion occurred in 60% of patients with a mean time to reperfusion of 35 min. A systemic lytic state was induced in all patients at this dose.

To summarize: it appears from the data of the limited number of patients treated with APSAC that this is a fibrin-specific agent whose use at doses effective at lysing coronary thrombi associated with acute myocardial infarction is accompanied by a systemic plasminemic state. Advantages to APSAC include the option of delivery by bolus i.v. injection and a relatively long plasma half life (75 min) which may mitigate against reocclusion., Disadvantages are related to its streptokinase moiety, and include the production of a systemic lytic state which may lead to bleeding complications, as well as dosage problems stemming from existing anti-streptokinase antibodies.

t-PA is undergoing extensive clinical trials that will lead to determination of optimal dosage regimens. Experience to date suggests that it is a relatively safe and effective thrombolytic agent when used for acute myocardial infarction. Advantages to t-PA include its ability to lyse coronary thrombi at doses that do not induce a systemic lytic state, and its short (8 min) plasma half-life, which would allow for immediate follow-up surgery if needed. Disadvantages include the necessity for intravenous infusion over long periods of time (30 min to 3 hours).

INTRAMUSCULAR INJECTION OF t-PA

I would now like to address recent efforts in our laboratory to administer plasminogen activators by means of intramuscular injection (Sobel et al, 1985). It has become apparent in animal experiments involving coronary artery thrombolysis that salutary effects are critically dependent on the rapidity of clot lysis after the onset of ischemia. This is the case in part because "aged" clots are more highly organized and harder to lyse with a given dose of drug and particularly because myocardium distal to the thrombus becomes irreversibly damaged soon after the onset of ischemia.

Treatment with the conventional activators, urokinase and strepto-kinase, and with the second generation compounds such as t-PA and APSAC, require administration by trained personnel in a hospital setting. It appeared to us that maximal benefit could be offered to patients with coronary disease if t-PA could be administered with automatic injectors by the patient or by paramedical personnel.

The following studies were undertaken to determine whether blood levels of t-PA sufficient for induction of coronary thrombolysis can be attained in rabbits and dogs given the drug by intramuscular injection.

Our initial studies were performed with anesthetized male New England white rabbits weighing 2 kg. Skeletal muscle from the hind legs was exposed bilaterally and an indwelling venous catheter was used to withdraw blood samples. Electrical field stimulation was used in some experiments to augment local blood flow. Human rt-PA in buffer (produced by Genentech) was administered in 1 ml aliquots in each of 4 sites at a dose of 1 mg/kg. Various absorption enhancing agents were added to the rt-PA/buffer solution immediately prior to injection. Blood collected into citrate vacutainer tubes at 0, 5, 15, 30 and 60 min after injection was centrifuged and the plasma frozen until assay. t-PA was assayed both immunoradiometrically using the assay of Rijken et al (1983) and functionally on fibrin plates using euglobulin fractions. Qualitatively similar results were obtained with both assays.

We found that a 2 mg total dose of rt-PA in buffer yielded plasma levels of 8-10 ng/ml. The addition of 1% to 3% dimethylsulfoxide, a compound known to enhance absorption of low molecular weight compounds provided little improvement (8-11 ng/ml). The addition of hydroxylamine-HCl (a compound known to dissociate t-PA from its naturally occurring inhibitor, to inhibit platelet aggregation, and to elicit smooth muscle relaxation), provided a significant enhancement of t-PA absorption in a dose-dependent fashion.

The time course for absorption was similar in all hydroxylamine doses tested, from 43.75 to 175 mg/4 ml dose. Peak levels of approximately 400 ng/ml were achieved at 5 min, with a rapid return toward baseline by 15 -30 min. A second broad rise in plasma t-PA was usually observed from 45 -60 min.

When the t-PA dose was varied from 0.5 to 2 mg/rabbit while holding hydroxylamine-HCl constant at 175 mg/4 ml dose, a similar dose-response relationship was obtained, again with peak plasma levels apparent at 5 min.

The above experiments were done with local electrical field stimulation to enhance blood flow. In a similar set of rabbits, electrical field stimulation was omitted. Findings were similar except that blood levels were on average two-fold lower. The time course for absorption and clearance of t-PA was unaltered.

Facilitation of absorption of t-PA by hydroxylamine-HCl was not due to the decrease in pH caused by the enhancer; we showed no differences in absorption by varying pH between 5.5 to 7.5 in the presence or absence of hydroxylamine. Systemic effects of hydroxylamine similarly were not responsible; when t-PA in buffer was injected into muscle in one leg and hydroxylamine in buffer into the contralateral muscle, results were similar to rt-PA in buffer alone.

We next showed that the therapeutic levels of t-PA achieved in rabbits could be attained in anesthetized dogs. We used a copper coil inserted in the left anterior descending artery to produce an occlusive clot. Once this was documented angiographically, we injected rt-PA at 3 mg/kg in buffer containing 0.63 M hydroxylamine-HCl ($\equiv$175 mg/4 ml), using electrical field stimulation. Coronary thrombolysis, observed angiographically, was initiated within 15 min of intramuscular t-PA administration, even though peak plasma t-PA levels at 5 min (120 ng/ml) where lower than those in rabbits.

We believe that these results demonstrate the feasibilty of administering t-PA by intramuscular injection with the aid of enhancing agents.

Hydroxylamine-HCl, although it greatly enhances absorption of t-PA from an intramuscular site, may not be an ideal enhancing agent when used alone because it elicits methemoglobinemia, and (in high doses) a decrease in blood pressure and injury at the injection site. We are currently investigating the ability of other analogs to serve as facilitators of absorption of t-PA, with the eventual aim of being able to limit myocardial damage by enabling patients at high risk to self administer t-PA immediately early after coronary occlusion occurs.

REFERENCES

Been, M., DeBono, D. P., Muir, A. L., Boulton, F. E., Hillis, W. S., and Hornung, R., 1985, Coronary thrombolysis with intravenous anisoylated plasminogen-streptokinase complex BRL 26921, Br. Heart J., 53:253.

Bergmann, S. R., Fox, K. A. A., Ter-Pogossian, M. M., Sobel, B. E., and Collen, D., 1983, Clot-selective coronary thrombolysis with tissue-type plasminogen activator, Science, 220:1181.

Brommer, E. J. P., 1984, The level of extrinsic plasminogen activator (t-PA) during clotting as a determinant of the rate of fibrinolysis; inefficiency of activators added afterwards, Thromb. Res., 34:109.

Browne, M. J., Dodd, I., Carey, J. E., Chapman, C. G., and Robinson, J. H., 1985, Increased yield of human tissue-type plasminogen activator obtained by means of recombinant DNA technology, Thromb. Haemostas., 54:422.

Collen, D., Topol, E. J., Tiefenbrunn, A. J., Gold, H. K., Weisfeldt, M. L., Sobel, B. E., Leinbach, R. C., Brinker, J. A., Ludbrook, P. A., Yasuda, I., Bulkley, B. H., Robison, A. K., Hutter, A. M., Jr., Bell, W. R., Spadaro, J. J., Jr., Khaw, B. A., and Grossbard, E. B., 1984, Coronary thrombolysis with recombinant human tissue-type plasminogen activator: a prospective, randomized, placebo-controlled trial, Circulation, 70:1012.

Dupe, R. J., English, P. D., Smith, R. A. G., and Green, J., 1984, Acyl-enzymes as thrombolytic agents in dog models of venous thrombosis nad pulmonary embolism, Thromb. Haemostas., 51:248.

Dupe, R. J., Green, J., and Smith, R. A. G., 1985, Acylated derivatives of streptokinase-plasminogen activator complex as thrombolytic agents in a dog model of aged venous thrombosis, Thromb. Haemostas., 53:56.

European Cooperative Study Group, 1985, Randomised trial of intravenous recombinant tissue-type plasminogen activator versus intravenous streptokinase in acute myocardial infarction, The Lancet, April 13.

Fox, K. A. A., Robison, A. K., Knabb, R. M., Rosamond, T. L., Sobel, B. E., and Bergmann, S. R., 1985, Prevention of coronary thrombosis with subthrombolytic doses of tissue-type polasminogen activator, Circulation, 72:1346.

Gold, H. K., Fallon, J. T., Yasuda, T., Leinback, R. C., Khaw, B. A., Newell, J. B., Guerrero, J. L., Vislousky, F. M., Hoyng, C. F., Grossbard, E., and Collen, D., 1984, Coronary thrombolysis with recombinant human tissue-type plasminogen activator, Circulation 70:700.

Hoffmann, J .J. M. L., Van Rey, F. J. W., and Bonnier, J. J. R. M., 1985, Systemic effects of BRL 26921 during thrombolytic threatment of acute myocardial infarction, Thromb. Res. 37:567.

Kasper, W., Erbel, R., Meinertz, T., Drexler, M., Ruckel, A., Pop, T., Prellwitz, W., and Meyer, J. 1984, Intracoronary thrombolysis with an acylated streptokinase-plasminogen activator (BRL 26921) in patients iwth acute myocardial infarction, J. Am. Coll. Cardiol., 4:357.

Marder, V. J., Rothbard, R. L., Fitzpatrick, P. G., and Francis, C. W., 1986, Rapid lysis of coronary artery thrombi with anisoylated plasminogen: streptokinase activator complex, Ann. Int. Med., 104:304.

Matsuo, O., Collen, D., and Verstraete, M., 1981, On the fibrinolytic and thrombolytic properties of active-site p-anisoylated streptokinase-plasminogen complex (BRL 26921), Thromb. Res., 24:347.

Ny, T., Elgh, F., and Lund, B., 1984, The structure of the human tissue-type plasminogen activator gene: Correlation of intron and exon structures to functional and structural domains, Proc. Natl. Acad. Sci. USA, 81:5355.

Pennica, D., Holmes, W. E., Kohr, W. J., Harkins, R. N., Vehar, G. A., Ward, C. A., Bennett, W. F., Yelverton, E., Seeburg, P. H., Heyneker,

H. L., Goeddel, D. V., and Collen, D. 1983, Cloning and expression of human tissue-type plasminogen activator cDNA in E. coli, Nature, 301, 214.

Rijken, D. C. and Collen, D., 1981, Purification and characterization of the plasminogen activator secreted by human melanoma cells in culture, J. Biol. Chem., 256:7035.

Smith, R. A. G., Dupe, R. J., English, P. D., and Green, J., 1982, Acyl-enzymes as thrombolytic agents in a rabbit model of venous thrombosis, Thromb. Haemostas., 47:269.

Smith, R. A. G., Dupe, R. J., English, P. D., and Green, J., 1981, Fibrinolysis with acyl-enzymes: a new approach to thrombolytic therapy, Nature, 290:505.

Sobel, B. E., Fields, L. E., Robison, A. K., Fox, K. A. A., and Sarnoff, S. J., 1985, Coronary thrombolysis with facilitated absorption of intramuscularly injected tissue-type plasminogen activator, Proc. Natl. Acad. Sci. USA, 82:4258.

TIMI Study Group, 1985, The thrombolysis in myocardial infarction (TIMI) trial, N. Engl. J. Med., 312:932.

Tiefenbrunn, A. J., Robison, A. K., Kurnik, P. B., Ludbrook, P. A., and Sobel, B. E., 1985, Clinical pharmacology in patients with evolving myocardial infarction of tissue-type plasminogen activator produced by recombinant DNA technology, Circulation, 71:110.

Van de Werf, F., Bergmann, S. R., Fox, K. A. A., de Geest, H., Hoyng, C. F., Sobel, B. E., and Collen, D., 1984, Coronary thrombolysis with intravenously administered human tissue-type plasminogen activator produced by recombinant DNA technology, Circulation, 69:605.

Van de Werf, F., Ludbrook, P. A., Bergmann, S. R., Tiefenbrunn, A. J., Fox, K. A. A., de Geest, H., Verstraete, M., Collen, D., and Sobel, B. E., 1984, Coronary thrombolysis with tissue-type plasminogen activator in patients with evolving myocardial infarction, N. Engl. J. Med., 310:609.

Walker, I. D., Davidson, J. F., Rae, A. P., Hutton, I, and Lawrie, T. D. V., 1983, Acyl-streptokinase-plasminogen activator complex in acute myocardial infarction (AMI), Br. J. Haematol. 53:344.

Walker, I. D., Davidson, J. F., Rae, A. P., Hutton, I., and Lawrie, T. D. V., 1984, Acylated streptokinase - plasminogen complex in patients with acute myocardial infarction, Thromb. Haemostas., 51:204.

Zamarron, C., Lijnen, H. R., and Collen, D., 1984, Influence of exogenous and endogenous tissue-type plasminogen activator on the lysability of clots in a plasma milieu in vitro, Thromb. Res. 35:335.

BIOSYNTHETIC HUMAN GROWTH HORMONE IDENTICAL TO AUTHENTIC MATERIAL

Thorkild Christensen, Jørli W. Hansen, John Pedersen, Henrik Dalbøge, Søren Carlsen, Ejner B. Jensen, Karin D. Jørgensen, Bo Dinesen, Povl Nilsson, Hans H. Sørensen, Johannes Thomsen, and Anne-Marie Kappelgaard

Nordisk Gentofte A/S, Niels Steensensvej 1
NK-2820 Gentofte, Denmark

INTRODUCTION

The major component of human growth hormone (hGH) is a protein with 191 amino acid residues, and a molecular weight of approximately 22,000 D (22K-hGH). A minor component which constitutes about 5% of the more abundant form has a molecular weight of approximately 20,000 D. The minor form is derived from the major by deletion of 15 amino acid residues (32-46 of the 22K-isomer). Both molecules are single stranded, and two disulfide bridges stabilizes the structure. The N-terminus as well as the C-terminus is phenylalanine (Chawla et al., 1983).

Human growth hormone is produced in the anterior pituitary gland throughout life. By monitoring plasma levels in healthy volunteers a circadian profile of hGH has been demonstrated (Christiansen et al., 1983) showing increased nocturnal hGH-levels. Daily s.c. administration of hGH to hypopituitary children leads to plasma levels of hGH which better imitates the plasma growth hormone profile in normal children as compared to an i.m. administration 3 times weekly. The s.c. regimen results in a relatively increased growth rate (Kastrup et al., 1983).

So far only few investigations have been carried out for improving formulation of hGH and the administration. One reason has been the scarce supply of hGH due to its manufacturing by extraction of pituitary glands from human cadavers. Introduction of recombinant DNA-technology hold promises that the shortage problem can be overcome. However, before a general use of biosynthetic human growth hormone can take place, the possible immunogeneity of this polypeptide has to be evaluated.

BIOSYNTHETIC HUMAN GROWTH HORMONE

Background and philosophy for the process design

A major problem for biosynthetic production of proteins has been to obtain the product without an amino terminal extension, in particular the amino acid methionine encoded by the translation initiation codon AUG. Since an extra methionine may influence the conformational structure and give rise to altered immunological properties (Aston et al, 1985), it is of obvious interest to produce pharmaca identical to the authentic protein. Finally the general trend on the market for polypeptide hormones tends to shift towards the use of products, identical to the main authentic component (e.g. from porcine to human insulin although the difference is only 1 amino acid, and no therapeutic benefit so far has been demonstrated).

For these reasons it was decided to produce biosynthetic human growth hormone identical to authentic 22K-hGH.

Owing to the nature of protein synthesis in living organisms, the N-terminal amino acid in the nascent preproteins is always methionine (or formylated methionine). In general, the resulting product is a preprotein which posttranslationally is processed enzymatically to the mature product. Consequently, it is necessary to take into account the very nature of the protein synthesis before deciding on a strategy for the manufacturing process of hGH with phenylalanine as N-terminus.

As hGH contains 3 methionines, it is not possible unambiguously to cleave amino extended hGH chemically by means of cyanogen bromide at the C-terminal of a methionine residue placed adjacent to the N-terminus of hGH.

As shown in table 1, three different approaches seem theoretically feasible in order to obtain the mature protein.

Table 1. Possible methods

Protein modification	Protein maturation
Signal peptide	Enzyme system of E.coli
Amino extension	Specific cleavage site for an endopeptidase
Amino extension	Amino extension removed by an exopeptidase

Only the method where an amino extension is removed by an exopeptidase will be emphasized in the following (schematically shown in fig. 1). Purified amino extended hGH is converted enzymatically to the mature B-hGH.

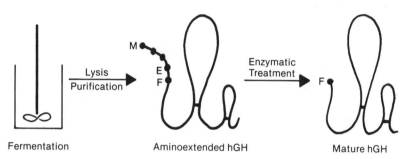

Fig. 1.   Process outline for enzymatic conversion of amino extended hGH to mature B-hGH.

Cloning

A gene encoding hGH and in addition 13 amino acids of the signal sequence was constructed by the combination of a hGH cDNA fragment (encoding amino acids 24-191), isolated from a human pituitary cDNA library using rat GH cDNA as probe, with a hGH gene fragment (encoding amino acids -13 to +23) isolated from a human placenta λ library. By means of an exonuclease, the 3'-5' activity contained in the Klenow fragment of DNA-polymerase I, the DNA coding for the 13 extra amino acids of the signal sequence was removed.

On four consecutive treatments using dTTP, dATP, dGTP and dATP it was possible to control the exonuclease digestion. To remove the plus strand overhang, the DNA was treated with nuclease S1, ending up with a blunt ended DNA-molecule. Synthetic DNA-linkers (Urdea et al., 1983) coding for the amino acid residues in the amino extension was blunt end ligated to the DNA-molecule coding for hGH.

In order to obtain transcription and translation, the above mentioned DNA fragment was attached to a synthetic constitutive promotor and a Shine Dalgarno Sequence. Furthermore the transcription terminator from phage fd was inserted after the hGH coding sequences (fig. 2). Several clones were constructed to obtain hGH forms with different amino extensions (X-hGH's) (Dalbøge et al., 1986). The genetic material was inserted in the non conjugative plasmid pAT 153. E.Coli MC1061 was used as host.

Fermentation

In order to carry out large scale fermentations it is of the utmost importance, that the clone in question is genetically stable and that a high expression level of amino extended hGH can be obtained.

It has turned up that the expression stability varies significantly between different amino extended hGH forms for cells grown at a number of generations. Furthermore it could be demonstrated that this variability in stability was due to differences in specific growth rates and that the growth rates correlated well with the observed expression levels.

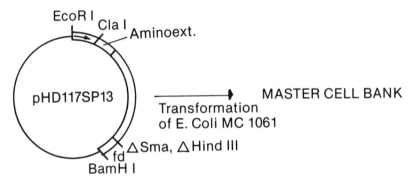

Fig. 2   Expression plasmid encoding amino terminal extended hGH.

These results show, that even small changes in the amino terminal part of chimeric molecules can lead to marked differences in specific growth rates, specific expression rates as well as genetic stability.

In fig. 3 is shown examples of genetic stability for clones expressing different types of amino extended hGH.

As demonstrated the two clones MFEE-hGH and MTEE-hGH show very high initial expression rates but are genetically unstable. However, it could be demonstrated, that the genetic instability was caused by loss of plasmids and not intra-plasmid modifications. Such clones are not applicable in large scale production because a large scale fermentation typically requires 30-40 generations of growth. Fermentation with instable clones will result in poor yields. Furthermore the regulatory authorities demands stability for at least 10 generations more than the number needed for production. Other clones such as MLE-hGH have excellent plasmid stability but suboptimal expression levels.

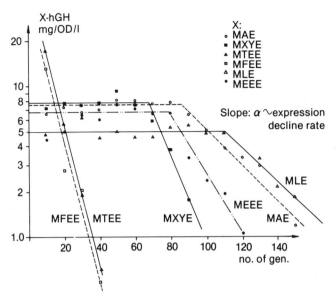

Fig. 3: Stability of different X-hGH clones without selection pressure.
(A: Ala, E: Glu, F: Phe, L: Leu, M: Met, T: Thr, X, Y: Amino Acids)

The physiological conditions in the cells during fermentation are very important for the expression levels. By composing the medium in such a way that the second limiting substrate component (after the C-source) is phosphate, it has been possible to develop a glucose fed batch process where biomass formation is blocked at a suitable level, whereas the metabolic conditions allow a continued X-hGH synthesis. By this cultivation procedure it has been possible to obtain X-hGH yields of 2000 mg/l even with X-hGH producing clones with moderate expression efficiency (see fig. 4).

The combination of using X-hGH producing clones with moderate expression efficiency and using cultivation conditions which allow late non-growth associated product formation results in a system with good genetic stability as well as high productivity (Carlsen and Jensen, 1986).

Protein chemistry

The final step in the fermentation process is a sterile filtration of lysed cells. From a very complex mixture of E.coli proteins, nucleic acids, carbohydrates, lipids, peptidoglycans, lipoproteins etc. amino extended hGH shall be isolated in high purity. The amino extension is removed enzymatically in vitro followed by further purification steps and the final formulation. In fig. 5 the process is shown schematically.

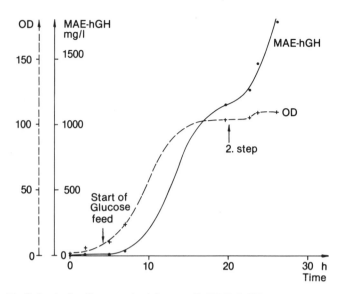

Fig. 4: Fed batch fermentation of MAE-hGH
1. step: Glucose feed rate = 3,6 g x l^{-1} x h^{-1}
2. Step: Phosphate limited phase with glucose feed rate = 5,4 g x l^{-1} x h^{-1}.

The first step is ion exchange chromatography carried out at pH 7. This step has a high purification factor and results in amino extended hGH of more than 95% purity. The next step is hydrophobic interaction chromatography, which removes substances with hydrophobic properties different from that of amino extended hGH. The third step is high performance ion exchange chromatography carried out at a pH different from the pH in the first purification step. Products with a net charge differing only one unit from amino extended hGH can be resolved.

The second amino acid in hGH is a proline. It is well known that certain aminopeptidases cannot cleave a peptide bond in which proline is involved. By use of the amino peptidase dipeptidylaminopeptidase I, (DAP I) which cannot cleave neither at the C-terminus nor at the N-terminus of a proline residue, the amino extension can be cleaved off very specifically. As a charged amino acid in the amino extension is positioned adjacent to the N-terminus of hGH, it is possible to separate, by means of ion exchange, the mature hGH (B-hGH) from contaminating bacterial proteins and any of the possible amino extended forms due to incomplete enzymatic conversion (Dalbøge et al., 1986).

The final 3 steps purifies B-hGH with respect to charge and size and removes any residual amino terminal extended forms.

Fig. 6 showns the enzymatic conversion of amino extended hGH to B-hGH as analyzed by ion exchange high performance liquid chromatography (IE-HPLC) also called FPLC.

310

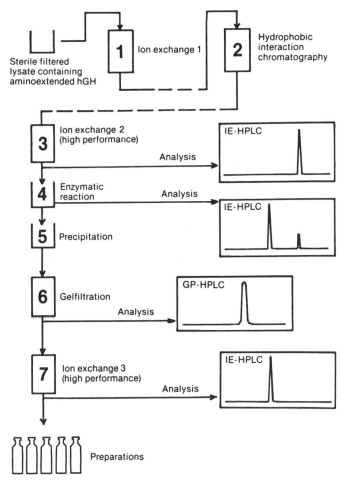

Fig. 5: Purification scheme of B–hGH. The inserts in the figure are schematic curves demonstrating the principle of charge shift from amino extended hGH to mature B–hGH.

The enzymatic conversion rate is dependent of temperature, concentration and amount of enzyme but also of the amino acid residues in the amino extension.

As discussed above the development of the process for manufacturing biosynthetic human growth has necessitated a set of compromises. Clones with high specific expression rates turned out to be genetically unstable. Clones with excellent genetic stability gave unsatisfactory yields. Certain amino extended forms were converted enzymatically to mature hGH at suboptimal rates.

When a clone has been selected, every step in the process from fermentation and throughout chromatographic purification has to be optimized.

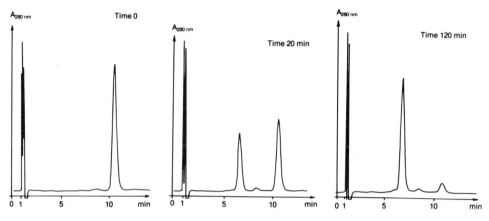

Fig. 6: Enzymatic   conversions   of   amino   extended   hGH
         followed by IE-HPLC.

IDENTITY AND PURITY

     As criterion for identity of hGH native polyacrylamide
gel electrophoresis (PAGE) has been used. Two major bands
occur, of which the upper band is the most abundant. The
lower band consists of deamidated hGH. PAGE of B-hGH and
22K-hGH are identical.

     Amino acid analysis of B-hGH gives a content of the
amino acids identical to the theoretical values within experimental error.
     Both N-terminus and C-terminus of B-hGH have been deter-
mined to be phenylalanine as in authentic hGH.
     A comparison of tryptic digests of B-hGH and 22K-hGH has
been carried out (Christensen et al., 1986) (fingerprint).
The HPLC chromatograms of the two digests were identical,
indicating correct primary structure. All fragments have
been collected and sequenced and found to be as expected by
comparing with the known sequence. Special attention was
paid to the cystein containing fragments, and the correct
placement of the disulfide bridges could thus be verified.

     The secondary structure has been determined by circular
dichroism. The spectra for B-hGH and 22K-hGH were indistinguishable indicating the secondary structure of B-hGH to be
identical to that of 22K-hGH.

     By ELISA (Dinesen and Dalbøge Andersen, 1984), using
polyclonal anti-hGH antibodies, no difference between B-hGH
and pituitary hGH could be detected.

A commercially available RIA-kit, using a monoclonal anti-hGH antibody (Gomez et al., 1984), being especially sensitive to changes in the amino terminal part of hGH, was investigated. The cross reactivity for B-hGH as well as for 22K-hGH was 100% as compared to the Kit-standard. Amino extended forms, including methionyl-hGH cross reacted to an extent of .05% or less as compared to the Kit-standard.

The immunological experiments do not indicate differences in tertiary structure between B-hGH and 22K-hGH.

The content of B-hGH and deamidated B-hGH is greater than 99% as judged by IE-HPLC (fig. 7) and no amino extended forms could be detected.

By means of an ELISA the final preparation of B-hGH was analysed for content of antigens from the host (E.coli). Less than 2 ppm (2ng/mg B-hGH) E.coli antigen is present.

The RNA/DNA content has been determined to be less than 1 ppm.

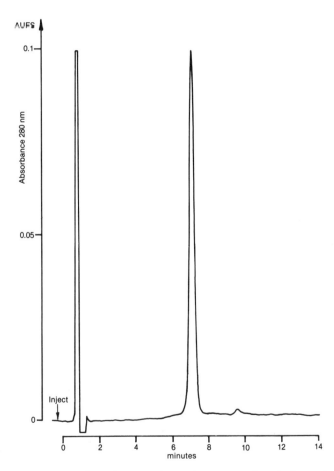

Figure 7: IE-HPLC of B-hGH. The minor peak with retention time approximately 9.5 min is a deamidated form of B-hGH.

POTENCY AND SAFETY

Pharmacodynamics

Comparative studies between B-hGH and pituitary human growth hormone drug (NORDISK, Nanormon[R]) has been carried out. The potency of B-hGH was found to be 84-119% of hGH of pituitary origin by the weight gain test and 66-114% by the tibia test.

Pharmacological profile

B-hGH was compared to pituitary human growth hormone in several in vitro and in vivo test systems. Pituitary 22K-hGH was included in the screening program. Studies of effect on naive behaviour, spontaneous activity, coordinated movements and temperature regulation, were carried out in experiments on mice. No drug induced changes were observed. Doses up to 25 IU/kg bw. were used, which is more than 100 times the human therapeutic dose.

Neuromuscular transmission was studied in anaesthetized rats and blood coagulation parameters in rats. In anaesthetized cats blood pressure, heart rate, ECG, respiration and ganglionic transmission was investigated. Guinea-pig ileum and vas deferens was studied in vitro.

In all tests, B-hGH, pituitary 22K-hGH, and pituitary human growth hormone behaved identically. No effect was observed on the autonomic nervous system, the parameters measured in the cats, and the coagulation parameters.

In the glucose tolerance test all 3 preparations as mentioned above caused a mild glucose intolerance. This implies that the well known diabetogenic effect of growth hormone is presumably linked to the 22K-molecule and that B-hGH can be expected to cause the same mild glucose intolerance in man that is observed after administration of human growth hormone of pituitary origin.

Toxicity

The acute toxicity of B-hGH is very low. 100 IE/kg bw given s.c. to rats caused no deaths, no clinical symptoms or adverse effects were observed within the 14 days observation period. Macroscopic pathology showed no changes though with the exceptions of some enlarged organs.

The 28 days toxicity tests in rats showed dose-dependent changes in body weight gain, food consumption and efficiency of food utilization that can be explained by the pharmacological action of B-hGH. No rats died, and there were no overt signs of reaction to treatment or changes of any toxicological significance in hematology, urinalyses or blood chemical values. B-hGH gave rise to increases in organ weights, to glandular hyperplasia of the mammary gland in female rats and to decidual reaction of the uterus, effects that are linked to the pharmacological effect.

CONCLUSION

Biosynthetic human growth hormone (B-hGH) has been manufactured using E.coli as the host. A product has been obtained identical to the 22K fraction of pituitary human growth hormome. The preparation is obtained in high purity. Biosynthetic human growth hormone has a physical, chemical and biological profile identical to human growth hormone of pituitary origin. Possible antigenicity has to be evaluated after clinical studies in humans.

REFERENCES

Aston, R., Cooper, L., Holder, A., Ivanyi, J., and Preece, M. (1985). Monoclonal antibodies to human growth hormone can distinguish between pituitary and genetically engineered forms. Molecular Immunology 22: 271.

Carlsen, S. and Jensen, E.B. (1986). Expression of amino extended human growth hormone in E.coli.Presented at Nordforsk Symposium 1986, Nyborg, Denmark, p. 56 (abstract).

Chawla, R.K., Parks, J.S., and Rudman, D. (1983). Structural variants of human growth hormone: Biochemical, genetic and clinical aspects. Ann. Rev. Med. 34: 519.

Christensen, T., Hansen, J.J., Sørensen, H.H., and Thomsen, J. (1986). RP-HPLC of biosynthetic and hypophyseal human growth hormone in "High performance liquid chromatography in biotechnology", ed. W.S. Hancock, John Wiley and Sons, Inc. (in press).

Christiansen, J.S., Ørskov, H., Binder, C., and Kastrup, K.W. (1983). Imitation of normal plasma growth hormone profile by subcutaneous administration of human growth hormone to growth hormone deficient children. Acta Endocrinologica 102: 6.

Dalbøge, H., Dahl, H-H.M., Pedersen, J., Hansen, J.W., and Christensen, T. (1986). A novel enzymatic method for production of authentic hGH from an E. coli produced hGH-precursor. Bio/Technology, accepted April 1986.

Dinesen, B. and Andersen, H.D. (1984). Monitoring the production of biosynthetic human growth hormone by micro enzymelinked immunosorbent assay. Anal. Chim. Acta. 163: 119.

Gomez, F., Pirens, G., Schaus, C., Closset, J., and Hennen, G. (1984). A highly sensitive radioimmunoassay for human growth hormone using a monoclonal antibody. J. Immuno assay 5: 145.

Kastrup, K.W., Christiansen, J.S., Andersen, J.K., and Ørskov, H. (1983). Increased growth rate following transfer to daily sc administration from three weekly im injections of hGH in growth hormone deficient children. Acta Endocrinologica 104: 148.

Urdea, M.S., Merryweather, J.P., Mullenbach, G.T., Coit, D., Heberlein, U., Valenzuela, P., and Barr, P.J. (1983). Chemical synthesis of a gene for human epidermal growth factor urogastrone and its expression in yeast. Proc. Natl. Acad. Sci. USA 80: 7461.

DELIVERY SYSTEMS FOR RECOMBINANT METHIONYL HUMAN GROWTH

Jerome A. Moore, Helga Wilking, and Ann L. Daugherty

Pharmacological Sciences
Genentech, Inc.

The advent of recombinant DNA technology has lead to an increased interest in convenient, effective pharmaceutical dosage forms for polypeptide drugs. It is well known that there are many obstacles to delivery of these compounds by conventional dosage forms. Large molecular weight, solubility problems, suseptibility to enzymatic degradation, sensitivity to pH and temperature, and short in vivo half life are some of the problems that must be confronted. For drugs with such complex biological activities as most therapeutic polypeptides one of the biggest obstacles to development of delivery systems is lack of information on the mechanism of action of the drug.

In order to design dosage forms for polypeptides one needs to ask some basic physiological questions:

How is the drug to be used?
What is the biological effect of the compound?
What is the target organ or cell population which mediates this effect?
What test systems are available for measuring the effects and
evaluating a dosage form?

For most products of recombinant DNA technology these questions are difficult to answer. Human growth hormone is an excellent model polypeptide to use to address these issues. It is used as replacement therapy in children suffering from hypopituitary dwarfism. Current therapeutic regimes require injections three times a week. Since the injections can be painful and inconvenient an alternate dosage form would be an improvement. As a result of the development of recombinant DNA methodology (Goeddel et al, 1979) plentiful supplies of this once scarce drug are now available to support a large scale research and development effort. A commercially available immunoradiometric assay makes determination of serum concentrations reliable and convenient. An efficacy model in rodents allows determination of biological activity.

This manuscript describes the test systems used to evaluate the absorption and efficacy of recombinant methionyl human growth hormone and discusses some of the efforts to deliver this polypeptide by alternate routes.

Test Systems

Serum concentrations of human growth hormone can be determined using an immunoradiometric assay (Tandem-R-HGH) produced by Hybritech, Inc. (La Jolla, CA). The assay uses a monoclonal antibody to methionyl human growth hormone coated onto a plastic bead. A second monoclonal antibody made to a different site on the met-hGH molecule is labeled with 125-I. Serum samples containing an unknown concentration of the hormone are incubated with both antibodies and excess labelled antibody is washed away. Radioactivity measured in a gamma counter is proportional to the concentration of met-hGH in the serum. Concentrations are computed by comparison of counts per minute to the linear regression of counts per minute versus growth hormone concentration for a set of standards.

The assay is highly specific for human growth hormone with negligible cross-reactivity from rodent growth hormones or other pituitary hormones. Only 100 microliters of serum is required for a single determination making it possible to take serial blood samples from a 100 gram rat. Sensitivity of 1 ng/ml makes this assay a valuable tool for determining circulating concentrations of hGH following administration by a variety of routes. Even routes of administration with low bioavailability are able to produce measurable concentrations with this assay.

Biological activity of human growth hormone can be determined in vivo using a method described by Wilhelmi (1973). Twenty-five to thirty day old female rats weighing approximately 100 grams have their pituitaries surgically removed resulting in cessation of growth. Following surgery body weights are monitored every two or three days. Rats with residual pituitary tissue will continue to grow about 1 gram per day. Animals which gain less than seven grams over a ten day period following surgery can safely be assumed to be hypophysectomized. Daily subcutaneous injections

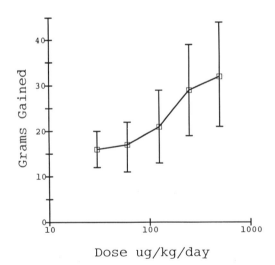

Figure 1. Mean weight gain (± standard deviation) of hypophysectomized rats after fifteen days of treatment versus the log of dose (μg/kg/day).

of human growth hormone produce body weight gain based on the dose of growth hormone. Growth is linear for about fifteen days and then starts to plateau. Figure 1 shows a plot of weight gain through fifteen days of treatment versus the log of the daily dose. The linear relationship shown in figure 1 makes it possible to compare preparations of drug or routes of administration to determine a relative potency value. A test substance and a standard are run at the same time in a parallel line bioassay to compute potency, confidence limits and index of precision as described by (Bliss,1956) .

These assays to determine serum concentrations and biological potency of the polypeptide are essential tools for the investigation of alternate delivery systems for hGH.

Continuous Subcutaneous Infusion

Human growth hormone is released from the anterior pituitary in a pulsatile pattern (Finkelstein, et al, 1972). Some of the delivery systems proposed for polypeptide drugs involve administration in temporal patterns very different from this natural secretion. Nasal and intestinal membrane barriers are not very permeable to high molecular weight compounds and may require prolonged exposure to permit absorption of therapeutically useful amounts of protein. It is important to determine the effect of sustained release of hGH on its efficacy.

A study was done to compare the potency of hGH given by single daily injection to that when given by continuous subcutaneous infusion. Alzet mini-osmotic pumps (Theeuwes and Yum , 1976) were filled with a solution of recombinant met-hGH at a concentration adjusted to infuse 5, 15, or 50 μg per day. The pumps were implanted subcutaneously in hypophysectomized female rats. Another group of rats received daily injections of the same solutions. Control animals received buffer solutions by the same routes. Daily body weights were measured for ten days. Figure 2 shows the gain in body weight over nine days versus the log of dose for the two routes of administration. The doses of hGH given by continuous infusion are based on measurements of the actual pumping rate of the infusion pumps rather than the rate stated on the manufacturer's package insert . The actual pumping rates were determined in a set of pumps from the same manufacturer's production lot and a group of rats identical to those used in the growth study. At two or three day intervals the pumps were removed, counted in a gamma counter, and replaced in the rats. Total hGH infused was estimated from loss in radioactivity from the pumps. The measured pumping rates were slightly greater in the first five days and a little slower in the last five days than the rate expected based on the manufacturer's information. In the growth study the pumps were filled with hGh at concentrations calculated to infuse the same total dose given to rats injected once daily assuming the pumps delivered the expected volume. Therefore the doses actually given by continuous infusion differed somewhat from those given as single daily injections. Through nine days of treatment the two groups had received the same amount of drug. A two way analysis-of-variance indicates that there was no difference in the weight gain based on the injection schedule. There are other issues that need to be considered in looking at continuous infusion such as immunogenicity, stability of hGH beyond the duration of this study, and other hormonal interactions but this experiment indicates that through nine days in this animal model continuous infusion of hGH is as effective as single daily injections.

The rat weight gain assay is a useful tool for these studies but it is somewhat time consuming taking five to ten days of treatment to produce a response that is well above background. A much more practical method would be to measure serum concentrations of hGH and then relate these to growth indirectly. This approach would also allow the experimenter the freedom to conduct studies in species useful for dosage form research such as the dog and the monkey in which a growth promoting model does not exist.

In order to collect data that would help define the relationship between serum concentrations and growth a study was conducted using the same treatment regimes described above for the continuous infusion study. Rats were given a single injection or a continuous infusion and killed at various times to collect samples of blood for serum hGH determination. Figure 3 shows the serum concentration versus time curves for both treatments. The low dose continuous infusion treatment was not performed in this study because the projected results would have been just at the sensitivity limits of the assay.

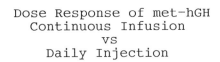

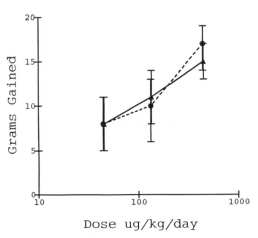

Dose ug/kg/day

Figure 2. Mean weight gain (± standard deviation) of hypophysectomized rats following subcutaneous administration of met hGH by single daily injection (triangle) or continuous infusion (circle).

Table 1 shows the peak heights and area under the curve for each dose tested by single injection and estimated steady state levels and AUC projected from these levels for the continuous infusion treatments. AUC for single injection animals is calculated by the trapezoid method (Notari,1980) and for continuous infusion by multiplying the steady state concentration by 1440 minutes. The steady state concentration is calculated from the mean of all measured values for the first 24 hours after implantation of the infusion pumps. The relationship between AUC and growth is roughly equivalent following single injection and continuous infusion with the possible exception of the high dose single injection group which is somewhat elevated. Whether this observation represents an actual difference in pharmacokinetics or merely statistical variation will be addressed more thoroghly in subsequent studies. Clearly many more doses will be required to completely define the relationship between serum concentration and growth but the data do help provide support for establishing a 'target' concentration that a delivery system under test should try to achieve.

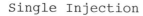
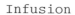

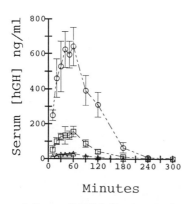
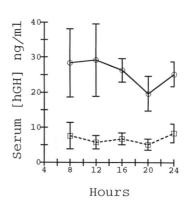

Figure 3. Serum [hGH] following single subcutaneous injection (left) of 500 μg/kg (circle), 150 μg/kg (square), 50 μg/kg (triangle) met hGH or during continuous infusion (right) of 500 μg/kg/24hr (circle) or 150 μg/kg/24hr (square).

Table 1. Relationship of serum concentrations to growth following treatment by single injection or continuous infusion of met-hGH.

Route	Dose	Maximum Concentration	Steady State Concentration	AUC	Growth
	μg/kg	ng/ml	ng/ml	ng-min/ml	grams/9 days
Daily	500	642		65100	15
Daily	150	156		13600	11
Daily	50	30		2400	3
Continuous	500		26	37400	17
Continuous	150		7	9800	10

Rectal Absorption

A number of reports in the literature have described compounds which may enhance the absorption of large water soluble molecules across biological membranes which would otherwise be barriers to the absorption of such drugs. Bile salts (Ziv et al,1981), lipid-bile salt mixed micelles (Muranishi et al, 1977 and Muranishi et al, 1980), enamine derivatives of amino acids and ethyl acetoacetate (Kamada et al, 1981 and Kim et al,1982), and salicylates (Nishihata et al,1982) have all been demonstrated to have absorption enhancing properties for high molecular weight compounds across the rectal mucosa. Some of these compounds were tested for enhancing properties with hGH across the rectal mucosa.

Acetyl salicylate, sodium salicylate, and an enamine derivative of phenylalanine and ethyl acetoacetate were mixed with human growth hormone in a cocoa butter base and rectally administered to 300 gram anesthetized rats. Blood samples were collected and serum hGH concentrations used to evaluate absorption. The concentration of enhancer was 4, 10, or 40 mg/g of cocoa butter and of met hGH was 5 mg/g. Suppositories weighed approximately 200 mg each making the dose of hGh about 3 mg/kg body weight. Table 2 shows the mean serum concentrations at various time points following rectal administration of hGH with three different concentrations of each of the three potential enhancers tested. Standard deviations are included with means for the highest concentration tested for each compound.

Both sodium salicylate and the enamine derivative enhanced absorption of hGH across the rectal mucosa of rats in a dose related manner. It is interesting to compare the serum concentrations following administration of 3 mg/kg hGH in rectal suppositories containing 40 mg/g sodium salicylate to those seen in figure 3 following subcutaneous injection of 150 μg/kg. While these studies were not specifically designed to determine bioavailability, it appears from the above comparison that the bioavailability of the rectal formulation tested was greater than 5%. It was important to determine if the hGH absorbed had biological activity. Sodium salicylate was used in a subsequent experiment to determine the growth promoting activity of hGH absorbed from rectal suppositories. Rectal suppositories were prepared as described above and administered to hypophysectomized rats daily for ten days. Control animals received suppositories containing sodium salicylate and the same excipients present in the growth hormone preparation.Body weights were measured daily. Figure 4 shows the weight gain of the two groups. Growth hormone treated animals gained significantly more weight than controls (t=4.26 , df=17, p<0.001). This study provides convincing evidence that the growth hormone being absorbed has biological activity.

Bile salts have been reported to promote absorption of insulin (Ziv et al, 1981) across the rectal mucosa. The hypophysectomized rat model employed above was a convenient model for testing the effects of bile salts on hGH absorption.

Rectal suppositories containing hGH and sodium glycocholate were prepared as before and administered to hypophysectomized rats. HGH was administered at daily doses of 100 μg or 500 μg per animal. Glycocholate doses were 200 μg and 1mg. Control groups included treatment with suppositories containing 500 μg hGH with no glycocholate and suppositories of cocoa butter alone. Body weight gains over ten days were compared to those of animals receiving daily intramuscular injections of

Table 2. Serum concentration of hGH following administration of met hGH with absorption promoters in cocoa butter based rectal suppositories.

	Serum [hGH] ng/ml								
Minutes After Treatment	Sodium Salicylate (mg/g)			Acetyl Salicylate (mg/g)			Enamine Derivative (mg/g)		
	4	10	40	4	10	40	4	10	40
5	42	102	181±90	14	0	3±6	4	40	148±83
10	62	129	179±91	0	4	0±0	10	50	185±105
20	54	91	181±97	2	2	8±14	6	26	107±76
30	37	65	184±107	4	5	8±14	2	13	61±44
45	0	19	219±155	0	0	12±20	0	5	29±27
60	10	32	178±128	0	0	0±0	0	11	18±17
90	7	19	174±135	0	0	5±8	0	0	10±9

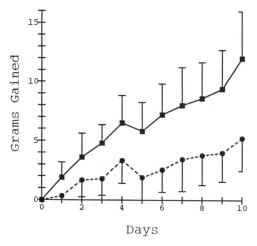

Growth of Hypophysectomized
Rats Given
Rectal Suppositories

Grams Gained

Days

Figure 4. Growth of hypophysectomized rats treated daily with rectal suppositories containing sodium salicylate and met hGH (square) compared to controls (circle). (circle).

10 μg or 50 μg hGH. Figure 5 shows the mean weight gained in the various treatment groups. The addition of sodium glycocholate does appear to have some effect on weight gain. As was the case with sodium salicylate growth following treatment with hGH and glycocholate was greater than that with no hGH. Treatment with hGH alone in cocoa butter did produce some growth but not as much as with the addition of the bile salt.

The technical aspects of administering cocoa butter based suppositories rectally to rats are far from optimized. Loss of drug from defecation or premature melting of the dosage form likely resulted in dosing below the prescribed level. The concentration of hGH in the suppositories , however, was high enough to provide the rats with a dose of hGH approximately twenty five times the injected dose that would have produced equivalent growth. Optimization of the concentrations of components in the dosage form and increased bioavailability are clearly required for making this a viable alternative for hGH therapy. Another concern is that the use of absoption enhancers leads to non-specific absorption of colonic contents.

Intestinal Absorption

Sodium salicylate was tested for absorption enhancing properties in higher levels of the gastrointestinal tract. Rats were anesthetized and a midline incision was made to expose the GI tract. Mixtures of hGH with or without sodium salicylate in an aqueous solution or suspended in mineral oil were injected directly into the stomach, duodenum, ileum or colon. The area around the injection was ligated to prevent leakage or migration of the injected material. Blood samples were collected and serum hGH was determined. Negligible absorption was seen in the stomach or duodenum regardless of the preparation tested. In the colon and in the ileum ,however, surprisingly high serum concentrations resulted from the combination of sodium salicylate with mineral oil. Figure 6 shows a plot of the hGH concentration versus time in the colon following injection of the four formulations. The area under the curve was cal-

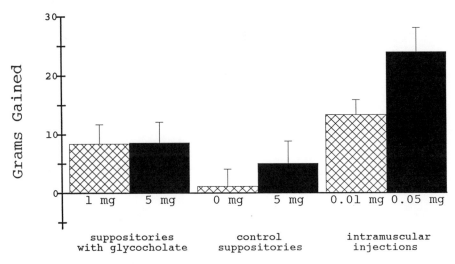

Figure 5. Growth of hypophysectomized rats given daily rectal suppositories compared to growth following intramuscular injections.

culated using the trapezoid method and compared to the area under the curve following intravenous injection in an identical group of animals. Table 3 shows the bioavailability determined for each preparation in each region of the GI tract. The table illustrates the fact that absorption from the lower levels of the GI tract using salicylate plus mineral oil is far greater than any other combination tested.

A two way analysis of variance was performed on the bioavailabilities testing for the presence or absence of salicylate and the presence or absence of mineral oil in the four regions of the GI tract. A significant interaction between the main effects was seen in the ileum ($F=5.36$, $df=1,20$, $p<0.05$) and in the colon ($F=10.89$, $df=1,16$, $p<0.01$). A significant interaction effect in such a test is an indication of interference or synergism (Sokal and Rohlf, 1981). Since the results here are in a positive direction, this study has shown that sodium salicylate and mineral oil act synergistically to enhance the absorption of hGH from lower levels of the GI tract of rats.

The mechanism of the synergistic relationship between sodium salicylate and mineral oil can only be speculated upon at this time. One possibility is that the mineral oil serves as a reservoir for sodium salicylate thus prolonging the effects of the enhancer.

An animal model useful for screening intranasal formulations has been reported by Hirai (1981) and adapted for use in the following studies. Male rats weighing 300 to 400 grams were anesthetized and placed on a heated pad to maintain body temperature. The nasal cavity was blocked at the back of the nasopharnx and the naso-palatine openings were sealed. Trachael intubation allowed the animal to continue breathing. Test formulations in carefully measured 70 microliter volumes were infused into the external nares with a pipet tip and the nares were sealed with polyacrylamide adhesive. At various times after dosing blood samples were collected via a catheter placed in the femoral artery and plasma concentration of hGH deter-

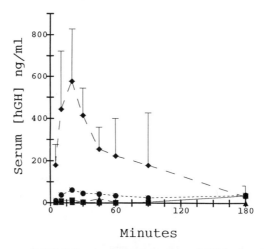

Figure 6. Mean serum [hGH] following injection of met hGH in four formulations into the colon. Formulations tested were aqueous buffer (triangles), salicylate in aqueous buffer (squares), mineral oil (circles), and salicylate in mineral oil (diamonds with standard deviation indicated).

Table 3. Bioavailability of met hGH from various levels of the GI tract of rats.

Formulation	Stomach	Duodenum	Ileum	Colon
Aqueous Buffer	<1	1.0±1.1	<1	<1
Salicylate & Buffer	<1	<1	<1	<1
Mineral Oil	1.0±0.5	2.9±3.7	2.3±2.4	1.6±2.3
Salicylate & Oil	<1	1.7±1.2	7.0±4.7	9.5±4.3

mined. This system is quite invasive but nevertheless serves as a useful preliminary screening method to study absorption across the nasal mucosa.

The effects of a non-ionic surfactant, polyoxyethylene 9-lauryl ether, and a bile salt, sodium deoxycholate, on intranasal absorption of hGH were tested using the animal model described above. Recombinant methionyl human growth hormone was reconstituted with a 1% aqueous solution of one of the surfactants to produce the proper concentration of growth hormone to provide a dose of 1, 2, or 3 mg hGH per kg body weight. All animals were treated with the same volume of test drug therefore the concentration of hGH varied from 4 mg/ml to 16 mg/ml depending on dose.

Figure 7 shows the plasma concentration versus time following intranasal administration of the surfactants. Both surfactants promote absorption of hGH. Higher doses of hGH lead to higher plasma concentrations. Bioavailability computed by comparing the AUC of the curves in figure 7 to the AUC following intravenous injection is shown in table 4.

Plasma concentrations following administration of hGH with no enhancer were undetectable at doses of 1 mg/kg or 2 mg/kg. Even at 3 mg/kg the bioavailability was less than 1%. A different pattern is observed with the two surfactants tested. The bioavailability with 9-lauryl ether is the same regardless of the dose of hGH. Since dose is taken into account when computing bioavailability this simply means that the AUC is directly proportional to the dose. In the case of deoxycholate, however, the bioavailability increases with increasing dose. Increasing flux across the nasal mucosa with increasing concentration of drug in the test formulation has been reported (Anik,et al 1984). As stated above the dosage volume remained constant in this study so the higher doses were administered at higher concentrations.

Speculation into the mechanisms of absorption enhancement leads to the discussion of tissue damage resulting from nasal administration of surfactants. This issue was addressed in the current study by treating animals with hGH in 1%

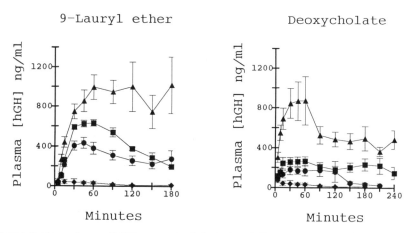

Figure 7. Mean plasma [hGH] ± standard deviation following intranasal administration of met hGH in 1% 9lauryl ether (left) or 1% sodium deoxycholate (right). Doses of met-hGH were 1 mg/kg (circles), 2 mg/kg (squares), or 3 mg/kg (triangles) with enhancer or 3 mg/kg without enhancer (diamonds).

Table 4. Effects of surfactants on the intranasal bioavailability of met hGH in rats.

Absolute Bioavailability			
Enhancer	Dose mg/kg		
	1	2	3
9-Lauryl Ether	45±15	45±15	41±22
Deoxycholate	17±9	21±13	36±21
Control	<1	<1	0.96±0.23

solutions of 9-lauryl ether or sodium glycocholate, killing by decapitation, and excising the nasal region of the skull. The specimens were fixed in 10% formalin, placed in decalcifying solution (Easy Cut, American Histology Reagent Co. , Stockton, CA), embedded in paraffin and cut in 4 to 6 micron sections. The sections were stained with alcian blue Periodic Acid-Schiff (PAS) to visualize goblet cells which contain mucin or with hemotoxylin and eosin to study mucous membrane structure.

Light microscopic histopathological examinations revealed significant tissue damage resulting from treatment with hGH in 1% 9-lauryl ether. Inflammation and multifocal necrosis was evident within 30 minutes of treatment. This treatment also induced reduction in numbers of PAS positive mucosal goblet cells as a result of cell loss and reduced staining of intact cells. Tissue damage resulting from treatment with hGH in 1% glycocholate was minor and indistinguishable from that caused by treatment with hGH alone.

It is highly likely in light of this histopathological information that the mechanism of absorption enhancement of 9-lauryl ether is through widespread disruption of the mucosal epithelium. Such effects even if transient are clearly unacceptable for human use. A number of mechanisms are possible for the absorption promoting activity of sodium deoxycholate such as mild membrane disruption as seen by another bile salt, sodium glycochoalte, in this study, formation of reverse micelles in the nasal membrane as described by Gordon et al (1985), or inhibition of proteolytic enzymes as described in the case of insulin by Hirai et al (1981b).

General Discussion

The experiments discussed above describe some promising possibilities for the delivery of polypeptide drugs. For a number of reasons, some practical and some physiological, human growth hormone is an excellent polypeptide to use in the development stages of this effort. The drug is very safe making concerns over day to day fluctuations in bioavailability much less serious than in the case of insulin. Test systems are available to determine serum concentrations and biological activity. Plentiful supplies of hGH are available for research and development projects.

Many of the fundamental elements of an alternate dosage form have been defined. Sustaining the release of the hormone to produced lower serum concentrations over a longer period of time is at least as effective as injecting it in a form which is quickly cleared from the circulation. Some preliminary pharmacokinetic data have been collected and assays have been described that will permit the determination of the relationship between serum concentrations and growth. It would appear, based on these studies, that absorption from an oral or intranasal formulation might be possible but would require the use of absorption promoting compounds. The use of such compounds would require extensive toxicological studies on tissue damage and effects of nonspecific absorption of bacterial proteins. Since studies such as the ones described here represent early attempts to develop alternate delivery systems the formulations have not been optimized. Enhancers have been used at concentrations that may far exceed those required in an optimized preparation.

While data such as those presented here show promise, many obstacles still stand between these biological phenomena and pharmaceutical realities. The major tasks which face the pharmaceutical industry involve physical chemistry and physiology. Careful characterization of the polypeptide in the dosage form is essential to the understanding of data such as those presented here. Relevant, reliable animal models are necessary to understand the physiological effects of the drug and evaluate the dosage form. The success of the industry in developing safe, effective and convenient dosage forms for polypeptide drugs will depend upon its success in coordinating the efforts of the physical chemist and the physiologist.

References

Anik, S.T., McRae, G., Nerenberg, C., Worden, A., Foreman, J., Hwang, J., Kushinsky, S., Jones, R.E. and Vickery, B., 1984, Nasal Absorption of Nafarelin Acetate, the Decapeptide [D-Nal (2)6] LHRH, in Rhesus Monkeys. *J. Pharm. Sci.* 73:684.

Bliss, C.I., 1956, Confidence limits for measuring the precision of bioassays. *Biometrics,* 12:491.

Finkelstein, J.W., Roffwarg, H.P., Boyar, R.M., Kream, J. and Hellman, L., 1972, Age related change in the twenty-four hour spontaneous secretion of growth hormone. *J. Clin. Endocrinol. Metab.* 35:665.

Goeddel, D.V., Heynecker, H.L., Hozumi, T., Arentzen, R., Itakura, K., Yansura, D.G., Ross, M.J., Miozzari, G., Crea, R., Seeburg, P.H., 1979, Direct expression in Escherichia coli of a DNA sequence coding for human growth hormone. *Nature,* 281:544.

Gordon, G.S., Moses, A.C., Silver, R.D., Flier, J.S. and Carey, M.C., 1985, Nasal Absorption of Insulin: Enhancement by Hydrophobic Bile Salts. *Proc. Nat'l. Acad. Sci. USA* 82:7419.

Hirai, S., Yashiki, T. and Mima, H., 1981a, Absorption of Drugs from the Nasal Mucosa of Rat. *Int. J. Pharm.* 7:317.

Hirai, S., Yashiki, T. and Mima, H., 1981b, Mechanisms for the enhancement of the nasal absorption of insulin by surfactants. *Int. J. Pharm.* 9:173.

Kamada, A., Nishihata, T., Kim, S., Yamamoto, M.,and Yata, N., 1981, Study of enamine derivatives of phenylglycine on the rectal absorption of insulin. *Chem. Pharm. Bull.,* 29:2012.

Kim, S., Kamada, A., Higuchi, T., and Nishihata, T., 1982, Effect of enamine derivatives on the rectal absorption of insulin in dogs and rabbits. *J. Pharm. Pharmacol.,* 35:100.

Muranishi, N., Kinugawa, M., Nakajima, Y.,Muranishi, S., and Sezaki, H., 1980, Mechanism for the inducement of intestinal absorption of poorly absorbed drugs by mixed micelles I. Effects of various lipid-bile salt mixed micelles on the intestinal absorption of streptomycin in rat. *Int. J. Pharm.,* 4:271.

Muranishi, S., Tokunaga, Y., Taniguchi, K.,and Sezaki, H., 1977, Potential absorption of heparin from the small intestine and the large intestine in the presence of monoolein mixed micelles. *Chem. Pharm. Bull.,* 25:1159.

Nishihata, T., Rytting, J., Kamada, A., Higuchi, T., Routh, M., and Caldwell, L., 1982, Enhancement of rectal absorption of insulin using salicylates in dogs. *J. Pharm. Pharmacol.,* 35:148.

Notari, R. E., Biopharmaceutics and Clinical Pharmacokinetics, Marcel Dekker, Inc., New York, 1980, p.86.

Sokal, R.R. and Rohlf, F.J., Biometry, W. H. Freeman and Co., San Francisco,1981, p. 329.

Theeuwes, F. and Yum, S.I., 1976, Principles of the design and operation of generic osmotic pumps for the delivery of semisolid or liquid formulations. *Ann. Biomed. Eng.* 4:343.

Wilhelmi, A.E., Growth hormone-measurement-bioassay. In: Berson, S.A., Yalow, R.S. (eds) Methods in Investigative and Diagnostic Endocrinology. North Holland, Amsterdam, vol 2A (1973) 296.

Ziv, E., Kidron, M., Berry, E. M.,and Bar-On, H., 1981, Bile salts promote the absorption of insulin from the rat colon. *Life Sciences,* 29:803.

ELEDOISIN AND CERULETIDE, TWO NATURALLY OCCURRING PEPTIDE DRUGS OF NONMAMMALIAN ORIGIN

Roberto de Castiglione

Farmitalia Carlo Erba SpA
Research & Development
Via dei Gracchi 35
20146 Milan, Italy

INTRODUCTION

Poor absorption and metabolic instability usually make the parenteral route of administration the sole practical one for peptide drugs. Restricted permeability of the blood-brain barrier to peptides may constitute another drawback. The availability of suitable delivery systems could possibly extend the field of application of these drugs. On the other hand, technical problems and uncertain forecast of return of investment often actually limit the studies in this area. This was also the case with eledoisin and ceruletide, two naturally occurring peptide drugs developed in our laboratories as a result of a long and continuous collaboration with Prof. V. Erspamer in the field of biologically active peptides of nonmammalian origin.

ELEDOISIN

Eledoisin is an undecapeptide of formula Glp-Pro-Ser-Lys-Asp-Ala-Phe-Ile-Gly-Leu-Met-NH$_2$, originally isolated from the methanol extracts of the posterior salivary glands of Eledone moschata and Eledone Aldrovandi, two Mediterranean molluscan species belonging to the octopod Cephalopoda (Erspamer & Anastasi, 1962; Anastasi and Erspamer, 1963).

Eledoisin is the prototype of tachykinins, a peptide family so named because of their prompt action on the smooth muscle, as opposed to the group of the slow-acting kinins, the bradykinins. Tachykinins include an increasing number of peptides from amphibian skin and from mammalian gut and brain (Harmar, 1984; Erspamer et al., 1985; and citations herein), characterized by the common COOH-terminal sequence Phe-X-Gly-Y-Met-NH$_2$, where X is a hydrophobic aliphatic or aromatic residue and Y is usually Leu (only in one case Y is Met) (Fig. 1). As expected, this evolutionary conservative sequence constitutes also the minimal structural requirement for bioactivity (Bernardi et al., 1964). Mammalian representatives are the well-known substance P and the recently discovered substance K and neuromedin K.

Molluscans:

Glp-*Pro*-Ser-Lys-*Asp*-*Ala*-*Phe*-*Ile*-*Gly*-*Leu*-*Met*-*NH*$_2$ Eledoisin

Amphibians:

Glp-Ala-Asp-Pro-Asn-Lys-*Phe*-Tyr-*Gly*-*Leu*-*Met*-*NH*$_2$ Physalaemin

Glp-Ala-Asp-Pro-Lys-Thr-*Phe*-Tyr-*Gly*-*Leu*-*Met*-*NH*$_2$ [Lys^5,Thr^6]-physalaemin

Glp-*Pro*-Asp-Pro-Asn-*Ala*-*Phe*-Tyr-*Gly*-*Leu*-*Met*-*NH*$_2$ Uperolein I

Glp-Ala-Asp-Pro-Lys-Thr-*Phe*-Tyr-*Gly*-*Leu*-*Met*-*NH*$_2$ Uperolein II

Glp-Asn-Pro-Asn-Arg-*Phe*-*Ile*-*Gly*-*Leu*-*Met*-*NH*$_2$ Phyllomedusin

Asp-Val-*Pro*-Lys-Ser-*Asp*-Gln-*Phe*-Val-*Gly*-*Leu*-*Met*-*NH*$_2$ Kassinin

Asp-Glu-*Pro*-Lys-Pro-*Asp*-Gln-*Phe*-Val-*Gly*-*Leu*-*Met*-*NH*$_2$ [Glu^2,Pro^5]-kassinin

Asp-Pro-*Pro*-Asp-Pro-*Asp*-Arg-*Phe*-Tyr-*Gly*-Met-Met-*NH*$_2$ Hylambatin

Mammals   :

Arg-Pro-Lys-Pro-Gln-Gln-*Phe*-Phe-*Gly*-*Leu*-*Met*-*NH*$_2$ Substance P

His-Lys-Thr-*Asp*-Ser-*Phe*-Val-*Gly*-*Leu*-*Met*-*NH*$_2$ Substance K (neurokinin α)

Asp-Met-His-*Asp*-Phe-*Phe*-Val-*Gly*-*Leu*-*Met*-*NH*$_2$ Neuromedin K (neurokinin β)

Fig. 1. Amino acid sequences of the tachykinin family

In addition to their spasmogenic activity on the extravascular smooth musculature, tachykinins display also potent vasodilating and hypotensive effects by a direct action on the smooth muscle, powerful stimulation of the salivary and lachrymal secretion by a direct action on the secretory cells (Erspamer and Melchiorri, 1973; Bertaccini, 1976; Holzer-Petsche et al., 1985), and variable effects on the central nervous system (CNS) and the anterior pituitary (Erspamer and Melchiorri, 1983).

Because of its vasodilating activity, eledoisin was initially proposed for clinical use in the treatment of peripheral vascular diseases such as Raynaud's disease, claudicatio intermittens, arteriosclerotic arteriopaty, and acute thrombosis of large arterial trunks. All systemic administration routes were used: intramuscular (i.m.), intravenous (i.v.), i.v. infusion, and intraarterial (i.a.). The best results were obtained by rapid i.v. injection and by i.v. infusion. By rapid i.v. route, doses of 5-10 ng/Kg caused a well evident hypotensive effect without any sign of intolerance. Doses ranging between 30 and 60 ng/Kg proved to be the upper limit of tolerance (Sicuteri et al., 1962). With slow i.v. infusion, the best posology appeared to be 100-200 mcg of the drug in 250 ml of saline solution, at the rate of 20-40 drops/min (Sicuteri et al., 1962).

The product was registered for systemic administration, under the trade name of Eloisin, as a 1 ml ampoule containing 50 mcg of active ingredient in aqueous solution. In spite of the positively favorable effects, however, it was never used routinely in this therapeutic indication, due to the extremely short-lasting action by the systemic route, practically observed only at the time of administration. Attempts to prolong the life of the drug by modifying either the chemical structure (synthesis of analogues) or the pharmaceutical formulation (choice of appropriate vehicles), or both, had limited succes (Stürmer and Fanchamps, 1965; Bernardi et al., 1967) and were not prosecuted.

Eledoisin, on the contrary, could find a well-defined, though limited, therapeutic allocation in ophthalmology by exploiting its stimulatory activity on the lachrymal secretion, exerted not only by the systemic route but also by topical administration. The peptide is currently used as eye-drops in all those pathological conditions in which lachrymal secretion is required, such as keratoconjunctivitis sicca, Sjögren's syndrome, senile xerophthalmia and hyposecretion due to irradiation or ablation of the main lachrymal glands. In normal individuals eledoisin is practically ineffective (Impicciatore et al., 1973). Particularly in the more severe diseases, such as Sjögren's syndrome, eledoisin is a unique drug, and its ethical value greatly outweighs any profitability consideration.

The drug is available as a 0.4 mg/ml collyrium to be reconstituted at the moment of the use from a freeze-dried mixture of eledoisin trifluoroacetate and mannitol. Doses are usually a drop (20 mcg) per eye by instillation in the lower conjunctival fornix 3 times a days.

No real attempts were made in order to increase the duration of action of the collyrium. A promising clue in this direction was provided by the observation that the lachrymal stimulating effect was not only greater, but lasted three times longer by combining the instillation of eledoisin with the application of a soft contact lens presoaked in the same solution (Bietti et al., 1976).

CERULETIDE

Ceruletide, international nonproprietary name (INN) proposed by the World Health Organization (WHO) for caerulein, is a sulphated decapeptide of formula Glp-Gln-Asp-Tyr(SO$_3$H)-Thr-Gly-Trp-Met-Asp-Phe-NH$_2$, first isolated from the methanol extracts of the skin of the Australian hylid frog Litoria (Hyla) caerulea (Anastasi et al., 1967). It belongs to a peptide family that has its mammalian counterparts in the different forms of gastrin and cholecystokinin (CCK), two gastrointestinal hormones present also in the CNS, where they play a neurotransmitter or neuromodulatory role (Fig. 2). Ceruletide, or a ceruletide-like peptide, is considered the common precursor from which both gastrin and CCK have evolved (Larsson and Rehfeld, 1977).

The peptides of this group share a common COOH-terminal pentapeptide and display very similar spectra of biological activity, differing only in the intensity of their effects. Discriminating in this regard is the presence and location of a sulphated tyrosine residue. The tetrapeptide amide (CCK-4) constitutes the biological active site of the larger molecular forms. Ceruletide closely resembles CCK-8 both in structure and biological properties, but is much more stable to degrading enzymes (Deschodt-Lanckman et al., 1981).

The gastrointestinal actions that can be regarded as physiological for CCK include stimulation of pancreatic enzyme secretion, stimulation of gallbladder contraction, relaxation of the sphincter of Oddi, inhibition of gastric emptying, trophic action on pancreatic growth, and stimulation of small intestinal and colonic activity (Solomon, 1983).

Amphibians:

$$\overset{\displaystyle SO_3H}{\overset{\displaystyle |}{Glp\text{-}Gln\text{-}Asp\text{-}Tyr\text{-}Thr\text{-}Gly\text{-}Trp\text{-}Met\text{-}Asp\text{-}Phe\text{-}NH_2}} \qquad Caerulein$$

$$\overset{\displaystyle SO_3H}{\overset{\displaystyle |}{Glp\text{-}Gln\text{-}Tyr\text{-}Thr\text{-}Gly\text{-}Trp\text{-}Met\text{-}Asp\text{-}Phe\text{-}NH_2}} \qquad Phyllocaerulein$$

$$\overset{\displaystyle SO_3H}{\overset{\displaystyle |}{Glp\text{-}Asn\text{-}Asp\text{-}Tyr\text{-}Leu\text{-}Gly\text{-}Trp\text{-}Met\text{-}Asp\text{-}Phe\text{-}NH_2}} \qquad [Asn^2, Leu^5]\text{-}caerulein$$

Mammals :

$$\overset{\displaystyle SO_3H}{\overset{\displaystyle |}{\ldots Asp\text{-}\mathbf{Arg}\text{-}Asp\text{-}Tyr\text{-}Met\text{-}Gly\text{-}Trp\text{-}Met\text{-}Asp\text{-}Phe\text{-}NH_2}} \qquad Cholecystokinin$$

$$\overset{\displaystyle R}{\overset{\displaystyle |}{\ldots Glu\text{-}Glu\text{-}Glu\text{-}Ala\text{-}Tyr\text{-}Gly\text{-}Trp\text{-}Met\text{-}Asp\text{-}Phe\text{-}NH_2}} \qquad \begin{array}{l} Gastrin \ \ I \ (R = H) \\ Gastrin \ II \ (R = SO_3H) \end{array}$$

Fig. 2. Amino acid sequences of caerulein-like peptides

On account of its CCK-like activity, ceruletide has found clinical application in diagnostics and in therapy under the registered trademark of Takus, Ceosunin, Cerulex and Tymtran. As a diagnostic agent ceruletide is currently used in cholecystography and cholangiography, X-ray examination of the bowel and testing of pancreatic exocrine function. Therapeutic applications are the treatment of intestinal atony and paralytic ileus.

The product is available either as a solution of ceruletide diethylamine salt containing sodium thiomalate as antioxidant (ampules dosed at 5 and 40 or 20 mcg) or as a freeze-dried formulation with lactose as bulking agent (vials dosed at 5 and 30 mcg). The more stable freeze-dried ampules were not developed for marketing reasons.

Posology varies according to indications and mode of administration. The drug is usually administered by slow i.v. injection (at the dosage of 0.050 mcg/Kg) in the radiological examination of the extrahepatic bile ducts with intraoperative cholangiography; by i.v. infusion (1-2 ng/Kg/min for 15 min to 2-3 hr) in the diagnosis of pancreatic diseases and in the treatment of diagnosed paralytic ileus; and by i.m. injection (at the dosage of 0.3 mcg/Kg) in the radiological examination of the gallbladder and alimentary tract, and in the treatment of postoperative intestinal atony and chronic fecal stasis.

Alternative routes of administration (namely intranasal, rectal and intragastric) have been tested in experimental animals and in humans. The intranasal route proved to be the most effective. In humans the cholecystokinetic response to a dose of 0.5 mcg/Kg of ceruletide as a spray was approximately matched by the response to doses of 0.5 and 0.05 mcg/Kg i.m. and i.v., respectively. Nasal absorption was confirmed in the dog, and the effect was found to be due only to absorption by the mucous membrane of the upper respiratory tract (Agosti and Bertaccini, 1969). In other studies in human volunteers, 1 mcg/Kg of ceruletide by spray produced about the same cholecystokinetic (Orlandini and Agosti, 1969) and gastric secretory effect (Agosti et al., 1969) as 0.5 mcg/Kg i.m.

Gastrointestinal absorption of ceruletide was indirectly evaluated in the guinea pig by measuring the cholecystokinetic activity in situ after intrarectal and intragastric administration of an aqueous solution by intubation. The intensity and duration of the effect was compared with that obtained by the i.v. route. Whereas for maximal contraction peak extremely high rectal and intragastric doses were required (1000-2000 and 2000-4000 times higher, respectively, than by rapid i.v. injection), the same contraction curve area for the two routes of administration was reached at doses which were only 75-100 and 100-300 times as high, respectively, as those required by a 2 hr i.v. infusion (di Salle and Ragazzi, 1976).

In a clinical study, the action of ceruletide on gastric secretion after administration by rectal route (suppositories dosed at 300 mcg) was compared with that obtained when the drug was administered i.m. (0.5 mcg/Kg body weight). The secretagogue effect was, on the average, less evident when ceruletide was administered by rectum. In duodenal ulcer patients, however, unlike in normal subjects, the difference between the secretory responses following the two routes of administration was minimal, probably as a consequence of a higher sensitivity of parietal cells to low blood concentration of secretagogue peptides in patients with duodenal ulcer than in normal subjects (Grossi et al., 1980).

Although the reported trials proved the efficacy of ceruletide by alternative routes of administration, particularly by nasal absorption, the present limited diagnostic and therapeutic applications did not justify further studies aimed at obtaining valid pharmaceutical formulations for practical medical use. On the other hand, the availability of such formulations would have probably extended the field of application of the drug in other directions, such as, e.g., the treatment of chronic pancreatitis (Pap et al., 1981).

The great expectations offered in recent times by ceruletide as an effective analgesic and antipsychotic agent have been revised. Although the efficacy of the peptide in selected schizophrenic patients is still under study and requires confirmation, the pain-relieving activity has been firmly established only in biliary colics, mainly due to relaxation of the sphincter of Oddi and the ensuing decrease of intracholedocal pressure and bile duct distension (Basso et al., 1985). True analgesia, on the contrary, is rather weak and probably masked by other central effects, such as sedation and other mood modifications (de Castiglione and Rossi, 1985).

MANUFACTURING

Both eledoisin and ceruletide are manufactured by chemical syntheses using classical solution methods, as outlined in Figs. 3 and 4. The two products are eventually obtained as hydrated trifluoroacetate and diethylamine salts, respectively. A number

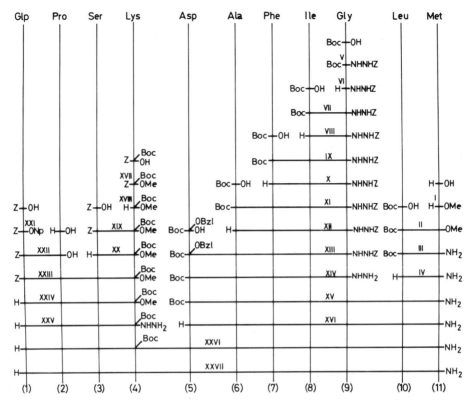

Fig. 3. Scheme of synthesis of eledoisin

of manufacturing, formulation and analytical problems have been encountered and solved during the development of the two drugs (de Castiglione, 1983). At variance with the reported publication, eledoisin is now directly obtained and purified as trifluoroacetate.

Both syntheses require a final coupling of two segments by the azide method (4+7, eledoisin; 6+4, ceruletide). In the case of eledoisin, also the COOH-terminal heptapeptide is obtained by this procedure. Quite unexpectedly for a peptide, it was observed, during the scale-up of the synthesis, that some lots of eledoisin trifluoroacetate presented a slightly positive activity in the in vitro Ames' mutagenic test, particularly with the Salmonella typhimurium TA 1535 strain without metabolic activation. This effect was proportional to the concentration of the sample and independent from the peptide purity (Castellino et al., in preparation). The responsible agent was water-soluble, since mutagenicity could be reduced by precipitation of the product from aqueous solutions. Complete removal could be achieved only when efficaceous washings were feasible, or by counter-current distribution in appropriate solvent mixtures. The last procedure, being the most effective and reproducible one, is currently used in the manufacturing of eledoisin.

This phenomenon is quite general, as similar mutagenic

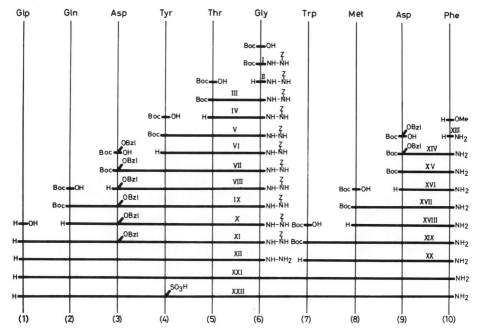

Fig. 4. Scheme of synthesis of ceruletide

activity was found also in other peptides obtained by final segment condensation by the azide method, and is probably attributable to trace amounts (p.p.m.) of azidic contaminants. The same peptides, in fact, synthesized through a different final coupling (e.g., by the mixed anhydride procedure) did not show any sign of positive reaction to the Ames' test (de Castiglione et al., 1981). In the case of ceruletide, due to the different work-up, a very slight mutagenicity can be detected only in the coupling reaction product (unsulphated decapeptide). Crude ceruletide is itself already free from mutagenic contaminants.

CONCLUDING REMARKS

Eledoisin and ceruletide are two hormone-like peptides of nonmammalian origin which are currently manufactured by chemical synthesis and have found a well-defined, although limited, use as therapeutic and diagnostic agents.

The potential applications of these two drugs (particularly in the therapeutic field, where repeated administrations or prolonged effects are required) have been drastically reduced by the same drawbacks common to most peptide drugs: low bioavailability after oral administration due to their non-lipophilicity and instability to peptidases in the gastrointestinal tract, which limit the route of administration to injections; and biological half-lives often so short that frequent administration is needed to maintain their action.

The present limited use and, most important in some cases, the lack of a real medical need have not justified in the past efforts aimed at realizing valid alternative delivery systems, which, however, if available, would have increased and extended the field of application of these two peptide drugs.

An observation made during the development of the synthesis of eledoisin, but of far larger extension, is worth mentioning. Hormone-like peptides are, almost by definition, non mutagenic. The synthetic replicates, however, when obtained by an azide coupling, can contain trace of azidic contaminants which are positive to the in vitro Ames' mutagenic test. These contaminants, which are water-soluble, can withstand purification by the usual chromatographic methods. We have been able to completely remove them by counter-current distribution in appropriate solvent systems (which are not, necessarily, the best ones for removal of peptide impurities). Whatever the meaning of the Salmonella thyphimurium mutagenic test for these contaminants (sodium azide belongs to the "false positive" group of mutagens) (Owais et al., 1983), this observation constitutes a general warning for peptide drugs obtained by procedures based on azide formation.

REFERENCES

Agosti, A. and Bertaccini, G., 1969, Nasal absorption of caerulein, The Lancet, March 15:580.
Agosti, A., Biasoli, S., and Naranjo, G., 1969, Azione della ceruleina sulla secrezione gastrica umana, Soc. Ital. Biol. Sperim., 45:778.
Anastasi, A., and Erspamer V., 1963, The isolation and amino acid sequence of eledoisin, the active endecapeptide of the posterior salivary glands of Eledone, Arch. Biochem. Biophys., 101:56.
Anastasi, A., Erspamer, V., and Endean, R., 1967, Isolation and structure of caerulein, an active decapeptide from the skin of Hyla caerulea, Experientia, 23:699.
Basso, N., Bagarani, M., Materia, A., Gizzonio, D., De Paolis, C., Praga, C., and Speranza, V., 1985, Effect of caerulein in patients with biliary colic pain, Gastroenterology, 89:605.
Bernardi, L., Bosisio, G., Chillemi, F., de Caro, G., de Castiglione, R., Erspamer, V., Glässer, A., and Goffredo, O., 1964, Synthetic peptides related to eledoisin, Experientia, 20:306.
Bernardi, L., de Castiglione, R., Fregnan, G.B., and Glässer, A.H., 1967, An experimental approach to long-lasting hypotensive eledoisin-like peptides, J.Pharm.Pharmac., 19:95.
Bertaccini, G., 1976, Active polypeptides of nonmammalian origin, Pharmacol.Rev., 28:127.
Bietti, G.B., de Caro, G., Pecori Giraldi, J., and Romani, E., 1976, Besondere Indikationen für die Anwendung weicher Kontactlinsen als Augentropfenreservoir (Drug release system), Klin.Mbl.Augenheilk., 168:33.
Castellino, S., de Castiglione, R., Galantino, M., Forino, R., Licci, S., and Perseo, G., Mutagenic contaminants in synthetic peptides obtained by an azide coupling, Manuscript in preparation.

de Castiglione, R., 1983, Exploitation and exploration of ceruletide and eledoisin, two peptides of nonmammalian origin, Biopolymers, 22:507.

de Castiglione, R., Faoro, F., Piani, S., Perseo, G., Santangelo, F., Arcari, G., di Salle, E., and Rossi, A., 1981, Synthesis and biological activity of dermorphin analogues, Poster presented at the "7th American Peptide Symposium", Abstract p. 53.

de Castiglione, R., and Rossi, A., 1985, Amphibian skin peptides with analgesic activity, in "8th International Symposium on Medicinal Chemistry, Vol. 1", R. Dahlbom and J.L.G. Nilsson, eds., Swedish Pharmaceutical Press, Stockholm, pp. 147.

Deschodt-Lanckman, M., Bui, N.D., Noyer, M., and Christophe, J., 1981, Degradation of cholecystokinin-like peptides by a crude rat brain synaptosomal fraction: a study by high pressure liquid chromatography, Regul.Peptides, 2:15.

di Salle, E., and Ragazzi, P., 1976, Evidenza dell'assorbimento della ceruleina dal tratto gastroenterico mediante valutazione dell'attività colecistochinetica nella cavia, Communication at the "XVIII Congresso Nazionale della Società Italiana di Farmacologia", Abstract p. 105.

Erspamer, V., and Anastasi, A., 1962, Structure and pharmacological action of eledoisin, the active endecapeptide of the posterior salivary glands of Eledone, Experientia, 18:58.

Erspamer, V., and Melchiorri, P., 1973, Active polypeptides of the amphibian skin and their synthetic analogues, Pure Appl. Chem., 35:463.

Erspamer, V., and Melchiorri, P., 1983, Actions of amphibian skin peptides on the central nervous system and the anterior pituitary, in "Neuroendocrine Perspectives, Vol. 2", E.E. Müller and R.M. Mac Leod, eds., Elsevier Publishers B.V.

Erspamer, V., Melchiorri, P., Falconieri Erspamer, G., Montecucchi, P.C., and de Castiglione, R. 1985, Phyllomedusa skin: huge factory of a variety of active peptides, Peptides, 6:suppl.3, 7.

Grossi, E., Vertemati, F., Casiraghi, M.A., Petrillo, M., and Bianchi Porro, G., 1980, Action of caerulein on gastric acid secretion. A comparative study between the rectal and i.m. routes, Il Farmaco-Ed.Pr., 35:504.

Harman, A.J., 1984, Three tachykinins in mammalian brain, TINS, 7:57.

Holzer-Petsche, U., Schimek, E., Amann, R., and Lembeck, F., 1985, In vivo and in vitro actions of mammalian tachykinins, Naunyn-Schmiedeberg's Arch.Pharmacol., 330:130.

Impicciatore, M., Maraini, G., and Bertaccini, G., 1973, Action of eledoisin on human lacrimal secretion in normal and pathological conditions, Naunyn-Schmiedeberg's Arch. Pharmacol., 279:127.

Larsson, L.-J., and Rehfeld, J.F., 1977, Evidence for a common evolutionary origin of gastrin and cholecystokinin, Nature, 269:335.

Orlandini, I., and Agosti, A., 1969, Azione colecistocinetica della ceruleina e sua utilizzazione nella metodica colangiocolecistografica, Soc.Ital.Biol.Sperim., 45:782.

Owais, W.M., Rosicham, J.L., Ronald, R.C., Kleinhofs, A., and Nilan, R.A., 1983, A mutagenic metabolite synthesized by Salmonella typhimurium grown in the presence of azide is azidoalanine, Mutation Res., 118:229.

Pap, A., Berger, Z., and Varrò, V., 1981, Trophic effect of cholecystokinin-octapeptide in man. A new way in the treatment of chronic pancreatis?, Digestion, 21:163.

Sicuteri, F., Franchi, G., and Anselmi, B., 1962, Proprietà farmacologiche e terapeutiche dell'eledoisina nell'uomo, Settimana Med., suppl.31 dic.:19.

Solomon, T.E., 1983, Structure-activity relationships of cholecystokinin-related peptides, in "2nd Hiroshima Symposium on Gut Peptides and Ulcer", A. Miyoshi, ed., Biomedical Research Foundation, Tokyo.

Stürmer, E., and Fanchamps, A., 1965, Eledoisin. Chemie, Pharmakologie, klinisch-experimentelle und vorlaufige therapeutische Erfahrung, Dt.med.Wschr., 90:1012.

CONSIDERATION OF THE PROTEINS AND PEPTIDES PRODUCED BY

NEW TECHNOLOGY FOR USE AS THERAPEUTICS

Darrell T. Liu, Neil Goldman, and Frederick Gates, III

Division of Biochemistry and Biophysics,
Office of Biologics Research and Review, CDB, FDA
8800 Rockville Pike, Bethesda, MD 20892 U.S.A.

INTRODUCTION

Proteins and peptides for use as therapeutics may be isolated and purified from appropriate natural sources, prepared by rDNA technology or chemically synthesized. In this report we shall address mainly our experiences in considering production, purification, and testing of biologicals derived from rDNA technology and briefly review available documents that relate to products produced by chemical synthesis. Regardless of the source of the proteins and peptides, ultimately it is the responsibility of the manufacturers to demonstrate consistency in the safety, potency, efficacy, and purity of their products.

The Office of Biologics Research and Review (OBRR) is taking a cautious but flexible attitude in guiding these products onto the consumer market. Our basic philosophy in regulating biologicals produced by new technology is consistent with that used to evaluate other biologicals and may be described simply by a few concepts:

Sound scientific principles

The majority of OBRR staff involved in regulatory tasks are scientists actively engaged in basic research who, by virtue of being on the National Institutes of Health campus, maintain close interactions with world-renowned scientists present on the same campus. These close interactions have a major effect of ensuring scientific competence of OBRR staff and assuring that the decisions made on regulatory issues are based on valid scientific criteria.

Flexibility

The frontiers of new technologies are constantly being extended, and regulatory work must keep up with the advance of new scientific findings.

Case-by-case approach

The clinical usages of biologicals differ from one product to another. Insulin is injected 1-3 times a day for many years, and immunogenicity is to be avoided. In contrast, a vaccine is injected into a normal person 1-5 times with the primary intention of immunization. Thus, although many aspects of control apply to all products, different properties of each product may require special consideration.

Good common sense

As practicing scientists, OBRR regulators should be able to formulate realistic requests for scientific data from manufacturers.

Risk vs. Benefit assessment

Regulators, academics, industry, users, and the general public, do not wish to run undue risks. However, if the benefits that can be derived from new technologies are to be realized, some potential risk cannot be avoided. It takes careful consideration of the scientific evidence, buttressed by sound judgment, to maintain appropriate risk:benefit ratios. The better each of these compounds can be defined, the better the ratio can be understood.

PRODUCTS DERIVED FROM rDNA TECHNOLOGY

The rapid advances in molecular genetics over the past few years have allowed us to isolate and clone just about any gene from a cell's genome. These gene cloning techniques combined with our ability to express cloned genes in cells growing in culture enable us to produce useful quantitites of specific protein products for use as vaccines or as replacement therapeutics in such diverse categories as hormones, enzymes, immunomodulators, serum proteins, and viral antigens. There is an impressive list of protein products derived from cloned genes currently being used or evaluated in humans or soon to be available for clinical trials. Specific products include insulin, human growth hormone, various interferons and interleukins, albumin, clotting factors, and the surface antigens of the hepatitis and herpes viruses.

This new wave of biological products has required a reassessment of the historical concerns over product purity, potency, safety, and efficacy. This reevaluation has resulted in the development of regulatory documents, entitled "Points to Consider..." which are not guidelines per se that carry the force of law, but are designed to convey the current consensus of the OBRR relating to product development and testing. These "Points to Consider..." documents will remain as dated "drafts" and will never be finalized. They will be updated as needed using input from industry, academia and other regulatory agencies both from within the U.S. and abroad.

Several "Points to Consider..." documents have been issued covering a number of specific topics, including most recently interferon (July, 1982), monoclonal antibodies for in vitro use (March, 1982), monoclonal antibodies for in vivo use (July, 1983), recombinant DNA (April, 1985) and cell lines used to produce biological products (June, 1984).

This series of documents has served a number of useful purposes. Within the OBRR, they help to maintain uniformity of regulatory review, and serve as the basis for policy discussion. Externally, they provide a forum for scientist-to-scientist communication between the industry and the regulatory authority. They facilitate academic input into the regulatory process and generate international scientific consensus. They are useful in strategic planning by manufacturers, and have been especially relevant for the newly formed biotechnology firms which have had limited interactions with regulatory agencies. These flexible and evolving "Points to Consider..." documents appear to have been well received by all interested parties and have had positive effects in facilitating the development of new drugs and biologics.

In the experiences of the Office of Biologics Research and Review, there are a number of scientific and safety issues related to rDNA derived products that deserve special attention, e.g., A, alterations in molecular structure and B, purity of the product and impurities associated with the product.

Alterations in Molecular Structure

Heterogeneity in amino terminal sequence. A number of mammalian proteins have been synthesized in Escherichia coli. While bacterial cells appear to possess many attributes for heterologous gene expression, certain problems may persist in generating products that are identical to the native protein. Most secretory or membrane proteins in eukaryotic cells are synthesized with leader peptides which are subsequently removed by specific proteases to yield native proteins. When mammalian proteins are synthesized in E. coli without that leader sequence, the resulting product may be homogeneous, but it is often a heterogeneous mixture of N-formyl-methionyl-protein, methionyl-protein, and protein missing one, two or more amino terminal residues. Proteins which are missing carboxyterminal residues have also been encountered. With the attachment of segments encoding bacterial or eukaryotic leader sequences to eukaryotic genes expressed in E. coli, the resulting proteins at times have been shown to have the correct amino terminal residues and are secreted into the periplasmic space (Talmadge et al. 1980; Pollitt and Zalkin, 1983).

The potential heterogeneity in amino terminal sequence is not limited to proteins expressed in E. coli, human α-interferon synthesized in the yeast Saccharomyces cerevisiae (Hitzeman et al., 1983) was found to be a heterogeneous mixture consisting of the mature protein, protein with the intact leader peptide, and protein with the leader sequence partially removed.

Chemical and physical alteration. Proteins produced by rDNA in E. coli are often found deposited in insoluble inclusion bodies. The resulting extraction and purification often necessitates the use of detergents to assure solubilization, and protease inhibitors to suppress proteolytic degradation. Such agents conceivably could alter the structure of the proteins. Most detergents are known to denature proteins to some degree, and when used in conjunction with reducing agents will almost certainly cause protein denaturation. Procedures designed to remove detergents and reducing agents may not allow all of the protein molecules to restore their natural conformation. Proteolytic enzyme inhibitors such as the widely used phenylmethylsulfonyl fluoride could chemically modify side chains of amino acids in the protein. These alterations, whether in conformation or in covalent structure, may induce the recognition of these proteins by the immune system, a process that may be detrimental to the health of the recipient either by limiting the clinical efficacy of the antigenic material itself, or by stimulating cross reactive autoimmune response to the natural homologue. The ability to express specific proteins at high yields (30-50% of total cell proteins) and to have them secreted extracellularly using cloned genes with an appropriate leader sequence may greatly facilitate purification of gene products of "native" structure for clinical use.

TABLE I

Oligosaccharides can have many more isomeric forms than peptides

Monomer composition	Product	Number of Isomers	
		Peptides	Saccharides[a]
X_2	Dimer	1	11
X_3	Trimer	1	176
XYZ	Trimer	6	1056

a Pyranose ring only. **Source:** Calculations by John Clamp [*Biochem. Soc. Symp.*, **40**, 3 (1974)]

Alteration due to non-glycosylation or glycosylation.
Oligosaccharides can have many more isomeric forms than peptides (Table I)
(Clamp, 1974). For instance, whereas there are only six different ways in
which a tripeptide can be formed from 3 different amino acids, the number
of trisaccharide that can be formed from 3 different hexoses through
pyranose ring structure is 1056.

Many of the hormones and plasma proteins isolated from human tissue
and plasma are glycoproteins. When these human proteins are synthesized
in E. coli they will not be glycosylated since E. coli can not make
glycoproteins. On the other hand, proteins produced by rDNA using
heterologous eukaryotic cells may have different carbohydrate composition
and structure from their natural counterparts because the complement of
enzymes required for the synthesis and processing of complex glycoproteins
vary from one eukaryotic cell to the other (Hsieh, et al., 1983).

For those products which are administered parenterally in large
amounts or repeatedly over long periods, non-glycosylated protein may
reveal new antigenic sites while glycoprotein with unnatural carbohydrate
structure may be antigenic. Proteins without the appropriate carbohydrate
moieties may have altered pharmacokinetics and tissue distribution and
also may cause other unknown and possibly adverse effects.

Protein folding and pairing of disulfide bonds. It is generally far
easier to insure and to ascertain the "intactness" of the primary
structure of a protein than to establish the natural conformation and the
correct pairing of disulfide bonds of a protein.

The number of possible ways in which a given number of half-cystine
residues can combine to form disulfide bonds (SS) upon oxidation is shown
in Table II (Anfinsen, 1968). These numbers show, for example, that in the
case of tissue plasminogen activator, the random chance of forming the
correct 18 SS bonds from the available 37 half-cystine is infinitesimally
small, less than one in 2×10^{20}. In the case of insulin which contains 6
half-cystines, 15 possible sets of 3 SS bonds can be made, only one of
which is the native structure. How does one determine the correct paring
of SS bonds in a rDNA derived protein? At present, the only realistic
method is the protein-based quantitative analysis which involves peptide
mapping in conjunction with compositional analysis and sequence analysis
of each of the SS containing peptides. For rDNA derived insulin, this was
exactly the way the 3 pair of SS bonds were established (Johnson, 1983).
The amount of protein samples required and the difficulty involved in
establishing the SS bonds of a protein increases dramatically with the

Table II

Source: Self-assembly of macromolecular structures, Anfinsen, C. B., 27th Symposium of the Society for Developmental Biology, Developmental Biology, Supplement 2, 1968, 1-20.

THE NUMBER OF WAYS IN WHICH $2n$ SULFHYDRYL GROUPS CAN COMBINE
TO FORM j DISULFIDE BONDS

Number of bonds	Number of combinations
1	1
2	3
3	15
4	105
5	945
6	10395
7	135135
8	2027025
9	34459425
10	654729075
11	13749310575
12	316234143225
13	7905853580625
14	213458046676875
15	6190283353629375
16	191898783962510625
17	6332859870762850625
18	221643095476699771875
19	8200794532637891559375
20	319830986772877770815625
21	13111307045768798860344 0625
22	563862029680583509947946875
23	25373791335626257947657609375
24	1192568192774434123539907640625
25	58435841445947272053455474390625

$$N_{2n}{}^j = \frac{(2n)!}{2^j (2n - 2j)! j!}$$

increase in the number of SS bonds. Moreover, even if the position of SS bonds are established for a rDNA derived protein, it will not be possible to ascertain if they are identical to the natural protein unless the positions of SS bonds for the natural protein have also been determined. In many instances this is not possible since the particular protein in question is not available in sufficient quantity to permit such an analysis.

Sufficient data (Anfinsen, 1968; and Liu, 1978) are now available to indicate, however, that the specific three-dimensional structure of a protein is dictated by the linear sequence of its amino acid residues and that the pairing of half-cystines in SS bonds in a protein is the consequence rather than a director of protein folding. This conversion from linearity to spacial organization appears to be a spontaneous process (Anfinsen, 1968). The native proteins that one finds in cells are polypeptide translation products of genetic information, arranged in a form possessing maximum thermodynamic stability under physiologic conditions.

An examination of the extent to which various "derived" multichained proteins produced by specific in vivo cleavages of single chained proteins (e.g. chymotrypsin, insulin) and naturally occurring multichained proteins formed by disulfide bonding of two or more separately synthesized chains (e.g. immunoglobulins) undergo reversible denaturation suggests that interruption of a single chained protein is generally not conducive to proper folding. Some multichained proteins, however, that are made up of identical or genetically related subunits may be reversibly denatured. Thus, whereas chymotrypsinogen, proinsulin, and immunoglobulins can be reversibly denatured, chymotrypsin and insulin are thermodynamically unstable and informationally insufficient to undergo spontaneous refolding of the molecules and the formation of the native pairs of disulfide bonds.

In the context of rDNA derived proteins, it would seem to be advantageous and, in some instances, necessary to synthesize human proteins containing multiple disulfide bonds in eukaryotic cells that can oxidatively form disulfide bonds. When such proteins are synthesized in cells (Pollitt and Zalkin, 1983) that lack the ability to oxidatively form disulfide bonds intracellularly (e.g. E. coli) (Pollitt and Zalkin, 1983) the resulting proteins are often found in the inclusion bodies of cytoplasm where their half-cystines remain in the reduced form. During the isolation and purification of such intracellular proteins, steps should be taken to preserve native protein conformation and avoid unwanted proteolytic cleavages so as to favor the spontaneous generation of native protein conformation.

Purity of the product and impurities associated with the product

In regard to the assessment of the "purity" of the final product and the testing for "impurities" in the product, the consensus view is that the sensitivity of the test method and the degree of product purity should be appropriate to the product's intended use; products which are given repeatedly or in large doses will require higher purity than those given only a few times or at low doses. Tests used to support claims of purity or absence of contaminants should be capable of accurately detecting and quantitating the expected substances.

The primary reasons for concern over the "purity" of the rDNA derived product are the safety questions involved in using certain types of cell substrates for producing biologics. Concern has been expressed over the use of continuous cell lines for the production of some biologics because continuous cell lines may have biological, biochemical, and genetic abnormalities. In particular, they may contain viruses, host cell components that may be antigenic in humans, and potentially oncogenic DNA. It is important, therefore, to assure that biological products derived from continuous cell lines are highly purified by employing methods for the extensive removal and/or inactivation of cellular DNA, host cell antigens, and adventitious agents.

Residual Cellular DNA (Noble, 1985). In considering potential risk from residual DNA, it should be pointed out that a number of different products are given by different routes, in different amounts, and according to different schedules. For those products that are given repeatedly in large doses it is especially important that procedures for production demonstrate that no unnecessary DNA molecules will be in the final product. It is not clear how much residual DNA contamination would be necessary to induce changes in normal cellular processes. Until more information on the determination of the biological activities of DNA becomes available, a level of unwanted DNA in the picogram range per dose appears reasonable to measure and to achieve by conventional purification techniques.

Pyrogenic and Immunogenic Contaminants (Van Metre, 1985). Contaminants may come from component of cell substrates (cell wall, cell membrane, mucopeptide, lipopolysaccharide, etc.), media constituents, affinity column components or may be derived from chemical modification of the proteins used in the manufacturing process. These residual contaminants may be a potential source of risk because they may be pyrogenic or recognized as antigens by the recipient of the product, and they may have direct undesirable biological effects. It is important to monitor the production process and the final product to make sure that their levels are in an acceptable range.

Recent experience with recombinant products has emphasized that biological pharmaceuticals may be pyrogenic in humans despite having

passed the Limulus Amebocyte Lysate test and the rabbit pyrogen test.
This phenomenon appears to be due to nonendotoxin contaminants which
demonstrate a marked species dependence in their pyrogenicity. To
attempt to predict whether the human subject will experience a pyrogenic
response, tests have been used in which human peripheral blood
mononuclear cells are cultured in vitro in the presence of the product.
The supernatant fluid from the treated cells is then injected into
rabbits (Dinarello, 1974). A fever in the rabbits indicate that the
substance had stimulated the cultured human mononuclear cells to produce
leukocytic pyrogen, the protein mediator believed to be involved in the
in vivo febrile response. We have successfully used this test to detect
the presence of pyrogenic materials in several preparations which have
been negative on both Limulus Amebocyte Lysate and rabbit pyrogen tests,
but which were pyrogenic in humans.

The possibility of developing a humoral or cellular immune response
to minor contaminants should be carefully assessed in both preclinical
and clinical studies particularly in products to be administered
chronically. Reliable and sensitive tests such as Western Blots are
needed to assay for trace contamination present in separate production
batches. Sensitive techniques such as radioimmunoassay and ELISA can be
used to measure the induction of specific antibodies in recipients in
response to microbial or cellular constituents likely to contaminate the
final product. In addition, periodic skin testing can be performed with
the product to rule out development of delayed type hypersensitivity.

Viral Contamination (Osborn, 1985). Techniques available to test for
the presence of viral agents in the cell substrate or in biological
products are neither simple nor straightforward in their applications.
This issue is further complicated by the difficulty in defining "viral
agents." Risks imposed by viral contamination range from known viruses
with predictable patterns of replication to as-yet-unknown infectious
agents (e.g. potential cause of Creutzfeldt-Jakob disease) which cannot
be recognized with currently available technology. Between these two
extremes are "visible" viruses such as type B retroviruses whose presence
can be demonstrated by electron microscopy but for which there is no
sensitive in vitro assay for infectivity; latent proviral components such
as viral DNA sequences integrated into the genome; and "unconventional
agents" such as scrapie which has been identified as a transmissible
pathogenic agent of unknown life cycle. Given the present state of
science, precise measures for the elimination of risks from scrapie-like
agents and as-yet-unknown viruses cannot be rationally proposed.

Because many pathogenic agents cannot be detected with great
sensitivity and assurance, characterization of the final product alone is
not sufficient to optimally assure safety. Initially, therefore, it is
necessary to fully characterize the individual components used in the
manufacturing process, especially the cell substrate. In all cases the
cell line should be established and evaluated using a master cell bank
system. Cells should be cultured to their furthest proposed passage
level to look for induction of latent viruses and instabilities of
genotype or phenotype. Judgment on the suitability of a cell line and
its properties may be made on a case-by-case basis considering both the
cell line and the potential clinical use of proposed products derived
from it. In any case, however, in the initial assessment of the
proposed purification techniques, demonstration of the elimination or
inactivation of a deliberately introduced viral contaminant whose
infectivity can be measured by a sensitive in vitro method, should
provide some assurance that the techniques employed may be effective
against unknown viruses of a similar nature.

A final point is that it is important to maintain surveillance of possible untoward effects because no matter how thorough the testing of products may be, there can always be unforeseen events. A long-term surveillance should be established and maintained relevant both to the cell lines themselves and to the proposed biological products.

The previously discussed considerations and tests to determine identity, safety, and purity will give some level of confidence that the rDNA product corresponds to the expected product. However, it should be remembered that structure and function of proteins may now be modified by means of genetic engineering thus it is possible to improve a desirable biological activity while eliminating undesirable toxic side effects associated with the natural product. Such a product is not identical with the natural product and may be observed to be immunogenic. Is such an altered product acceptable? The answer to that question is not a simple "yes" or "no" but will depend on a careful assessment of the new benefits of this product as compared to the risks identifiable during its preclinical and clinical evaluations. Requirements for long-term animal testing, including tests for carcinogenicity, teratogenicity, and effects on fertility, will depend upon the availability of animal models and should be based upon the intended use of the product, its mode of action and metabolic fate. Specific preclinical toxicity evaluations are best addressed on a case-by-case basis. Clinical trials will be necessary for all products derived from rDNA technology to evaluate their safety and efficacy.

SYNTHETIC PEPTIDES

Synthetic peptides are being introduced in increasing variety and frequency for human use as hormones and growth factors (Synthetic peptides:toxicity tests and control, NIBSC, 1984). In some instances, it appears to be commercially more attractive to synthesize peptides of up to 30-40 residues than to obtain them from biological sources or by rDNA technology. Examples include calcitonin, pentagastrin, and tetracosa ACTH peptide. In addition, new peptide analogues with unnatural amino acid substituents designed for selected pharmacological activities, and/or improved therapeutic ratio (efficacy:safety) can only be produced via chemical synthesis.

Since each of the steps involved in the chemical synthesis of a polypeptide will not be complete (Finn and Hofmann, 1976; Barany and Merrifield, 1979) (i.e. < 100% yield) the resulting product will not likely be "pure." A major concern for synthetic peptides for use as therapeutics is, therefore, the possible significance of the impurities associated with the product. Impurities may be comprised of truncated or partial sequences, of peptides with deletions, substitutions or modified (e.g., residually blocked) functional groups, of enantiomers, or molecules with altered conformation (Finn and Hofmann, 1976; Barany and Merrifield, 1979; Wünsch, 1983; Moser et al., 1985). The amount and the complexity of such peptide impurities vary from batch to batch and, in general, increase with the length of the polypeptide chain. Polypeptides synthesized by a route not involving stepwise assembly of purified fragments will, most likely, be less pure.

Sophisticated multi-dimensional analytical methods available today, such as high performance liquid chromatography, isoelectric focusing, peptide mapping, ELISA, peptide microsequencing and fast atom bombardment mass spectrometry, are powerful but may not identify, quantitate, or detect all such impurities associated with synthetic peptides. Evidence for the purity of a synthetic peptide must necessarily depend on the careful evaluation of biological activities as well as the use of a variety of analytical systems based on differing physicochemical principles. The ability to detect peptide impurities does not, by itself, imply that practical methodology could be developed to remove them during purification of the product.

For the reasons given above, products consisting of synthesized polypeptides should not be treated a priori as a simple chemical whose identity, purity, and/or safety can be shown by chemical and physical methods alone. As with rDNA-derived products, specific preclinical toxicity evaluation, and long-term animal testing for of synthetic peptide products are best addressed on a case-by-case basis.

REFERENCES

Anfinsen, C.B. (1968). Self-assembly of macromolecular structures in the 27th Symposium of the Society for Developmental Biology, Developmental Biology Supplement 2, 1-20.

Barany, G. and Merrifield, R.B. (1979). Solid Phase Peptide Synthesis, in "The Peptides," Vol. 2, Eds. A.E. Gross and J. Meienhofer, Academic Press, New York, NY.

Clamp, J.R. (1974). Analysis of glycoproteins, in "The Metabolism and Function of Glycoproteins," Biochem. Soc. Symp. 40: 3.

Dinarello, C.A. (1974). Endogeneous Pyrogen, in "Methods for Studying Mononuclear Phagocytes," Eds. D. Adams, P. Edelson, and H. Koren, 629, Academic Press, New York, NY.

Finn, F.M. and Hofmann, K. (1976). The synthesis of peptides by solution methods with emphasis on peptide hormones, in "The Proteins," Eds. H. Neurath and R.L. Hill, 3rd Ed., Vol. 2, Academic Press, New York, NY.

Hitzeman, R.A., Leung, D.W., Perry, L.J., Kohr, W.J., Levine, H.L., and Goeddel, D.V. (1983). Secretion of human interferons by yeast. Science 219: 620.

Hsieh, P., Rosner, M.S., and Robbins, P.W. (1983). Host-dependent variation of asparagine-linked oligosaccharides at individual glycosylation sites of sindbis virus glycoproteins. J. Biol. Chem. 258: 2548.

Johnson, I.S. (1983). Human Insulin from recombinant DNA technology. Science 219, 632.

Liu, T.-Y. (1978). The role of sulfur in proteins, in "The Proteins," 3rd Ed., Eds. H. Neurath and R.L. Hill, Vol. III, Academic Press, New York, NY.

Noble, G.R. (1985). Biological risk of residual cellular nucleic acid, in "In Vitro," Monograph 6: 173.

Moser, R., Klauser, S., Leist, T., Langen, H., Epprecht, T., and Gutte, B. (1985). Application of synthetic peptides, Angewandte Chemie 24: 719.

Osborn, J.E. (1985). Biological risk of viral agents endogeneous to cell substrates, in "In Vitro," Monograph 6, 174.

Pollitt, S., and Zalkin, H. (1983). Role of primary structure and disulfide bond formation in β-lactamase secretion. J. Bact. 153: 27.

Talmadge, K., Kaufman, J., and Gilbert, W. (1980). Bacteria mature preproinsulin to proinsulin. Proc. Natl. Acad. Sci. 77: 3988.

Van Metre, T.E. (1985). Biological risk of residual cellular proteins, in "In Vitro," Monograph 6, 172.

Wünsch, E. (1983). Peptide factors as pharmaceuticals:criteria for application. Biopolymers 33:493.

Synthetic Peptides: Toxicity Tests and Control. (1984). British National Institute for Biological Standards and Control, Division of Hormones. Document V9 24. ii.

KEY ISSUES IN THE DELIVERY OF PEPTIDES AND PROTEINS

E. Tomlinson[*], S.S. Davis[+] and L.Illum[++]

[*]Ciba Geigy Pharmaceuticals, Wimblehurst Road, Horsham
West Sussex, England, [+]Pharmacy Department, University of
Nottingham, University Park, Nottingham, England
[++]Royal Danish School of Pharmacy, 2 Universitetsparken
Copenhagen, Denmark

During the workshop the delegates were assigned to small syndicate
groups that met to discuss two assigned topics that represented key
issues in the delivery of peptides and proteins. Each syndicate reported
on their deliberations at the end of the meeting and this final chapter
is based largely on these reports.

IMMUNOGENICITY - THE EXTENT OF THE PROBLEM AND POSSIBLE TECHNICAL
SOLUTIONS

The administration of a peptide or protein can be expected to lead
eventually to an immune response, although the resultant antibodies may
not be neutralising. The frequency and route of administration as well
as the delivery system are important factors. The causes and extent of
immunogenicity can be mediated by new epitopes formed upon alteration of
primary structure such as the addition, subtraction or substitution of
amino acids and/or the alteration of secondary and tertiary structures
leading to different conformational isomers. Furthermore, novel epitopes
can be induced as a consequence of degradation or modification of the
peptide/protein due to storage, formulation, processing and even the mode
of administration. Impurities, such as contaminating bacterial proteins,
represent another source of immunogenic material. Some types of
formulation and routes of administration are likely to predispose an
individual to an immune reaction. The administration of peptide/proteins
in colloidal vehicles, (e.g. liposomes, emulsions), might lead to an
enhancement of the presentation of the material to lymphoid tissues.
(Indeed, the adjuvant properties of these formulations are sometimes
exploited in the development of vaccines).

The extent of the problem of immunogenicity will be related to the
nature of the response. For a humoral response the production of a
neutralising antibody may result in the drug being non-effective. With
non-neutralising antibodies the drug could be cleared more rapidly and
although in theory the dose could be increased to compensate for this
effect there is the danger of the formation of a (toxic) immune complex.
For a cellular response, this may occur more for large proteins than for
lower molecular weight peptides. Variations in immunogenicity will occur
for different proteins/peptides, with acute versus chronic treatment and
certainly with different patients. For a proportion of patients,
immunogenicity may not be a significant problem due to immunostat
variation within the population.

Attempts to prevent immunogenicity should commence with the identification of the correct native structure. This can now be accomplished by analytical methods that allow the authentic structure to be identified, and for this to be compared with chemically modified, synthesised, stored, formulated or administered material. Protection against immune response, (and also possible enzymatic degradation or modification), can be achieved by the choice of an appropriate method of formulation and administration. Examples include site-specific delivery and the masking of recognition sites from the immune system (perhaps through the use of tolerogens such as the polyethylene glycols, dextrans etc). Improvements in synthesis and purification, together with a rational choice of mammalian cells and the development of methods to detect and remove impurities such as DNA, viruses, endotoxins and immune adjuvants could also have a significant impact in reducing immune responses. Other strategies might include the induction of tolerance by using low doses initially and the suppression of the immune system, perhaps by blocking Ia receptors.

OPPORTUNITIES FOR THE ORAL ADMINISTRATION OF PEPTIDES AND PROTEINS

Two main problems can be established, namely the stability of the molecule to degradation/metabolism and transport across critical (membrane) barriers. Antibody sequestration and unfavourable solubility characteristics represent other possible limitations to oral delivery.

Problems of stability can be circumvented by the production of more stable analogues, the use of enzyme inhibitors and protection of the drug during its passage through the different regions of the gastrointestinal tract, (e.g. enteric coating).

The passive absorption and subsequent membrane transport of peptides/proteins represent a major challenge since the inherent physicochemical properties of peptides and proteins are unsuitable, and the exploitation of active transport mechanisms is only possible for di- and tripeptides. Resolution of the problem might be achieved through a greater understanding of receptor mediated and facilitated transport mechanisms, coupled with studies on the uptake of dietary factors as well as the mechanism responsible for the passage of, for example, viruses. The anomalous absorption of cyclosporin deserves further attention, as also does the role of the M cells situated in the Peyer's Patch regions of the small intestine.

Finally, an elucidation of the mechanisms by which certain absorption enhancers (adjuvants) act, could lead to the development of materials that provide both selectivity and low toxicity.

ROUTES OF PREFERENCE

The chosen route for a peptide or protein will be related to the type and chemical character of the molecule, the target site, the convenience factor and the cost effectiveness. In general terms, an injectable (parenteral) form will normally be required in all instances, while the nasal route appears to have early potential and could well be acceptable in a number of therapeutic situations. It is stressed that no universal system for administration (or indeed site-specific delivery) is likely nor perhaps desirable. In choosing a delivery system, the therapeutic index of the drug must be considered carefully, as must also the paracrine/endocrine-like nature of many mediators. The questions of novel dose-response relationships and chronopharmacological effects also require attention.

352

As mentioned above, further studies are required on absorption enhancers before their safe utility can be deemed possible in anything other than acute therapy.

Subdermal implants and injected particles (e.g. microspheres) have a potential for improved dosage regimens due to their sustained release characteristics. Furthermore, they can be designed with constant release profiles ranging from hours to months, and also have the possibility for pulsed release. Limitations of this route include the stability of the peptide or protein over the long term, the necessary dose/carrier size and the total carrier capacity of the system. Once administered the chance of "dose dumping" through the failure of the depot cannot be ignored. The converse problem of the formation of a fibrous capsule that will act as a barrier to the release of high molecular weight molecules also needs to be addressed. Candidate peptides or proteins for early exploitation by this route include calcitonin, LHRH, soluble vaccines and growth hormones.

The intranasal route is judged to have the advantage of being a possible alternative to injectable formulations. However, limitations include the prospect of low and variable bioavailability, a lack of data on the toxicity of many of the proposed absorption enhancers, and the question that untoward immunogenic effects might arise with this route. Nevertheless the nasal route has already been used for a number of therapeutic applications with peptides that demonstrate good bioavailability and are administered on an acute rather than a chronic basis.

Surprisingly, the pulmonary route has received little attention except for brief mention in the patent literature. It is to be expected that the absorption of peptides and proteins from this route will be similar to that for intranasal administration, but there could be a greater opportunity for untoward reactions.

Buccal, vaginal and rectal modes of delivery all have definite advantages, particularly with regard to the avoidance of first-pass metabolism. The vaginal route is obviously limited in its applicability, and the practicability of rectal dosing in many countries depends on the acceptability-to-benefit ratio. As for nasal administration, the use of absorption enhancers for other transmucosal routes could well lead to an increase in bioavailability, but such materials are yet to be proven in terms of safety.

The results presently available for the transdermal delivery of peptides are not encouraging. However, this is not surprising considering their high molecular weights. Penetration enhancers and electrotransport (iontophoresis) are reasonable strategies, but the chances of commercial success may be very limited.

The delivery of peptides and proteins by the oral route is also a rather poor prospect. Much more needs to be understood about relevant and exploitable transport processes. Consequently the route represents a long-term goal.

POTENTIAL FOR SITE SPECIFIC CARRIERS

The ability to direct peptides and proteins to designated sites is a worthy objective in that it will deliver the drug to the site where the therapeutic effect is needed, thereby leading to a reduction in toxic and/or side effects. Moreover, it will protect the drug from undesirable modification or degradation. Other perceived advantages include the temporal delivery of the drug in response to certain physiological states and to provide access to previously inaccessible compartments. Such an approach could be used as a tool to discover new drugs whose activity might have been overlooked in the absence of site specific delivery.

The form of the carrier can be of two types; soluble (bio)conjugates and insoluble particulates. Their use in site-specific delivery can be direct administration of a peptide of protein into a discrete anatomical region, (e.g. intra-articular injection, aerosolisation into the lungs), or through transport in body fluids, followed by a site-specific uptake at the target. This second process may require any one or all of the following phases:- carrier transport, passive or active localisation, cellular processing (including, for example, transcytosis), site specific activation, and passive or activated release. With regard to the last point drug release can be controlled by the specific action of enzymes, (i.e. proteases, amidases, sulphatases) or through a process of deglycosylation.

The prime advantages and disadvantages of the proposed carrier systems are summarised in Table 1.

Table 1   Advantages and disadvantages of soluble (bio)conjugates and particulate systems

	SOLUBLE (BIO)CONJUGATES	PARTICULATES
ADVANTAGES	- nonparenteral delivery possible - protection (e.g. as PEG conjugates) - extravasation possible by specific targeting mechanism	- load and release adjustable - circulating sustained release - anatomical localisation - could extravasate if taken up by macrophages
DISADVANTAGES	- low load - release non-adjustable - caution with murine Ab as ligands being possibly immunogenic, consider chimeric Ab	- usually no extravasation - toxicity, eg RES ablation, release of monokines (TNF,IL-1 etc) - only parenteral administration -can enhance immunogenicity

Attainable uses for site-specific carrier systems include targeting to lung, liver, bone marrow and ex vivo treatment, (e.g. bone marrow clean up to remove cancer stem cells via the use of specific immunotoxins). In addition, gene therapy could rely upon ex vivo gene transfer into bone marrow stem cells and in vivo gene transfer via virus-derived carriers.

In order to develop these site-specific delivery systems properly, a better definition of the target(s) is required from the standpoints of their biochemistry, physiology and cell biology, as well as the pathogenesis of the disease. From this can follow a judgement as to whether a site-specific carrier would be a rational mode of delivery, as well as indicating the constraints arising with respect to the accessibility of the target, the payload to be delivered and the acceptable therapeutic index.

Major difficulties with particles could be the potential for their indiscriminate uptake by the various elements of the reticuloendothelial system.

REGULATORY ISSUES

It is apparent that the current states of knowledge on delivery systems for peptides and proteins are unprecise, and consequently it is important to continue the existing approaches in which testing is evaluated on a case-by-case basis. The route of administration and the carrier system are of particular importance.

Among the more obvious issues that are difficult to resolve is the nature of long-term toxicity studies that will be required for peptides and proteins intended for chronic use. The assessment of immune responses and the selection of appropriate species for immunotoxicity (and efficacy) testing will be key issues. A final plea is for uniformity in the practices of regulatory bodies in the various countries.

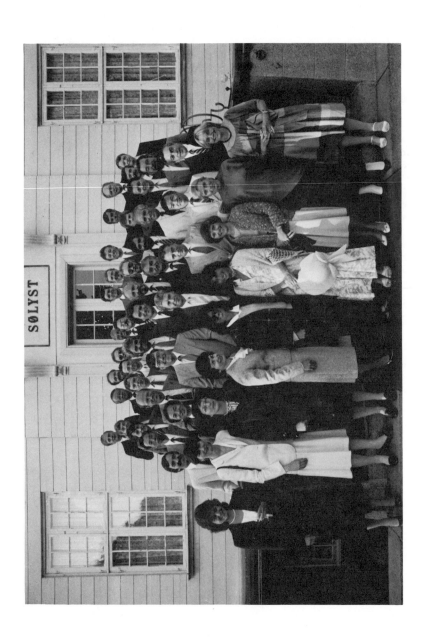

Alberetto, M., Istituto Scientifico Ospedale San Raffaele, Clinica Medica
    and Clinica Ortopedica, Universita de Milano, Milano, Italy

Anders, R., Pharmazeutisches Institut der Universität, Pharmazeutische
    Technologie, D-5300 Bonn 1, Germany

Augustine, M., Pharmacy Research and Development, Rorer Group, Inc.,
    Tuckahoe, N.Y. 10707, USA

Barry, B.W., Postgraduate School of Pharmacy, University of
    Bradford, Bradford DB7 1DP, England.

Baughman, Jr., R.A., Genentech, Inc., South San Francisco, CA, USA

Benet, L.Z., School of Pharmacy,
    University of California, San Francisco, CA and Genentech, Inc.,
    South San Francisco, CA, U.S.A.

Bibus, C., Biocenter, University of Basel, Klingelbergstrasse
    70, CH-4056 Basel, Switzerland.

Bundgaard, H., Royal Danish School of Pharmacy, Department of
    Pharmaceutical Chemistry AD, 2 Universitetsparken, DK-2100 Copenha-
    gen, Denmark

Cahill, J., Pharmacy Research and Development, Rorer Group, Inc.,
    Tuckahoe, N.Y. 10707, USA

Calderara, A., Istituto Scientifico Ospedale San Raffaele, Clinica Medica
    and Clinica Ortopedica, Universita di Milano, Milano, Italy

Campanale, K.M., Pharmaceutical Research Department, Division of CNS and
    Endocrine Research, and Toxicology, Lilly Research Laboratories,
    Eli Lilly and Company, Indianapolis, IN 46285, USA

Carlsen, S., Nordisk Gentofte A/S, Niels Steensensvej 1, DK-2820
    Gentofte, Denmark

Castiglione, R. de, Farmitalia Carlo Erba SpA, Research &
    Development, Via dei Gracchi 35, 20146 Milan, Italy.

Christensen, T. Nordisk Gentofte A/S, Niels Steensensvej 1, Dk-2820
    Gentofte, Denmark

Daemen, T., Laboratory of Physiological Chemistry, University of
    Groningen, Medical School, Bloemsingel 10, 9712 KZ Groningen, The
    Netherlands

Dalbøge, H., Nordisk Gentofte A/S, Niels Steensensvej 1, DK-2820
    Gentofte, Denmark

Daugherty, A.L., Pharmacological Sciences, Genentech, Inc., 460 Point San
    Bruno Boulevard, S. San Francisco, CA 94080, USA

Davis, S.S, Department of Pharmacy, University of Nottingham,
    University Park, Nottingham, NG7 2RD, England.

Dinesen, B., Nordisk Gentofte A/S, Niels Steensensvej 1, DK-2820
    Gentofte, Denmark

de Boer, O., Laboratory of Physiological Chemistry, University of
    Groningen, Medical School, Bloemsingel 10, 9712 KZ Groningen, The
    Netherlands

Emtage, S, Molecular Biology Division, Celltech Limited, 250
    Bath Road, Slough SL1 3DY, Berks, England

Eppstein, D.A. Institute of Bio-Organic Chemistry, Syntex Research, Palo
    Alto, CA 94304, U.S.A.

Falk, K.-E., Physical Pharmacy, AB Hässle, S-431 Mölndal, Sweden.

Felgner, P.L., Institute of Bio-Organic Chemistry, Syntex Research, Palo
    Alto, CA 94304, USA

Furr, B.J.A., Pharmaceutical Department and Research Department, Imperial
    Chemical Industries, PLC, Pharmaceuticals Division, Mereside,
    Alderley Park, Macclesfield, Cheshire SK10 3TG, England

Garcia-Anton, Laboratory of Peptides, Biological Organic Chemistry De-
    partment, C.S.I.C., Jorge Girona Salgado 18-26, 08034 Barcelona,
    Spain.

Gates, III, F., Division of Biochemistry and Biophysics, Office of
    Biologics Research and Review, CDB, FDA, 8800 Rockville Pike,
    Bethesda, MD 20892, USA

Gazdick, G., Pharmacy Research and Development, Rorer Group, Inc.,
    Tuckahoe, N.Y. 10707, USA

Gloff, C.A., Triton Bio-Sciences, Inc., Alameda, CA 94501, USA

Goldman, N., Division of Biochemistry and Biophysics, Office of Biologics
    Research and Review, CDB, FDA, 8800 Rockville Pike, Bethesda, MD
    20892, USA

Gries, C.L., Pharmaceutical Research Department, Division of CNS and
    Endocrine Research, and Toxicology, Lilly Research Laboratories,
    Eli Lilly and Company, Indianapolis, IN 46285, USA

Hansen, J.W., Nordisk Gentofte A/S, Niels Steensensvej 1, DK-2820
    Gentofte, Denmark

Hanson, M., Pharmacy Research and Development, Rorer Group, Inc.,
    Tuckahoe, N.Y. 10707, U.S.A.

Harris, A.A., Ferring AB, P.O. Box 30561, S-200 62 Malmö,
    Sweden

Humphrey, M.J., Department of Drug Metabolism, Pfizer Central
     Research, Sandwich, Kent CT13 9NJ, England.

Hutchinson, F.G., Pharmaceutical Department and Research Department,
     Imperial Chemical Industries PLC, Pharmaceuticals Division,
     Mereside, Alderley Park, Macclesfield, Cheshire SK10 4TG, England.

Illum, L., Department of Pharmaceutics, Royal Danish School of Pharmacy,
     2 Universitetsparken, DK-2100 Copenhagen, Denmark

Jensen, E.B., Nordisk Gentofte A/S, Niels Steensensvej 1, DK-2820
     Gentofte, Denmark

Jørgensen, K.D., Nordisk Gentofte A/S, Niels Steensensvej 1, DK-2820
     Gentofte, Denmark

Kappelgaard, A.-M., Nordisk Gentofte A/S, Niels Steensensvej 1, DK-2820
     Gentofte, Denmark

Kerchner, G.A., Pharmaceutical Research Department, Division of CNS and
     Endocrine Research, and Toxicology, Lilly Research Laboratories,
     Eli Lilly and Company, Indianapolis, IN 46285, USA

Lee, V.H.L., University of S. California, School of Pharmacy,
     Los Angeles, CA 90033, U.S.A.

Liu, D.T., Division of Biochemistry and Biophysics, Office of Biologics
     Research and Review, CDB, FDA, 8800 Rockville Pike, Bethesda, MD
     20892, U.S.A.

Löfroth, J-E., Physical Pharmacy, AB Hässle, S-431 83 Mölndal, Sweden

Longenecker, J.P., California Biotechnology Inc., 2450 Bayshore
     Frontagea Road, Mountain View, CA 94043, U.S.A.

Malefyt, T.R., Smith Kline & French Laboratories, 709 Swedeland Road,
     Swedeland, PA 19479, USA

Manganelli, V., Istituto Scientifico Ospedale San Raffaele, Clinica
     Medica and Clinica Ortopedica, Universita di Milano, Milano, Italy

McMartin, C., Horsham Research Centre, Ciba-Geigy Pharmaceuticals,
     Horsham, W.Sussex RH12 4AB, England.

McRae, G.I., Syntex Research, Palo Alto, CA, USA

Mendelsohn, L.G., Pharmaceutical Research Department, Division of CNS and
     Endocrine Research, and Toxicology, Lilly Research Laboratories,
     Eli Lilly and Company, Indianapolis, IN 46285, USA

Merkle, H.P., Pharmazeutisches Institut der Universität, Pharmazeutische
     Technologie, D-5300 Bonn 1, W.Germany.

Mishky, P.B., Syntex Research, Palo Alto, CA, USA

Moore, J.A., Pharmacological Sciences, Genentech, Inc. U.S.A.

Murakami, M., Kyoto Pharmaceutical University, Misasagi, Yamashina,
     Kyoto, Japan

Muranishi, S., Kyoto Pharmaceutical University, Misasagi, Yamashina, Kyoto, Japan

Nilsson, P., Nordisk Gentofte A/S, Niels Steensensvej 1, DK-2820 Gentofte, Denmark

Pajetta, E., Istituto Scientifico Ospedale San Raffaele, Clinica Medica and Clinica Ortopedica, Universita di Milano, Milano, Italy

Pedersen, J., Nordisk Gentofte A/S, Niels Steensensvej 1, DK-2820 Gentofte, Denmark

Peters, G., Horsham Research Centre, CIBA-GEIGY Pharmaceuticals, Horsham, W.Sussex RH12 4AB, England

Pontiroli, A.E., Istituto Scientifico Ospedale San Raffaele, Cattedra di Clinica Medica, Universita di Milano, Milano, Italy.

Pozza, G., Istituto Scientifico Ospedale San Raffaele, Clinica Medica and Clinica Ortopedica, Universita di Milano, Milano, Italy

Regts, D., Laboratory of Physiological Chemistry, University of Groningen, Medical School, Bloemsingel 10, 9712 KZ Groningen, The Netherlands

Reig, F., Laboratory of Peptides, Biological Organic Chemistry Department C.S.I.C., Jorge Girona Salgado 18-26, 08304, Barcelona, Spain

Robinson, A.K., Cardiovascular Division, Washington University School of Medicine, St. Louis, Missouri, U.S.A.

Roerdink, F.H., Laboratory of Physiological Chemistry, University of Groningen, Medical School, Bloemsingel 10, 9712 KZ Groningen, The Netherlands.

Sanders, L.M., Syntex Research, Palo Alto, CA, U.S.A.

Sandow, J., Hoechst AG, D-6230 Frankfurt aM 80, Germany

Scherphof, G.L., Laboratory of Physiological Chemistry, University of Groningen, Medical School, Bloemsingel 10, 9712 KZ Groningen, The Netherlands

Schryver, B.B., Institute of Bio-Organic Chemistry, Syntex Research, Palo Alto, CA 94304, USA

Schurr, W., Abteilung Innere Medizin VI, Universitätspoliklinik, D-6900 Heidelberg, Germany

Sobel, B.E., Cardiovascular Division, Washington University, School of Medicine, St. Louis, MI, USA

Soike, K.F., Delta Regional Primate Center, Tulane University, Covington, LA 70433, USA

Sternson, L.A., Smith Kline & French Laboratories, 709 Swedeland Road, Swedeland, PA 19479, U.S.A.

Su, K.S.E., Pharmaceutical Research Department, Division of CNS and Endocrine Research, and Toxicology Division, Lilly Research Laboratories, Eli Lilly and Company, Indianapolis, IN 46285, U.S.A.

Sørensen, H.H., Nordisk Gentofte A/S, Niels Steensensvej 1, DK-2820 Gentofte, Denmark

Takada, K., Kyoto Pharmaceutical University, Misasagi, Yamashina, Kyoto, Japan

Tessari, L., Istituto Scientifico Ospedale San Raffaele, Clinica Medica and Clinica Ortopedica, Universita de Milano, Milano, Italy

Thomsen, J., Nordisk Gentofte A/S, Niels Steensensvej 1, DK-2820 Gentofte, Denmark

Tomlinson, E., Ciba Geigy Pharmaceuticals, Wimblehurst Road, Horsham, W.Sussex, England

Valencia, G., Laboratory of Peptides, Biological Organic Chemistry Department, C.S.I.C., Jorge Girona Salgado 18-26, 08304 Barcelona, Spain

Veninga, A., Laboratory of Physiological Chemistry, University of Groningen, Medical School, Bloemsingel 10, 9712 KZ Groningen, The Netherlands

Vitale, K.M., Syntex Research, Palo Alto, CA, USA

van der Pas, M.A., Institute of Bio-Organic Chemistry, Syntex Research, Palo Alto, CA 94304, USA

Wilking, H., Pharmacological Sciences, Genentech, Inc., 460 Point San Bruno Boulevard, S. San Francisco, CA 94080, USA

Yoshikawa, H., Kyoto Pharmaceutical University, Misasagi, Yamashina, Kyoto, Japan

FAB-mass spectrometry, 76, 41, 348
Factor VIII, 201, 296
Fermentation, 308
Fibrin, 295
Fibronectin, 296
First pass effect, 10, 139, 177,
        191, 205, 221
Fluorometric detection, 42
Folding, 6, 39, 344
Formulation, 139, 249, 351
  buccal systems, 170
Fusidic acid, 212
Fusion proteins, 25

Gamma scintigraphy, 196, 207
Gastrin, 88, 95, 337
Gastrointestinal tract, 159
  permeability, 10
Gastrointestinal absorption, see
        Absorption
Gelling formulations, 209
Gels for nasal administration, 94
Gene expression, 24
Gene therapy, 354
Gene-fusion, 109
Genetic stability, 308
Glass-transition temperature, 118
Glucagon, 243
Glycocalyx, 141
Glycopeptides, 76
Glycoprotein, 206
Glycosylation, 29, 33, 36, 105,
        344, 354
Golgi apparatus, 105, 107
Gonadotropin releasing hormone
        (GRH), 233
Gramicidin A, 7
Growth hormone (GH), 23, 27, 35,
        88, 243, 255, 305-315,
        317-328, 342, 353
  biosynthesis, 306
Growth hormone releasing factor
        (GHRF), 194, 205, 221

Hairy cell leukemia, 282
Half-life, 80
Histological examination of
        nasal mucosa, 223
Histopathology, 229, 327
Homopolymers of lactic and
        glycolic acid, 115
Horseradish peroxidase, 12, 140,
        260
HPLC, 4, 35, 38, 76, 119, 222, 256,
        310, 348
Hydrogels, 161
Hydrolysis, 7, 49, 52, 153, 281,
        287 (see also Stability)
Hydrophilicity of polymers, 117
Hydrophobic interactions, 6, 73
Hydrophobicity, 72

Hydroxylamine, 302
Hypophysectomized rats, 318

Identity, 312
Immune complex, 351
Immune response, 352
Immune system, 343
Immunoassays, 37
Immunogenicity, 2, 6, 11, 12, 14,
        33, 116, 282, 305, 341, 346,
        348, 351, 354
Immunoglobulins, 87
Immunological adjuvants, 279
Immunological differences, 313
Immunological effects, 1 (see also)
        Immunogenicity)
Immunomodulators, 282, 342
Immunotoxins, 354
Implants, 8, 116, 280, 353
Impurities, 343, 346, 351
Instability, see Stability
Insulin, 2, 7, 23, 35, 84, 89, 139,
        155, 169, 188, 209, 211,
        233, 243, 260, 327, 341
  gelling, 7
  nasal administration, 93
Interferon, 2, 23, 29, 81, 95, 180,
        188, 221, 277-283, 285, 342
  medical applications, 282
  intramuscular injection, 83
Interleukin, 2, 9, 342, 354
Intestinal absorption, see
        ' Absorption
Intestinal permeability, 1, 139
Intracellular sorting, 105-111
Intramuscular administration, 255,
        278
Intranasal administration, see
        Nasal administration
Intrinsic factor, 11
Iontophoresis, 273, 353
Irritation,
  buccal mucosa, 160
  nasal mucosa, 195, 214
Isoelectric focusing, 348

Kupffer cells, 9, 286

Labelled peptides, 256
Lactic/glycolic acid polymers, 117
Laureth-9, 214, 245
Leaching of drug, 119
Leader sequences, 110
Leuprolide, 98, 140
Leutinising hormone releasing
        hormone (LHRH), 6, 83, 84,
        116, 118, 155, 192, 205,
        221, 243, 266, 280, 353
LHRH, see Leutinising hormone
        releasing hormone
Lipophilicity, 51, 56, 95, 145